D1597228

Biology of the Periodontal Connective Tissues

Biology of the Periodontal Connective Tissues

P. Mark Bartold, BDS, BSCDENT(HONS),
PHD, DDSC, FRACDS(PERIO)
Professor of Periodontology
Department of Dentistry
University of Queensland
Australia

A. Sampath Narayanan, PHD
Research Professor
Department of Pathology
University of Washington
Seattle, Washington

quintessence
books

Quintessence Publishing Co, Inc
Chicago, Berlin, London, Tokyo, Paris, Barcelona,
São Paulo, Moscow, Prague, and Warsaw

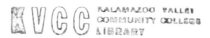

Library of Congress Cataloging-in-Publication Data

Bartold, P. Mark.
        Biology of the periodontal connective tissues / P. Mark Bartold,
    A. Sampath Narayanan.
            p.   cm.
        Includes bibliographical references and index.
        ISBN 0-86715-340-7
        1. Periodontium—Physiology.   2. Periodontium—Molecular aspects.
    3. Periodontal disease.   I. Narayanan, A. Sampath. II. Title.
        [DNLM: 1. Periodontium—physiology.   2. Connective tissue—
    physiology.   3. Periodontal Diseases—physiopathology.   WU 240
    B292b   1998]
    QP88.6.B37   1998
    617.6'32—dc21
    DNLM/DLC
    for Library of Congress   98-17716
                                                                        CIP

© 1998 by Quintessence Publishing Co, Inc

Quintessence Publishing Co, Inc
551 Kimberly Drive
Carol Stream, Illinois 60188

Editor: Betsy Solaro
Production: Timothy M. Robbins
Cover design: Michael Shanahan

Printed in the USA

Contents

Foreword

The art and science of periodontics are currently undergoing a paradigm change.

The prevalence of moderate to severe periodontitis is much lower than previously believed and is decreasing. We now know that while bacteria are essential for the causation of periodontitis, they are insufficient. Host susceptibility may be equally or more important than bacteria in determining whether clinical disease occurs and, when it does, its final outcome.

Determinants of host susceptibility are now becoming clear. Pathways through which alveolar bone and components of the extracellular connective tissue matrix are destroyed have been elucidated, and they are shared by all forms of periodontitis. These pathways are modified by environmental, acquired, and hereditary risk factors, which are the major determinants of disease occurrence and outcome. Tobacco smoking accounts for a portion of enhanced susceptibility at least as great as the bacterial factor. Heredity alone accounts for roughly 50% of susceptibility for periodontitis, and several specific genes have recently been linked to enhanced susceptibility. Notably, a genetic test that identifies individuals at enhanced risk for periodontitis now exists and is commercially available.

Diagnosis and therapy for periodontitis are also in the midst of revolution. We are turning from procedures arrived at through empiricism and trial and error to diagnostics and therapies based on scientific evidence and sound biologic principles. Traditional therapies, aimed almost exclusively at controlling the pathogenic bacteria, are being modified to include efforts to significantly reduce the level of risk. We now understand the pathways of destruction of bone and connective tissue sufficiently to begin to devise and use new therapies aimed at modification of host responses. The use of anti-inflammatory drugs and agents that inhibit the enzymes responsible for degradation of the extracellular matrix are examples.

The goals of periodontal therapy have also changed. Patients are no longer satisfied with treatments that only arrest progression of their disease; they are demanding and we are attempting to provide treatments that result in regeneration of periodontal tissues destroyed by disease. Achieving these goals requires a much greater depth of understanding of biologic phenomena than was the case previously.

An entirely new aspect of periodontics, the strong relationship between oral status and systemic health, is currently being born. For example, periodontitis in a pregnant woman clearly has direct and significant effects upon her fetus. Severe periodontitis also directly affects such common diseases as atherosclerosis, cardiovascular disease, and stroke.

This new paradigm in periodontics has dramatically altered the nature and level of understanding of genetics and molecular and cellular biology required to adequately perceive and deal successfully with the clinical problems dentists and periodontists face day to day. It is from this viewpoint that this book by Bartold and Narayanan must be considered.

Biology of the Periodontal Connective Tissues is targeted toward residents, graduate students, and investigators in periodontics. The book appears not only to meet the emerging needs of this audience admirably but will likely appeal to a much broader audience. The overall goal of the book is to draw together the fundamentals of molecular and cellular biology and basic information about compo-

sition of extracellular matrices. This body of fundamental information is then applied to normal and diseased connective tissues of the periodontium and to clinical problems. Because the amount of information is so enormous, this is a daunting undertaking. Nevertheless, the authors have been successful in selecting the key portions of information and weaving them into an easily readable and understandable fabric.

The authors bring complementary talents, expertise, and knowledge to their task. Both are well known in the field of biochemistry, with Bartold having contributed in an important way to knowledge in the proteoglycan area and Narayanan recognized as a leader in the area of extracellular matrix collagens. Both are broadly knowledgeable in the area of pathologic alterations of the extracellular matrix, and Bartold is a recognized expert in clinical periodontics and periodontal pathology.

This unique book appears at a propitious time. It reflects the new paradigm in periodontics and will be a valuable single source of information for years to come.

Roy C. Page, DDS, PhD
Professor of Periodontics
School of Dentistry
Professor of Pathology
School of Medicine
University of Washington
Seattle, Washington

Acknowledgments

The production of this book has been both a labor of love and, at times, a very difficult task. To try to gain a snapshot of the field of periodontal connective tissue biology, and distill it into a form suitable for use by those who may not be so familiar with the field, has been a challenging task. The fact that the two of us remain best of friends and still talk to each other, despite the problems of communicating from opposite sides of the globe and never physically meeting during the entire process of writing this book, is a mark of a very accommodating long-standing friendship.

We are particularly indebted to those individuals responsible for the conceptualization of this book—graduate students in periodontics. Without graduate students to stimulate us and to teach us their needs in the field of periodontics, we would be in a predicament. In particular, we would like to thank our current graduate students who took the time to read the many drafts of the chapters and gave us valuable feedback, often meeting deadlines that interfered with their own schedules.

We would also like to thank our many colleagues and friends who took time to read the draft chapters. These included: Leigh C. Anderson (Oral Biology, University of Washington, Seattle, Washington), Peter Byers and Beverley Dale (University of Washington, Seattle, Washington), Rod Marshall (Periodontology, University of Queensland, Australia), David R. Morris (Biochemistry, University of Washington, Seattle, Washington), Roy C. Page (Periodontics and Pathology, University of Washington, Seattle, Washington), Frank Roberts (Periodontics, University of Washington, Seattle, Washington), Thomas N. Wight (Pathology, University of Washington, Seattle, Washington), Dan Williams (Pathology, University of Washington, Seattle, Washington), William G. Young (Oral Biology, University of Queensland, Australia). In addition, the expert help with many of the illustrations by Kumar Narayanan, Madhu Narayanan, and Andrew Gordon-Macleod is gratefully acknowledged.

The final form of this book would not have been possible without the outstanding secretarial work provided by Glenda Maher and Theo Heinz. Their patience and attention to detail have, at times, been a real bonus and has been truly appreciated by both authors.

All of the authors' original work referred to in this book has been variously funded by research grants from the National Institutes of Health (USA) (DE-08229 and DE-10491) and the National Health and Medical Research Council of Australia.

Finally, we wish to record our sincere thanks to our families who have tolerated the considerable amount of time we have spent on this project. We acknowledge that much of this time was theirs, and we thank them for their patience and understanding.

Introduction

Many diseases common in our society are associated with alterations to either the connective tissue matrices, their resident cells, or both. The periodontium is no exception. Under diseased conditions, the periodontal tissues manifest all of the classic signs and symptoms of a tissue undergoing significant degradative and remodeling changes, which lead to either impaired tissue function or repair of the damage. With the above in mind, the objective of this book is to introduce the reader to the molecular and cellular interactions of connective tissues in general, and the periodontal tissues in particular.

The periodontium is a unique anatomical site that includes four discrete connective tissues, namely: gingiva, periodontal ligament, cementum, and alveolar bone. By virtue of the constant masticatory forces and bacteria in the mouth, these tissues are under continual mechanical and chemical abuse, yet for the most part, they manage to maintain their functional and structural integrity. However,

if the delicate balance between host defense and bacterial virulence is upset, then disease and associated tissue destruction ensue. Upon removal and control of the offending agents, tissue repair follows and health may be restored to the periodontium.

Because the responsiveness of the affected tissues to treatment is paramount to the successful outcome of various periodontal therapies, an understanding of the basic biology of these systems (as well as establishing the mechanisms involved in their failure) will permit us to be better positioned to influence these adverse processes during clinical management.

One important feature of the periodontal diseases is that they occur in a relatively small and well-localized region. As a result, studies of the local reactions have been easily performed following excisional biopsy of the affected areas and histologic assessment. The general features of normal and inflamed periodontal tissues have thus been examined in detail. There is little doubt that the components of the extracellular matrix of the periodontium are significantly affected during inflammation. During the development of gingivitis, the tissue changes are confined to the gingiva and include altered histochemical staining patterns of the affected matrix components, as well as infiltration of inflammatory cells such as polymorphonuclear leukocytes, macrophages, lymphocytes, and plasma cells.

In addition to changes in the matrix itself, significant changes are brought about by inflammation-mediated effects on the resident fibroblasts. Studies analyzing cultured fibroblasts isolated from normal and inflamed gingival tissues have proven invaluable in studying these relationships. Recent advances in molecular and cell biology have now allowed detailed assessment of the regulatory mechanisms and secretory pathways associated with matrix deposition (and degradation).

The clinical implications of research into the connective tissues of the periodontium are many and varied, and include pharmacological approaches to disease control, new approaches to tissue management and regenerative therapies, as well as development of diagnostic aids. Currently, major efforts are being placed on the development of agents that might block some of the mediators of tissue destruction, including prostaglandins, various cytokines, and enzymes. The future for many of these agents looks promising.

A major biologic response critical to survival of the dentition is repair of damaged tissue. However, once the destructive phases reach the deeper periodontal structures, repair in the form of tissue regeneration is less predictable. This feature of damaged tissues is not restricted to the periodontium. Indeed, mammals in general evince little regeneration of most organs or appendages in response to tissue destruction. Commonly, the repair process in humans, where severe tissue damage has occurred, leads to additional problems of scarring. Therefore, a clearer understanding of the composition of developing dental matrices, together with an understanding of the molec-

ular signals associated with tissue repair and regeneration, will lead to rational regenerative therapies based on sound biologic principles.

Connective tissue elements also have considerable potential for use in monitoring tissue changes and, as such, may be developed as an aid to periodontal diagnosis. At present, there are no consistently reliable diagnostic tests that accurately measure periodontal destruction with active periodontitis. Possible parameters that could provide this information would include ongoing loss of attachment or loss of alveolar bone. The gingival crevicular fluid contains many components of break-down products from the diseased periodontium, such as plasma proteins, bacterial and leukocytic enzymes, and inflammatory mediators. As a result, many studies have focused on analyzing components of this inflammatory exudate in the hope of finding an indicator of active periodontal breakdown. Unfortunately, one serious drawback of each of these potential markers is that they reflect the processes occurring in the gingiva. Thus, no distinction can be made between gingivitis and periodontitis. However, it is now apparent that there is some site specificity of various connective tissue extracellular matrix components within the periodontium. Therefore, the development of an assay that could detect components unique to either bone or periodontal ligament would be of significant use.

In writing this book, it has been our intention to provide a broad overview of connective tissue biology. One of our main objectives is to bring forth new principles that have evolved, and are emerging, as they apply to diseases of the periodontium. We have attempted to identify recent important concepts of growth regulation, gene expression, as well as inflammation, and to apply these to contemporary periodontics. We have drawn parallels, when necessary, to other diseases.

The book is targeted toward graduate students in dental (oral) sciences and those interested in pursuing research in these fields, and is intended to provide adequate biochemical, biologic, and pathologic background to this audience. The object is to discuss overall principles and provide adequate references to which the reader can turn when advanced and additional information is necessary. The text has been divided into four broad sections covering the fundamental principles of connective tissue biology; the molecular composition of extracellular matrices; the development, normal structure, and pathologic changes of the periodontal tissues; as well as a consideration of two major clinical implications of research into the connective tissues of the periodontium. In doing so, we wanted to highlight the overriding importance of the periodontal connective tissues in the manifestation, pathology, and responses of the periodontal tissues to disease and regeneration.

From a large body of fundamental and applied research, it is now apparent that all reactions (pathologic, reparative, and regenerative) occur within a complex environment that is exquisitely sensitive to disruption as a result of matrix destruction or interference of fibroblast metabolic activity. The fundamental responses of treatment rely on a sound understanding of these responses and allow us to recognize what constitutes an acceptable clinical outcome.

Part I

Fundamental Principles of Connective Tissue Biology

1

Gene Expression and Regulation of Protein Synthesis

Introduction

The properties and functions of a cell are determined by the types and amounts of its constituent proteins. In multicellular organisms, the requirements for proteins change continually during development and growth because of the need for different proteins to carry out and coordinate various morphogenetic events. These changing requirements are met by switching the genes that code for specific proteins on and off in a spatially and temporally programmed fashion. In adult organisms, however, proteins are needed mostly to replace molecules lost during normal homeostasis or due to injury; therefore, the pattern of gene expression remains relatively stable and only undergoes up- or down-regulation as needed. Gene transcription in eukaryotic cells is regulated by complex interactions between various physiological and environmental factors, and involves cell–cell and cell–matrix interactions. In contrast, prokaryotic gene regulation is relatively simple because these cells modify protein synthesis mainly to accommodate changes in their nutritional environment.

Structural information for proteins and instructions for their expression are encoded in genes. A gene is a hereditary unit that carries information for a specific function, and represents the portion of DNA that produces one RNA molecule. The RNA product that encodes proteins is messenger RNA (mRNA), in which codon sequences of three nucleotides each specify a different amino acid. In eukaryotic cells, the genes are packaged as complexes of DNA with histones and other chromosomal proteins. This structure, chromatin, consists of beadlike subunits, called nucleosomes, in which pieces of DNA approximately 200 nucleotides in length are wrapped around a core made up of two copies each of H2A, H2B, H3, and H4 histone molecules. These beads are connected by short stretches of linker DNA containing the H1 histone. The chromatin is further organized into chromosomes, each of which is a linear DNA molecule representing hundreds to thousands of genes. The number, size, and shape of the chromosomes are the same for one species, but they differ from species to species, even among related species.

The arrangement of genes varies significantly between eukaryotes and prokaryotes. Bacteria contain a single, large, circular chromosome in which the genes are organized such that those devoted to a single metabolic function are clustered together in a contiguous linear array. This arrangement into functional groups, called operons, generates a continuous mRNA molecule that carries the message for the series of related proteins involved in a specific function. Each section of this mRNA represents a gene encoding one protein. In contrast, eukaryotic genes for related functions, and even the genes for subunits of the same protein, are often physically separated on different chromosomes and are transcribed separately. In these genes, protein coding sequences (called exons, for expressed sequences) are separated by other sequences not present in the mature mRNA. The latter are called intervening sequences, or introns.

DNA that is tightly folded and condensed into chromatin structures is transcriptionally inactive, and it must first be modified to become available for transcription by RNA polymerases. This is the first step of gene expression and the most important regulatory point that determines whether a protein is expressed or not. In differentiated tissues this decision has already been made, and the gene is open for transcription. Once protein synthesis is initiated, the process of decoding nucleotide sequences into functional proteins involves the following reactions:

1. The gene is transcribed to RNA.
2. The RNA transcription product is processed into functional mRNA by adding a poly(A) tail and splicing away intron sequences.
3. The mRNA is then transported to its cytoplasmic destination.
4. Ribosomes associate with the mRNA, and the mRNA is read and translated into the amino acid sequence of encoded protein. The order in which amino acids are added to a growing polypeptide chain is determined by the order of codons present in the mRNA.
5. The newly synthesized polypeptide chain undergoes posttranslational modification as it folds into a three-dimensional structure, and sugar residues or other chemical groups are added as needed. Some amino acids may be chemically modified at this stage.
6. Completed protein molecules are then transported to destination sites by specific targeting amino acid sequences. The placement of proteins may be in the cytosol or in the cell's organelles, nucleus, or plasma membrane, or the proteins may be secreted into the extracellular space. Some secreted proteins are further modified by removal of portions of the protein molecule.

This chapter summarizes the major biochemical events involved in protein synthesis and how the reactions that affect the quality and quantity of proteins are regulated. Although emphasis is on mechanisms operating in eukaryotes, relevant information from prokaryotic cells is also included where necessary. For a more detailed treatise, see Lewin (1994), Lodish et al (1995), and Watson et al (1992).

Biosynthesis of Proteins

Gene Transcription

The purpose of gene transcription is to generate single-stranded RNA. Three classes of RNA are transcribed: mRNA, ribosomal RNA (rRNA), as well as transfer RNA (tRNA) and other small RNA species. Completion of transcription requires the template DNA with its regulatory sequences, the enzyme catalyzing the transcription, other accessory proteins, and several RNA species that aid in the transcription.

Protein factors. A number of proteins participate in gene transcription; among these, the most important component is RNA polymerase, which catalyzes the transcription reaction. In prokaryotes, a single RNA polymerase carries out the transcription, whereas three separate enzymes are involved in eukaryotic systems. The three eukaryotic enzymes RNA polymerases I, II, and III, synthesize rRNA (I), mRNA (II), and tRNA and other small RNAs (III). The prokaryotic RNA polymerase is made up of two copies of α and one copy each of β, β', σ, and ω protein subunits. The eukaryotic enzymes, which are structurally related and believed to have evolved from the prokaryotic species, are also multisubunit proteins composed of two large and 12 to 15 smaller polypeptide chains. Some of the small subunits are common to all the three enzymes. The three eukaryotic polymerases can be distinguished from each other by their sensitivity to α-amanitin, a bicyclic

octapeptide from the mushroom *Amanitis phalloides*. This compound inhibits RNA polymerase II completely and polymerase III moderately, while polymerase I and prokaryotic RNA polymerase are insensitive to this agent.

Another family of proteins that regulate transcription are the transcription, or *trans*-acting, factors. These are proteins that bind to specific regulatory DNA sequences called *cis*-elements. These proteins have been divided into three groups, based on their action. The first group assembles around the transcription start site, and positions the transcription initiation complex on the DNA molecule to be transcribed. The role of these proteins, called basal factors or general factors, is to initiate transcription at the correct site. Examples of basal factors are the TATA box-binding protein (TBP) and polymerase II transcription factors TFIIA, TFIIB, TFIIE, TFIIF, TFIIH, and TFIIJ. The second group of proteins are called upstream factors because they recognize specific DNA elements located upstream of the transcription start site. These are ubiquitous proteins that facilitate and augment the efficiency of transcription. The inducible factors form the third group of transcription factors (Papavassiliou 1995). These are the most important regulators of gene transcription in the context of development and wound repair, because most environmental ligands, such as hormones, influence gene expression through their action on inducible factors (Aran et al 1995; Benvenisty and Reshef 1991; Maniatis et al 1987; Orkin 1995; Vellanoweth et al 1994; Wedel and Ziegler-Heitbrock 1995). Regulation by these proteins may be either positive or negative.

Transcription factors contain discrete amino acid sequence domains that bind to target DNA sequences and interact with other transcription factors (Johnson and McKnight 1989; Klug 1995). Based on structural features, these proteins have been classified into several families such as zinc finger proteins, leucine zipper proteins, homeodomain pro-

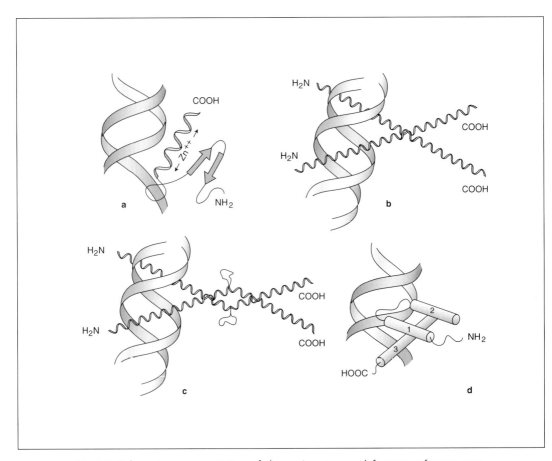

Fig 1-1 Schematic representation of the major structural features of some transcription factor classes. **(a)** A model of a zinc finger protein with an α helix and β sheets held together by a Zn^{++} ion and coordinated by a Cys$_2$-His$_2$ motif. An example of this type of zinc finger protein is the transcription factor TFIIIA. In steroid receptors the zinc is bound to four cysteines, whereas in yeast Gal4 two Zn^{++} ions are held by six cysteines. **(b)** Model of yeast GCN4 leucine zipper protein. In this structure, the carboxy terminal residues are packed together as a coiled coil. They diverge so that the basic amino terminal end binds to two adjacent half DNA major grooves. **(c)** HLH proteins are dimers in which a nonhelical loop separates two α helices in each subunit. The amino terminal domain with basic residues binds to DNA, while the carboxy terminal side is involved in hydrophobic interactions between the subunits. **(d)** A model of a homeodomain protein containing the helix-turn-helix feature. In this structure, one helix at the carboxy end (helix 3) contacts DNA, while two other helices (1 and 2) that lie across it contact other proteins. Redrawn with permission from Harrison 1991 (a), Ellenberger et al 1992 (b), Ferré-D'Amaré et al 1993 (c), and Wolberger et al 1991 (d).

teins, and helix-loop-helix family (HLH) proteins. The zinc finger proteins are characterized by the presence of a zinc finger motif. This motif is a domain of 30 to 70 amino acids; it contains one zinc ion (Zn^{++}) bound to two cysteines and two histidines (Fig 1-1a).

The zinc finger recognizes specific DNA sequences and is one of the most common DNA binding motifs in eukaryotic transcription factors. The transcription factors TFIIIA and SP1 (pregnancy specific β-1 glycoprotein), containing nine and three fingers, respectively, are examples of zinc finger proteins (Berg 1990; Harrison 1991). Steroid receptors are also zinc finger proteins; in these, the Zn^{++} is coordinated by four cysteines (Truss and Beato 1993). In the yeast transcription factor Gal4, the finger domain contains two zinc ions bound to six cysteines (Harrison 1991).

The DNA binding motif in leucine zipper proteins is a basic-region leucine zipper (called bZIP). The leucine zipper domain contains repeats of four or five leucines at every seventh position; the basic DNA binding domain is at its amino terminal end. These proteins are dimers with subunits that form continuous α helices. The carboxy ends form a parallel coiled coil that diverges towards the amino terminal domains and grips the DNA molecules at two adjacent major DNA grooves like scissors (see Fig 1-1b). The dimeric structure of these proteins is essential for binding to DNA. Because each of the two subunits can bind to different DNA sequences, they can form different homo- and heterodimers among a group of similar proteins; thus, the repertoire of DNA binding specificity of these proteins is high. CCAAT enhancer binding protein (C/EBP), the products of c-*fos* and c-*jun* proto-oncogenes, and yeast GCN4 transcription factor belong to this family.

Helix-loop-helix (HLH) transcription factors are characterized by bipartite DNA binding regions and are structurally related to leucine zipper proteins. The HLH motif consists of two amphipathic α helices of 40 to 50 amino acids linked by a loop, hence the name. This structure is responsible for dimerization, and immediately N-terminal to the HLH region is a highly basic domain (~15 residues) that binds to DNA. The HLH motif is flexible, allowing one helix to fold back and pack against the other; thus, one protein molecule can bind to DNA, as well as to the HLH motif of a second HLH protein (see Fig 1-1c). HLH proteins are found in eukaryotes ranging from yeast to mammals, and they are impor-

tant in the regulation of metabolism, cell differentiation, and development. MyoD, the muscle differentiation factor, and c-*myc* proto-oncogene product belong to this group of DNA binding proteins. Some HLH proteins do not contain a basic region, therefore they cannot bind to DNA; these proteins serve as negative regulators of the HLH transcription factors that contain the basic region.

Homeodomain proteins are another family of transcription factors with the helix-turn-helix motif. This motif is a segment of about 20 amino acids and helices that cross at a 120-degree angle. One helix acts as the recognition helix and is placed in a DNA major groove (see Fig 1-1d). A second helix, which lies across the first, interacts with other protein factors. Many prokaryotic transcription factors and eukaryotic homeodomain proteins belong to this group. The amino acid sequence in these domains is highly conserved among prokaryotes and vertebrates, including humans.

Regulatory DNA sequences. A gene destined to be transcribed contains the template sequence for the RNA product as well as the *cis*-elements involved in regulation of transcription. Regulation is mediated through specific transcription factors that bind to the *cis* sequences. These sequences are classified as either *promoters* or *enhancers*. Promoters are DNA sequences that determine the site of transcription initiation by RNA polymerase. These sequences are located toward the 5′ end (upstream) from the transcription initiation site (also called the cap site). Three common promoter-sequence motifs have been described. The first is the TATAA sequence (called the TATA box) located approximately at −25 to −30 nucleotides relative to the cap site; it is needed for positioning the RNA polymerase on the DNA molecule to be transcribed. The other two promoter motifs are located further upstream at −40 to −100 nucleotides; these are the CAAT box (CCAAT sequence located at ~ −80) and the GC box

Table 1-1. Some Promoter and Enhancer Sequence Motifs That Bind to Transcription Factors*

Sequence	Type	Transcription factor
TATAAA	TATA box, promoter	TATA box binding protein
CCAAT	CAAT box, promoter	CTF/NFI, CPI, C/EBP
GGCGGG	GC box, promoter	SP1
ATTTGCAT	Octomer, promoter	Oct-1, Oct-2, Oct-6
GGGACTTTCC	Enhancer[‡]	NFκB
TGTACAGGA<u>TGTTCT</u>AT[†]	GRE[‡], enhancer	glucocorticoid receptor
TGACTCA	TRE[‡], enhancer	AP1 (activator protein 1)
CCATATTAGG	SRE[‡], enhancer	SRF (serum response factor)
AGGTCATGACCT	RARE[‡], enhancer	Retinoic acid receptor
TGACGTCA	CRE[‡], enhancer	CREB[§]

* From Boulikas (1994).
† Those underlined are the essential nucleotides.
‡ RE: response element.
§ CREB: cyclic AMP response element binding.

(GGGCGG sequence). Location of the GC boxes is variable, but it is always farther away than the TATA box.

Enhancers are DNA sequences that regulate the rate of gene transcription. Like promoters, their effect is mediated through binding to specific protein factors. Enhancers have many different characteristics and differ from promoters in several respects. For example, their location, unlike that of the promoter, is highly variable, and they may be present upstream or downstream of the transcription start site, or even within introns. The enhancers are longer and placed farther away than the promoters, and are active even when thousands of base pairs (bp) away. They may consist of random repeats and are often active in the 5′ and 3′ orientations. Some enhancers may contain more than one functional domain acting synergistically, while others can function as both promoters and enhancers. Sequences that bind to one transcription factor may be present in several genes in the same cells, or restricted to a single gene. In the former case, the effect of the transcription factor on different genes will depend upon its affinity to different sequences. When the same regulatory sequence is active in different cell types, its action will depend upon the presence of other cell and tissue specific factors.

The primary function of enhancers is to bind to cellular transcription factors; this binding results in either positive or negative regulation of gene expression. In differentiated cells, enhancers may be constitutively active throughout the life of the cell. The enhancers are the major regulatory elements that determine the cell and tissue specificity of gene expression (Boulikas 1995; Gossen et al 1993; Johnson and McKnight 1989; Vellanoweth et al 1994). The sequence motifs of some DNA regulatory elements are given in Table 1-1.

RNA species. Protein synthesis requires the participation of several RNA species. These include the mRNA, rRNA, and tRNA and other small RNA types. While mRNA is the template for polypeptides, rRNA is the major component of ribosomes, in which translation takes place. The small RNAs play accessory roles in transcriptional and translational

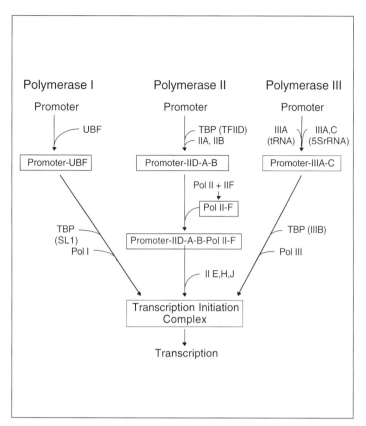

Fig 1-2 Formation of a transcription initiation complex by eukaryotic RNA polymerases. For transcription by RNA polymerase I, first the upstream binding factor (UBF) binds to the promoter, followed by the TBP subunit of factor SL1. Binding by the polymerase completes the transcription initiation complex and transcription begins. For polymerase II, first the TBP subunit of TFIID binds to the promoter, and then TFIIA and TFIIB. The transcription initiation complex is formed when the polymerase-TFIIF binds to this complex along with TFIIE, TFIIH, and TFIIJ. For transcription of small RNA species, the gene first binds to TFIIIA and TFIIIC (only TFIIIC for tRNA), and then to TFIIIB and polymerase III; thus the transcription initiation complex is formed and transcription begins. Promoter elements for all the three polymerases bind to the TBP subunit of transcription factors (SL1, TFIID, and TFIIIB, respectively, for polymerases I, II, and III).

reactions; for example, tRNAs serve as carriers for amino acids during polypeptide synthesis, and other small RNA types make up the ribonucleoprotein particles (RNPs).

Transcription. Transcription starts with the binding of a molecular complex of RNA polymerase and other accessory factors to the DNA segment to be transcribed (Lewin 1994; Lodish et al 1995; Watson et al 1992). The binding locally separates DNA strands and exposes the template sequence to be transcribed to the RNA polymerase. The polymerase then moves along the DNA, generating a growing RNA chain in the 5′ to 3′ direction by stepwise addition of ribonucleotide triphosphates. In prokaryotes, transcription is initiated by the binding of the σ subunit of RNA polymerase, which recognizes promoter sequences; it is released after polymerization of about 10 ribonucleotides,

then the core polymerase (made up of α, β', β, and ω subunits) takes over and completes the transcription. Eukaryotic genes are transcribed in a similar fashion. However, their transcription is more complex; it involves three different polymerases, and many more promoter elements and accessory factors.

Transcription of mRNA. The first step in mRNA transcription is the formation of a transcription initiation complex by RNA polymerase II. Assembly of this complex begins when the TBP subunit of TFIID binds to a TATAA promoter sequence, to which transcription factors TFIIA and TFIIB are added. Then a preformed complex consisting of RNA polymerase II and TFIIF binds to this complex, followed by factors TFIIE, TFIIH, and TFIIJ. Transcription then begins (Fig 1-2). The TBP binds to the TATAA element; the role of TBP binding is to position the RNA polymerase so that transcription can begin approximately 25 to 35 bases downstream of the TBP binding domain. Other accessory factors that bind to upstream elements increase the efficiency of transcription. Some genes do not contain a TATA box; these are recognized through other sequences.

Transcription begins most frequently at an adenine base at the +1 location preceded by a cytosine at −1. The consensus sequence for transcription initiation is pyridine$_2$ ANTpyridine$_2$ (where "N" is any base). After synthesis of about 30 nucleotides, the transcript is modified at its 5′ end by capping. Capping involves 5′-to-5′ linkage of 7-methylguanine by the enzyme guanyl transferase. The 5′-to-5′ linkage places the added G residue in the reverse orientation of the other nucleotides. The transcript is methylated at the 7- and 2′-O-positions of the penultimate A or G (which was the first base transcribed), and additional methylation may occur at other internal adenines. The enzyme catalyzing the methylation requires *S*-adenosylmethionine as a cofactor. Capping appears to be necessary for recognition of mRNA by the nuclear transport apparatus for transport to the cytoplasm, and it also renders the mRNAs resistant to nucleases.

Termination of transcription by RNA polymerase II is poorly understood, and it appears to occur at a loosely specified location downstream of the polyadenylation site. After termination, an endonuclease generates a 3′ end, which is polyadenylated (see Processing of mRNA, p. 11). Newly made transcripts become immediately associated with proteins to form heterogeneous nuclear ribonucleoprotein particles (hnRNP).

Transcription by RNA polymerases I and III. RNA polymerase I synthesizes 18S, 28S, and 5.8S rRNA. The transcription units are arranged in the gene in tandem arrays in the order 18S–5.8S–28S. The promoter for transcription is a single core sequence spanning from roughly −45 to +20. First the transcrip-

tion factor UBF (upstream binding factor) binds to the upstream promoter element, followed by the TBP subunit of the transcription factor SL1; it then combines with polymerase I to form the transcription initiation complex, and transcription begins (see Fig 1-2). Termination of rRNA transcription occurs approximately 1000 bp downstream of the 3′ end and requires a roughly 18-bp termination sequence and a protein factor. Transcription of tRNA and other small RNA species is catalyzed by RNA polymerase III. This enzyme requires a combination of bipartite promoter sequences located downstream as well as upstream of the start site. Binding of the transcription factors TFIIIC for tRNA, and TFIIIA and TFIIIC for 5S rRNA, is followed by binding of the TBP subunit of factor TFIIIB. Then RNA polymerase III binds to form the transcription initiation complex, and transcription begins (see Fig 1-2). Termination of polymerase III transcription occurs at the second U within a sequence of four U bases embedded in a GC-rich region.

Transcription of mitochondrial DNA. Mitochondria contain a roughly 16-kb circular DNA sequence that codes for some mitochondrial proteins, rRNA, and tRNA. This DNA is transcribed by a separate mitochondrial RNA polymerase, and a protein subunit similar to the bacterial σ factor initiates its transcription. The mitochondrial gene has two related 15-bp promoters, one on each DNA strand; both strands are transcribed entirely, and transcription requires mtF1, an accessory factor. Mitochondrial transcription products are processed to mRNA, tRNA, and rRNA.

Processing of Transcription Products

Transcription products of eukaryotic RNA polymerases undergo modification before they become functional. The modification reactions may involve removal of introns, addition of bases, or chemical modification of certain nucleotides. Products of all three eukaryotic polymerases are modified, although rRNA and the small RNA species are processed less extensively than is mRNA.

Processing of mRNA: endonuclease cleavage and polyadenylation. In addition to capping, described earlier, the transcription product of mRNA, referred to as pre-mRNA, undergoes additional tailoring reactions before it is converted into a mature translatable form. These reactions take place in the nucleus. The pre-mRNA is longer by at least 1000 bases at its 3′ end, and it has a AAUAAA sequence motif 10 to 30 bases to the 5′ side of the putative polyadenlyation site (Sachs 1993; Wahle and Keller 1996). This sequence, which is highly conserved among different mRNA molecules, is necessary for recognition by an endonuclease that removes the extra 3′ sequence, as well as for polyadenylation. An additional GU-rich region located within a few hundred bases downstream of the polyadenylation site also appears to be necessary for the endonuclease and polyadenylation.

Immediately after the endonuclease action most eukaryotic mRNAs, with the exception of histone mRNAs, are rapidly polyadenylated by the addition of about 200 adenines. Polyadenylation generates a poly(A) tail, and is carried out by the enzyme poly(A) polymerase in a two-step reaction (Wahle and Keller 1996). First, a short sequence of 10 A residues is added slowly. This reaction depends on the recognition of AAUAAA sequence by the poly(A) polymerase. Subsequently, 200 to 250 A residues are added rapidly. This step does not require the AAUAAA sequence. The mature poly(A) tract immediately associates with a poly(A)-binding protein. The mRNA, together with its poly(A) tail, is designated as poly(A)$^+$ mRNA.

What precise role the poly(A) tail plays is unclear, although mRNA without it is rapidly degraded. Removal of the poly(A) tail also inhibits translation in vitro, and during embryonic development, polyadenylation of a particular mRNA parallels its translatability. Recent studies indicate that a complex of the poly(A) tail with poly(A)-binding protein is involved in the recruitment of the 40S ribosomal subunit to the mRNA (Tarun and Sachs 1995).

Nuclear splicing. Splicing is the process by which intron sequences are removed from the pre-mRNA, and it takes place in the nucleus (McKeown 1992). It involves two transesterification reactions in which ester groups are exchanged and the exon ends are combined together. Introns start with the sequence GU at their 5′ junction with the preceding exon, and end with AG at the 3′ end. They contain a branch point A about 20 to 50 bases downstream of the 5′ splice site. The first transesterification involves nucleophilic attack of the 5′ phosphate of the intron guanidine at the 5′ splice site by the 2′ OH group of the branch site adenine. This results in releasing exon 1 and formation of a lariat structure in the intron due to a chemical bond between a 5′ G and branch site A (Fig 1-3a). During the second transesterification, the ester bond of the 5′ phosphate of exon 2 to 3′ O of the intron is transferred to the 3′ O of exon 1, which was freed in the first reaction; as a result, the intron is released. The released intron with the lariat structure is debranched and then degraded. The branch site is believed to identify the nearest 3′ splicing site.

Splicing requires the formation of a spliceosome complex where the actual splicing takes place. The spliceosome is formed by the association of small nuclear ribonucleoprotein particles (snRNPs, each snRNP contains RNA species U1, U2, U5, and U4/U6, and several protein-splicing factors) with the splice site in the precursor RNA.

Splicing offers a mechanism by which several isoforms of a protein can be produced from one mRNA. For example, molecules of varying sizes can be generated by including or

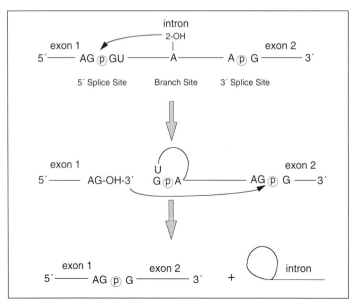

Fig 1-3a

Fig 1-3 Reactions involved in splicing of pre-mRNA. **(a)** The introns start with the sequence GU and end with AG. First the 5′ end of the intron is hydrolyzed and it is ligated to the A at the branch site by transesterification, and a lariat is formed in the intron. During the second transesterification, the 3′ end of the intron is liberated and the 5′ end of exon 2 is ligated to 3′ of exon 1. The lariat is then debranched and degraded. **(b)** Organization of the gene and alternative splicing of mRNA transcripts to produce tissue-specific isoforms of α-tropomyosin. Exons selected in most cells are shown as black or white boxes. The alternatively spliced tissue-specific exons are striped. Introns are shown as lines (Reproduced with permission from Nadal-Ginard et al 1990).

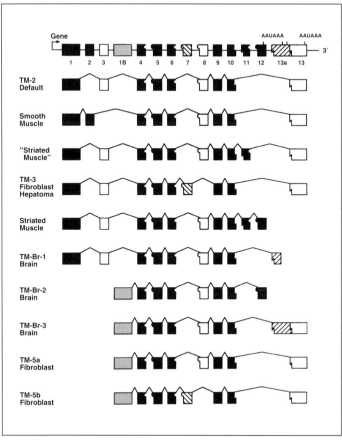

Fig 1-3b

excluding exons, some of which may contain alternate start and stop codons. In addition, functional domains of a protein molecule can be mixed and matched by splicing; this process, called alternative splicing, offers a mechanism by which tissue-specific variants of a protein can be synthesized. This is illustrated by the generation of a broad range of α-tropomyosin isomers in various tissues (see Fig 1-3b) (Nadal-Ginard et al 1990). Among the matrix proteins, different fibronectins are produced by alternative splicing; this is discussed in Chapter 5.

While most eukaryotic pre-mRNAs are spliced as described above, certain fungal, mitochondrial, and other gene products called group I and II introns autosplice themselves by transesterification catalyzed by the presence of secondary structures. Alternatively, mRNA in certain species such as the parasite *trypanosomes* undergo *trans*-splicing in which it is spliced with portions of a foreign donor RNA. RNAs of these species contain a common 35-nucleotide leader sequence not coded by the parent gene, but provided instead by a spliced leader RNA (SL RNA) (Bonen 1993).

Processing of rRNA and small RNAs. The product of polymerase I, pre-rRNA, is larger (45S) and includes 18S, 5.8S, and 28S species arranged in this order, separated by spacer sequences. In a process that requires snRNPs, the 45S species undergoes cleavage to form individual 18S, 5.8S, and 28S components, and then the spacer sequences are degraded. Specific bases in these RNAs are also methylated. After assembly with protein components of the ribosome, mature 40S and 60S ribosomal subunits are exported to the cytosol, where they participate in protein synthesis.

The precursor of tRNA, pre-tRNA, is also larger, and, in some eukaryotic species, tRNAs may have intron sequences as well. These introns are first excised at both ends by cleavage, and then the exon ends are ligated. Extra sequences present at the 5′ end are removed by a ribonuclease. Certain bases in the tRNA are chemically modified, and the processed tRNA is then transported to the cytoplasm.

Transport of mRNA to the Cytoplasm

Fully processed mRNA forms complexes with proteins and then is transported to the cytoplasm as mRNPs through nuclear pores. Its 5′-cap structure is believed to be a recognition signal for the transport machinery. After reaching their destination, the mRNPs dissociate releasing their protein components, freeing the proteins for return to the nucleus for recycling. The mRNA then binds to poly(A) binding protein and other cytoplasmic proteins. Certain viral proteins, such as E1B and E4B of adenovirus, facilitate the transport of mRNAs across the nuclear pores; however, these viral components favor the transport of viral mRNAs over the host species.

The final location of the mRNA may be perinuclear, near plasma membranes, or in any other geographical location within the cytoplasm. Placement at these locations appears to be specified by the 3′-untranslated regions of mRNAs and proteins that bind to this region (Hesketh 1996; Rings et al 1994).

Translation of mRNA and Polypeptide Synthesis

General concepts. Polypeptide synthesis takes place in ribosomes located either free in the cytoplasm or bound to membranes in rough endoplasmic reticulum (RER). The ribosomes are compact ribonucleoprotein particles consisting of a large and small subunit of size 50S and 30S, respectively, in bacteria, and 60S and 40S in eukaryotes. Each of the ribosomal subunits is made up of many proteins associated with rRNA. The smaller subunit contains separate sites for harboring aminoacyl-tRNA and the growing polypeptide chain. These A- and P-sites (for acceptor and

Table 1-2. Codons for Amino Acids in mRNA

Amino Acid	One-Letter Designation	Number of Codons	Codon Sequence*
Alanine	A	4	GCU, GCC, GCA, GCG
Arginine	R	6	CGU, CGC, CGA, CGG, AGA, AGG
Asparagine	N	2	AAU, AAC
Aspartic acid	D	2	GAU, GAC
Cysteine	C	2	UGU, UGC
Glutamic acid	E	2	GAA, GAG
Glutamine	Q	2	CAA, CAG
Glycine	G	4	GGU, GGC, GGA, GGG
Histidine	H	2	CAU, CAC
Isoleucine	I	3	AUU, AUC, AUA
Leucine	L	6	UUA, UUG, CUU, CUC, CUA, CUG
Lysine	K	2	AAA, AAG
Methionine (start)	M	1	AUG
Phenylalanine	F	2	UUU, UUC
Proline	P	4	CCU, CCC, CCA, CCG
Serine	S	6	UCU, UCC, UCA, UCG, AGU, AGC
Threonine	T	4	ACU, ACC, ACA, ACG
Tryptophan	W	1	UGG
Tyrosine	Y	2	UAU, UAC
Valine	V	4	GUU, GUC, GUA, GUG
Stop	...	3	UAA, UAG, UGA

* In the gene, the nucleotide for U is T.

peptide) are present in both prokaryotes and eukaryotes, whereas prokaryotes contain an additional E-site through which free tRNA is released. In eukaryotic cells, each molecule of the translating mRNA remains associated at any one time with several ribosomes. The number of ribosomes in these polyribosomes (also called polysomes) vary depending upon many factors, such as the efficiency with which ribosomes are loaded and the length of the mRNA. A ribosome attaches to the mRNA molecule at the 5′ end, and moves along its length in the 3′ direction; en route it translates triplet codons into corresponding amino acids. Translation begins at an AUG initiation site, and peptide synthesis proceeds from the amino to the carboxy end. Although the mRNA can be read at all three frames of its codon sequence, only one frame translates into a continuous and complete peptide chain; alternate reading frames usually contain several stop codons so that translation is terminated prematurely. GTP is an important cofactor necessary for many translation reactions. Several protein factors participate in the translation and, depending upon their function, they are called as initiation, elongation, termination, or release factors (IF, EF, TF, and RF respectively; for the eukaryotic factors the names start with an "e").

The amino acids for polypeptide synthesis are presented as aminoacyl-tRNAs. These tRNAs have a characteristic cloverleaf structure consisting of stems and unpaired loops to which amino acids are covalently linked. This linking is accomplished by a specific enzyme that recognizes the amino acid and its tRNA. Each tRNA contains a three-nucleotide anticodon sequence complementary to the corresponding codon for the particular amino acid it specifies. There are 64 possible codons and one amino acid may be specified by one or more codons (Table 1-2). Three codons, however, do not specify any amino acids, and these function as stop codons to terminate translation. The amino acids specified by codons are the same in all organisms. There is a separate tRNA for initiation of peptide synthesis. This tRNA species, initiator tRNA (tRNA$_i$), is charged with methionine in eukaryotes, and is formylated to *N*-formylmethionine in bacteria. Thus the first amino acid synthesized on a nascent polypeptide is methionine. The tRNA$_i$ is structurally different from generic elongator tRNAs (the first base pair of the amino acid acceptor stem, and presence of three GC pairs in the stem that precedes the codon are two differences among several), and its special structural features prevent it from occupying the A-site.

Initiation of translation. Initiation begins when an initiation factor (eIF2 in eukaryotes and IF2 in bacteria) forms a ternary complex with a molecule of GTP and tRNA$_i$. It combines with a 43S complex composed of small ribosomal subunit and eIF3, and then with mRNA. The mRNA binds as a complex consisting of cap-binding protein (CBP; this is initiation factor eIF4E) and factors eIF4G, eIF4A, and eIF4B. The complex then migrates to the AUG start codon. Factors eIF2 and eIF3 are released from the complex and, with the aid of eIF5 and eIF6, the mRNA -43S complex now associates with the larger 60S ribosomal unit (Fig 1-4) (Pain 1996). The cap structure in mRNA appears to be necessary for translation of eukaryotic mRNAs, and interference with the cap structure (during poliovirus infection, for example) results in blockage of translation. In eukaryotic cells, presence of certain nucleotides surrounding the initiator AUG sequence facilitates its recognition as the first codon; this sequence, called the Kozak sequence, is 5'-ACCAUGG.

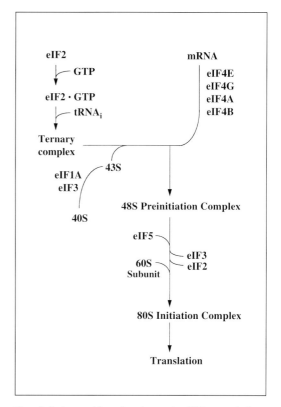

Fig 1-4 Assembly of eukaryotic 80S translation-initiation complex. First a ternary complex is formed between eIF2, one molecule of GTP, and tRNA$_i$. This together with the smaller (40S) ribosomal subunit bound to eIF1A and eIF3, and a complex formed from mRNA, eIF4E, eIF4G, eIF4A, and eIF4B, form the 48S preinitiation complex. This then moves to the first AUG codon, where it combines with the 60S ribosomal subunit to form the 80S translation initiation complex. This last reaction requires eIF5 and the release of the factors eIF2 and eIF3 from the complex (adapted from Pain 1996).

Elongation. Peptide chain elongation involves elongation factors eEF1A, eEF1B (EFTu in bacteria), and eEF2. These protein factors form a complex with GTP and aminoacyl-tRNA, and enter the A-site. A peptide bond forms between the first methionine, which is present at the P-site, and the aminoacyl-tRNA at the A-site (Fig 1-5a). Formation of peptide bond is catalyzed by the enzyme peptidyl transferase and other cofactors localized in the

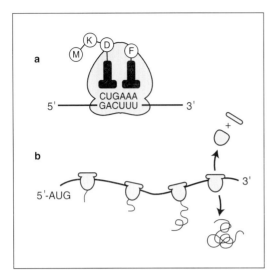

Fig 1-5 (a) A model of a ribosome in which a growing peptide (Met-Lys-Asp)- and phenylalanyl-tRNA are attached to Asp (GAC) and Phe (UUU) codons, respectively, through anticodons CUG and AAA. **(b)** Polypeptide chain elongation. Ribosomes move from the 5'-AUG in the mRNA toward the 3' end, adding amino acids to the peptide as they move along. One amino acid each is added as the ribosomes are displaced by a triplet codon. When the ribosomes reach a stop codon, further amino acid addition stops, and the polypeptide and ribosomal components are released. In eukaryotic cells at any one time, the mRNAs exist as polysomes in which several ribosomes are actively synthesizing protein.

large ribosomal subunit. Once a peptide bond is formed, the ribosome moves to the next codon, transferring the peptidyl tRNA to the P-site and releasing the deacylated tRNA. This sequence of reactions is repeated as the ribosomes move along the mRNA in the 5'-to-3' direction (see Fig 1-5b).

Termination of peptide elongation occurs when ribosomes recognize the termination codons UAG, UAA, or UGA, to which there are no corresponding tRNAs. Termination involves releasing the completed polypeptide chain from the tRNA, and free tRNA from the ribosome. This process requires proteins referred to as release factors.

Despite the large number of steps involved, polypeptide synthesis is relatively fast. In bacteria, about 15 amino acids per second are added at 37°C, completing an average polypeptide in 2 to 3 minutes. It is slower in eukaryotic cells, where the elongation rate is about 2 residues per second. Translation has an error rate of only 1 in 10^4 amino acids, and fidelity is maintained by the elongation factor, which allows correct codon-anticodon pairing, and by the aminoacyl-tRNA syn-

thetases, which recognize and remove incorrect amino acids attached to tRNAs.

The initiation factor eIF2 is one of the key regulators of overall eukaryotic protein synthesis rate. This factor becomes inactive when its α subunit is phosphorylated. Growth factors and a variety of conditions, such as cell cycle phase and stress, affect protein synthesis through phosphorylation of eIF2.

Posttranslational Processing and Protein Targeting

Targeting or sorting. The placement of newly synthesized proteins in target cell organelles is achieved either by synthesis at the required locations, as is seen in mitochondria and chloroplasts, or by translocation if proteins are synthesized elsewhere (von Heijne 1990; Walter and Johnson 1994). The movement of proteins from the site of synthesis to a different destination is referred to as targeting or sorting.

Glycolytic enzymes, skeletal proteins, and certain signaling molecules such as ras and src

Table 1-3. Some Protein Targeting Signals

Destination Site	Signal Features	Peptide Location	Examples*
ER	One or more basic amino acids followed by a core of hydrophobic amino acids	N-terminus, removed	Lys-Trp-Val-Thr-**Phe-Leu** **-Leu-Leu-Leu-Phe-Ile-Ser** **-Gly-Ser-Ala-Phe**-Ser-[†]
Mitochondria	3–5 nonconsecutive Arg or Lys, and Ser and Thr; no Glu or Asp	N-terminus, removed	**-Ser-Arg**-Lys-**Arg**...**Ala-Ile** **-Leu-Ala-Ala-Thr-Ser**-Ser-Val -Ala-**Tyr**-Leu-Asn-Trp[‡]
Peroxisome	Ser-Lys-Leu	C-terminus	—
Nucleus	Basic amino acid cluster	Internal	**-Lys-Lys-Lys-Arg-Lys**-[§] **-Arg-Lys-Lys-Arg-Arg**-Asn **-Arg-Arg-Arg**[‖]
Lysosomes	Mannose-6-phosphate	N-linked oligosaccharide	...

* Bold letters indicate the needed residues.
† Preproalbumin.
‡ Yeast cytochrome b_2.
§ SV40 large T antigen.
‖ HIV tat protein.

proteins, are synthesized on free ribosomes and released directly into the cytosol. In contrast, proteins targeted to nucleus are instructed to move to this site by a 7 to 9 basic amino acid sequence (Boulikas 1993), while the carboxy terminal triplet sequence of Ser-Lys-Leu places proteins such as catalase in the peroxisomes (Table 1-3). A leader sequence of approximately 25 amino acids, containing stretches of neutral and basic amino acids, provides the signal for the polypeptide to traverse through membranes in chloroplasts and mitochondria; once the polypeptide passes through the membrane, this sequence is cleaved off. Proteins destined to be anchored within the membrane contain this sequence followed by another stretch of uncharged amino acids.

Translocation. The movement of polypeptides across membranes of organelles and RER is known as translocation. In eukaryotic cells, secretory proteins, together with those to be placed on the endoplasmic reticulum (ER), Golgi, and plasma membranes, are synthesized at the RER. The amino terminus of these proteins contains a signal sequence consisting of 15 to 30 hydrophobic and one or more positively charged amino acids. When ribosomes initiate protein synthesis, this signal sequence binds to a signal recognition particle (SRP). Binding to the SRP, a ribonucleoprotein, stops protein synthesis temporarily, and the SRP-bound ribosome attaches to a receptor on the ER membrane. Translation then resumes and the signal sequence attached to the polypeptide enters the ER membrane. The SRP is then dissociated and the nascent polypeptide enters into the ER lumen. A signal peptidase subsequently removes the signal peptide and translation continues (Walter and Johnson 1994).

Some proteins are anchored into membranes; these proteins are called integral membrane proteins. These proteins can be located such that part of the molecule stretches into or outside of the cytosol. This is achieved by positioning an anchoring sequence at an appropriate location in the protein molecule. If the anchoring sequence is near the N-terminus, the N-terminus traverses through the membrane and is placed outside. How far it traverses through the membrane depends upon where the anchoring sequence is placed on the polypeptide. However, if the signal sequence is present internally or at the carboxy terminus, the amino end of the polypeptide becomes exposed to the cytosolic side (Glick et al 1992).

Nascent polypeptide chains are delivered to the lumen of the ER and transported to the Golgi apparatus via transport vesicles. Two key events occur in the Golgi apparatus: protein folding and glycosylation. Folding of nascent polypeptides into three-dimensional conformations proceeds from the amino to the carboxy end, and this process is usually assisted by accessory proteins, as well as by disulfide linkages. Formation of disulfide bonds is catalyzed by the enzyme protein disulfide isomerase. Protein folding is aided by molecular chaperones. These are a set of conserved proteins that bind with nascent polypeptides translocated into the ER lumen, facilitate their transport, and prevent their degradation (Hendrick and Hartl 1995; Hartl 1996). They also prevent misfolding proteins under normal conditions and during heat shock. One prominent chaperone is BiP, a homologue of the heat-shock protein Hsp70. Polypeptide chains then undergo posttranslational modifications in the ER lumen, and the modification may continue after they reach the Golgi apparatus. Some modifications, such as hydroxylation of proline and lysine residues in collagen, can occur only on unfolded polypeptides.

N-Glycosylation (addition of sugar to the NH_2 group of asparagine) begins at the ER and continues in the Golgi apparatus. This occurs through an oligosaccharide consisting of *N*-acetylglucosamine, mannose, and glucose on a dolichol phosphate carrier, and sugar residues are added to the amino acid sequence Asn-X-Ser/Thr (where X is any amino acid except proline). Mannose is added at the ER, while O-glycosylation (addition of sugars to the -OH of serine, threonine, or hydroxylysine), appears to occur exclusively at the Golgi apparatus. Glycosylation occurs in the cisternae of the ER where it progresses from the *cis* (ER) face towards the *trans* (plasma membrane) side. Glycosylation is believed to facilitate the movement of proteins to the cell surface, to be necessary for secretion, and to prevent degradation. The sugar mannose-6-phosphate targets proteins to lysosomes. Once addition of the sugar residues is completed, proteins targeted to plasma membranes and for secretion are packaged into vesicles. Vesicles are formed from membranes through a series of steps, involving several proteins and GTP hydrolysis (Rothman 1994).

Secretion of proteins may be *continuous* or *regulated*. Plasma membrane glycoproteins, collagen, and other matrix proteins, and other secretory proteins such as albumin in liver are secreted constitutively and continuously, and these proteins are transported to the plasma membrane from the *trans* Golgi network via non–clathrin-coated vesicles. In contrast, insulin and other specialized proteins are stored in storage vesicles, and are secreted through clathrin-coated vesicles in response to secretory signals. Some secreted proteins are present as inactive precursors within the cells, and their activation requires proteolytic cleavage of a portion of the protein molecule either immediately after secretion or after reaching their destination. The prefixes prepro- and pro- designate protein precursors with and without signal sequence, respectively. The pro- forms of proteolytic enzymes are often called zymogens.

The biosynthetic reactions involved in protein synthesis are illustrated schematically in Fig 1-6.

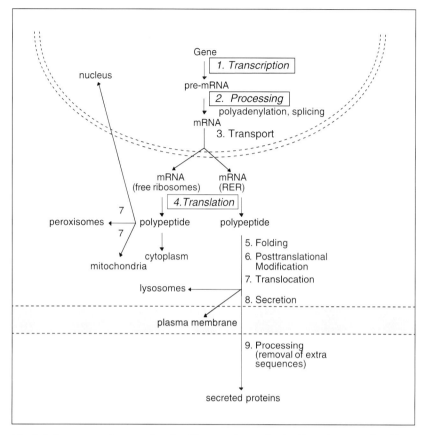

Fig 1-6 Summary of events involved in protein synthesis. Gene is transcribed into complementary RNA and capped at the 5′ end **(1)**. The pre-mRNA product formed is acted on by endonuclease and the free 3′ end generated is polyadenylated. It is then spliced to mature mRNA **(2)**, and transported to cytoplasmic locations **(3)**. Proteins targeted to intracellular organelles are translated on free ribosomes, while those destined for lysosomes, plasma membrane, and secretion are synthesized on the RER **(4)**. Nascent polypeptides undergo folding **(5)**, sugar and other residues are added **(6)**, and the polypeptide is translocated to destination sites **(7)**. Extracellular proteins are secreted into the matrix **(8)**; these proteins may undergo additional proteolytic cleavage to convert precursors into active forms **(9)**. Major regulatory points are shown in italics and boxed.

Protein content is also determined by the extent of degradation, which may be intracellular or extracellular. Intracellular degradation can occur by lysosomal and nonlysosomal pathways, and may be ubiquitin mediated.

Inhibitors of Protein Synthesis

Protein synthesis is affected by numerous compounds that may inhibit any of the reactions involved in transcription and translation processes. These inhibitors have proved valuable as therapeutic agents and in defining protein synthesis reactions in experimental systems. For example, α-amanitin inhibits protein synthesis, as described previously, by preferentially binding to RNA polymerase II and thereby blocking mRNA synthesis. Cycloheximide inhibits peptidyl transferase and prevents peptide translocation in the ribosomes.

Table 1-4. Some Antibiotic Inhibitors of Protein Synthesis

Inhibitor	Effective Species*	Affected Step	Action
α-amanitin	Eukaryotes	Transcription	Inhibits RNA polymerase II
Chloramphenicol	Prokaryotes	Translation	Binds to 50S ribosomal subunit
Cycloheximide	Eukaryotes	Translation	Binds to 60S ribosomal subunit; Inhibits peptidyl transferase
Erythromycin	Prokaryotes	Translation	Binds to 50S ribosomal subunit
Puromycin	Prokaryotes Eukaryotes	Elongation	Accepts peptidyl-tRNA, causes Premature termination and release
Streptomycin	Prokaryotes Eukaryotes	Initiation	Binds to 30S ribosomal subunit
Tetracycline	Prokaryotes	Initiation	Binds to 30S ribosomal subunit, blocks A site

* Drugs effective in prokaryotes also inhibit mitochondrial protein synthesis.

The antibiotic puromycin has a chemical structure resembling the adenosine-terminal end of aminoacyl-tRNA; therefore, in ribosomes, polypeptides attached to peptidyl-tRNA are transferred to the amino group of puromycin. Because the antibiotic is not anchored onto the A-site, peptidyl puromycin is released from the ribosomes, thus terminating the protein synthesis prematurely. The type and action of these and other protein inhibitors are listed in Table 1-4.

Regulation of Protein Synthesis

In eukaryotic cells, the quality and quantity of proteins synthesized are precisely regulated under healthy conditions. The necessity for accurate regulation is illustrated by conditions such as hypertrophic scar and keloid formation, in which protein synthesis continues unregulated during wound repair, resulting in an accumulation of connective-tissue matrix proteins and loss of tissue function.

Regulation of protein synthesis can occur at one or more steps during transcription and translation. In theory, the production of proteins can be regulated by any of the biosynthetic reactions outlined in Fig 1-6, however, the major regulatory step is the rate of gene transcription. Information for the initiation and activation of transcription is processed at the regulatory elements in each gene; this information is read through the transcription factors that bind to these elements. The synthesis of protein isoforms to suit specific functional needs of each cell and organ represents another level of regulation; this is achieved either through alternative splicing, or by utilizing alternative transcription initiation sites and termination codons. The content of proteins can also be regulated by degradation. Under normal conditions, degradation is primarily involved in the removal of defective and nonfunctional molecules; however, it becomes significant under certain physiological conditions, such as involution of the uterus, and during inflammation and wound healing when dead and damaged tissues are to be removed.

The biosynthetic events that participate in regulation of gene expression can be divided broadly into two types—those that influence protein production and those that affect protein content.

Mechanisms That Regulate Protein Production

DNA methylation. Many genes show patterns of methylation by which cytosines at CpG islands in the DNA molecule are converted reversibly to 5-methylcytosine. The methylated genes are usually inactive because promoter activity requires the presence of unmethylated sites. DNA methylation appears to be a major mechanism that determines whether certain genes are expressed or not. For example, genes undergo dramatic changes in methylation during development; global demethylation occurs from the eight-cell to the blastocyst stages in preimplantation mouse embryos, whereas immediately after implantation, global de novo methylation begins (Martienssen and Richards 1995; Monk 1995; Razin and Shemer 1995). The importance of DNA methylation in development is illustrated by the fact that mouse embryos expressing low levels of DNA methyltransferase do not fully develop to term and die at the 5 to 20 somite stage. Changes in methylation patterns have been a consistent finding in cancer cells (Eden and Cedar 1994; Martienssen and Richards 1995).

Regulation through transcription factors. Although information for regulation of gene expression is present on the DNA, it is interpreted by the transcription factors. Transcription factors are the primary agents that regulate gene transcription rates. Most environmental and physiological mediators affect gene transcription by modifying the synthesis and activities of transcription factors by one or more of the following mechanisms (Maniatis et al 1987; Vellanoweth et al 1994):

1. Synthesis of new species that are normally absent. This is a major mechanism in multicellular organisms by which a specific gene is expressed by a particular cell at a specific time during development. Examples are activation of metallothionein gene expression by Zn^{++} and Cd^{++}, and the regulation of expression of liver-specific genes. Liver produces the serum protein α-fetoprotein during fetal life, whereas albumin and phosphoenolpyruvate carboxykinase are expressed only at birth. C/EBP, a leucine zipper protein, determines the expression of albumin, which is expressed only by liver, fat, intestinal cells, and some brain cells (Benvenisty and Reshef 1991). The expression patterns of homeoproteins during *Drosophila* development is also regulated in this manner. Different combinations of transcription factors operate in tissue-specific expression of proteins.

2. The activity of transcription factors is often modulated by covalently modifying certain amino acids. Phosphorylation and dephosphorylation at specific tyrosine, serine, or threonine residues are the most common modifications (Boulikas 1995). These modifications may affect either the binding of transcription factors to corresponding DNA elements, or the activity of the transcription factors directly. For example, phosphorylation activates heat-shock transcription factor and facilitates its dimerization with Fos protein to form active HSTF-Fos dimers. Many hormones and cytokines that affect gene expression act by phosphorylation of AP1, a transcription factor that is commonly a dimer of Fos and Jun. Modifications may also change the conformation of transcription factors; for instance, phosphorylation of Stat1α by interferon-γ (IFN-γ) induces the formation of its homodimer. This dimer binds to DNA target sequences and affects the expression of target genes (Vellanoweth et al 1994).

3. Binding to a ligand is a major mechanism by which steroid receptors regulate gene expression. Corticosteroids, sex hormones, vitamin D, retinoic acid, and thyroid hormones bind to their respective cytoplasmic DNA binding receptors, and the resulting

hormone-receptor complex translocates to the nucleus. There it binds to specific DNA response elements and activates the transcription of target genes (Truss and Beato 1993).

4. Releasing an inhibitor from inactive transcription factor–inhibitor complexes. For example, the transcription factor NFκB is a family of at least five proteins. It consists of two subunits of 65 kd and 50 kd, and it normally exists as inactive complex with its inhibitor, IκBα. In response to pathogenic stimuli or cytokines such as IL-1 and TNF-α, oxygen free radicals are generated and the IκBα is phosphorylated. Phosphorylation of IκBα releases it from the NFκB complex, and the free NFκB migrates to the nucleus and activates the transcription of target genes. The liberated IκBα is rapidly degraded.

5. Changes in the subunit composition of dimeric transcription factors. This is a common mechanism by which the function of HLH proteins is modified. The HLH proteins form homo- and heterodimers, and the activity of the transcription factors is determined by which units come together. For example, the homo- and heterodimers of MyoD and E2A induce myogenesis. However, in the presence of another factor, Id, both MyoD and E2A form complexes with Id and formation of a MyoD-E2A dimer is prevented (Rudnicki and Jaenisch 1995).

Stability and degradation of mRNA. In addition to the rate of gene transcription, the abundance of mRNA depends upon the extent of mRNA degradation. Thus, the stability of the mRNA can determine the amount of proteins produced. Bacteria modify protein synthesis patterns in response to changes in their environment, and prompt response requires fast turnover of mRNA by degradation; therefore, the life of prokaryotic mRNA is typically short, with a half-life of only a few minutes. In contrast, eukaryotic mRNA is much more stable. The average half-life of mammalian mRNA, although it may vary by several orders of magnitude for individual species, is approximately 6 hours.

Many factors affect the stability of mRNA. The cap structure, in which the 5-5'-phosphodiester bond is resistant to ribonucleases, the poly(A) tail, and certain secondary structures confer stability to the mRNA molecule. In contrast, the presence of destabilizing nucleotide sequences lead to its degradation, and such sequences are found throughout the length of the mRNA. Specific proteins are believed to bind to and mask AU-rich 3' sequences in mRNA and protect it from degradation of the mRNA. Protein factors often unmask these destabilizing elements, and thus regulate the rate of mRNA decay. Most notable among the destabilizing sequences are the AU-rich domains present at the 3'-untranslated region (Peltz et al 1991; Ross 1996; Sachs 1993). These are AUUUA motifs repeated once or more within a U-rich region. Several cellular mRNAs, such as those for lymphokines and growth factors, contain this sequence. Deadenylation of the poly(A) tail appears to be a prerequisite for mRNA degradation, and degradation does not begin until the poly(A) tail is shortened to less than 10 bases. Complete deadenylation leads to rapid degradation of mRNA.

Many hormones and growth factors, as well as conditions such as starvation, hypoxia, and infection, affect mRNA stability. For example, the casein mRNA concentration in mammary cells increases 100-fold in response to the hormone prolactin, although the transcription rate is enhanced only threefold; this is due to an increase in the half-life of casein mRNA. Some eukaryotic mRNAs such as c-*myc* and c-*fos* are very short-lived, and two complementary mechanisms are responsible for the short half-life. These mRNAs are expressed transiently at specified times for brief periods, and, in addition, they also have multiple AUUUA sequences at their 3' ends.

Alternative splicing. While the concentration and stability of mRNA determine the amount of protein translated, alternative splicing provides a mechanism by which different functional domains can be shuffled to meet specific protein requirements in different tissues (Bonen 1993; Nadal-Ginard et al 1990; Sharp 1994). There is no variation in the translated protein product when only a single mRNA is produced; however, alternative splicing makes it possible to skip certain exons and include others. The size and type of proteins produced vary accordingly. Extracellular proteins, fibronectins, and collagens are designed in this manner (Chapters 4, 5, and 6; Ffrench-Constant 1995). Alternative splicing involves differential use of splicing junctions; thus, one site (5′ or 3′) remains common while the other is variable. Often, one of the exons may contain a stop codon, and including this exon will result in the production of a truncated form of protein, which may be nonfunctional. This form of regulation occurs in *Drosophila melanogaster* sex determination. Different mRNAs translatable into different protein isoforms can also arise by utilizing alternative transcription initiation sites. The alternate start and stop sites can be located anywhere in the gene, even within introns.

RNA editing. This is a mechanism by which bases in gene transcripts are altered prior to their maturation into translatable mRNA (Scott 1995). RNA editing is widespread in mitochondria and protozoa, however, it is relatively rare in higher eukaryotes. An example in mammals is tissue-specific expression of apolipoprotein β isomers. Full length apo-β100 is a ~500-kd molecule produced by hepatocytes. This molecule is capable of binding low-density lipoprotein (LDL) and transporting cholesterol and triglycerides. In intestinal cells, C_{6666} of the mRNA is converted to U by RNA editing, so that the codon CAA (glutamine) is changed to UAA (stop codon). As a result, a smaller, roughly 240-kd molecule that cannot bind (LDL) or transport choles-

terol is produced, although this molecule can still catalyze dietary lipid absorption. The editing is carried out by cytidine deaminase, and it requires AU-rich binding sites on the mRNA. Similar RNA editing occurs in neurons by site-specific adenosine deamination in pre-mRNA for a glutamate receptor B subunit. In this case the codon for glutamine (CAG) is edited to arginine (CGG), and the latter amino acid reduces Ca^{++} permeability across ion channels. The glutamine-to-arginine editing requires a double-stranded RNA structure produced by exonic and intronic sequences (Melcher et al 1996).

Translational and posttranslational mechanisms. The translational component of protein synthesis is a multistep process that involves several accessory factors, thus regulation can be exerted at several levels (Hershey et al 1996). For example, the rates of initiation (a rate-limiting step) and elongation are affected by cell cycle, infection, and many other conditions, and heat-shock activates the translation of heat shock mRNAs but represses other mRNAs. One mechanism by which these effects are mediated is through modification of accessory protein factors. For example, phosphorylation of several initiation factors (eg, eIF2B, eIF4B, eIF4E and eIF4G) promotes translation while it has the opposite effect in eIF2. Regulation of translation may also occur through *cis*-elements present in the mRNA; many mRNAs contain these sequences in the 5′- and 3′-untranslated regions. These elements can affect the translation either directly or through *trans*-acting factors that bind to these sequences. Regulation of translation can occur by structural features of the mRNA, and by the presence of initiating codons and sequences at the upstream open reading frames of mRNAs (Geballe and Morris 1994). Multiple start and stop codons can give rise to alternate protein isoforms.

The rate of protein production can also be regulated at the translational level by specific

RNA binding proteins. For example, in erythrocytes at low Fe^{++} concentration, iron response element–binding protein (IRE-BP) binds to 5′-ends and blocks the translation initiation of ferritin- (iron-binding protein) and 5-aminolevulinate-mRNAs; therefore, Fe^{++} remains within cells, is not utilized for heme production, and is available for other essential processes. At high Fe^{++} concentrations, the IRE-BP becomes inactive and the mRNAs are translated (Theil 1993). The abundance of tRNA species and presence of translational-inhibitory peptides can also affect the rate of translation; this mechanism has been identified for matrix proteins, however, to what extent they are physiologically significant is unclear.

Regulation can occur posttranslationally through modification reactions; interference with these reactions often decreases the stability of the polypeptides produced and affects their secretion. Defective protein molecules are degraded.

Mechanisms Affecting Protein Degradation

Protein degradation is a negative regulatory mechanism by which cellular proteins are removed during normal homeostasis and under pathologic conditions. It may occur intra- or extracellularly, and within the cells, degradation may be mediated by lysosomal or nonlysosomal pathways (Ciechanover and Schwartz 1994; Lee and Marzella 1994). Proteins entering cells from the extracellular space by endocytosis or by pinocytosis, as well as those under heat shock and other stress conditions, are degraded in lysosomes. Nonlysosomal protein degradation is mediated through the ubiquitin pathway. Ubiquitin is a highly conserved 76–amino acid polypeptide that attaches covalently to target proteins through consensus amino acid sequences in an ATP-dependent reaction. Proteins that are ubiquitinylated at multiple sites, not those with only one attached ubiquitin molecule, are targeted to be destroyed. A protease complex of approximately 700 kd, called macropain or 20S proteosome, degrades the ubiquitinylated proteins liberating free ubiquitin, which is then recycled (Ciechanover and Schwartz 1994; Wilkinson 1995). The primary purpose of ubiquitin-mediated degradation appears to be to remove defective, misfolded, and denatured proteins as well as alien molecules. Ubiquitin-mediated degradation is believed to play a significant role in cell cycle and division, stress response, DNA repair, and other cellular processes. It is a key component of degradation of cellular proteins such as Fos and cyclins.

The number of ubiquitin conjugates increase in carcinomas, Alzheimer's disease, and other pathologic conditions, however whether this is a cause for pathologic protein degradation is unclear. At least three peptide-sequence motifs have been identified that serve as recognition signals for degradation by ubiquitin as well as by nonubiquitin pathways. These sequences are PEST, KFERQ (for one-letter amino acid codes, see Table 1-2) and the cyclin-destruction box present in cyclins (Rechsteiner and Rogers 1996). The PEST amino acid motif is present in proteins that turn over rapidly, such as IκBα, ornithine decarboxylase and Fos, while the KFERQ motif is found in RNase A. Interestingly, molecular chaperones also appear to participate in and stimulate protein degradation (Hayes and Dice 1996).

Degradation of collagen, elastin, and other matrix proteins occurs predominantly in the extracellular space. Degradation of these proteins is minimal under healthy conditions; however, it becomes prominent during involution of the uterus, inflammation, tissue remodeling, and tumor invasion. Degradation of collagen and elastin requires special enzymes because these proteins are resistant to most common proteinases. Such enzymes are produced by tissues and inflammatory cells, and their production is influenced by the hormones estrogen and progesterone, numerous cytokines, and growth factors. The activity of these enzymes is also regulated through various tissue and serum inhibitor proteins that bind to these enzymes and inactivate them (see Chapter 4).

Summary

Gene expression and protein synthesis are two processes vital for the survival and propagation of all cells; they are also essential for the reconstitution of tissues after injury. The inability to synthesize the right proteins is one major reason why tissues containing differentiated cells are not restored by regeneration, but repaired. The general principles of synthesis and regulation apply to periodontal tissues and diseases affecting the periodontium. Understanding the mechanisms of gene expression and its regulation is necessary to elucidate the biochemical basis for normal tissue turnover, and to define biochemical alterations under pathologic conditions. A variety of growth factors and cytokines capable of affecting cellular functions are present in normal and inflamed periodontal tissues. These substances mediate their influence through their effect on gene transcription rates. How these substances affect the structure and turnover of matrix components is described in the following chapters, and how some of these substances contribute to diseases and repair of the periodontium is discussed in Parts II and III.

References

Aran A, Casuto H, Reshef L. Co-operation between transcription factors regulates liver development. Biol Neonate 1995;67:387.

Benvenisty N, Reshef L. Regulation of tissue- and development-specific gene expression in the liver. Biol Neonate 1991;59:181.

Berg JM. Zinc fingers and other metal-binding domains. J Biol Chem 1990;265:6513.

Bonen L. Trans-splicing of premRNA in plants, animals and protists. FASEB J 1993;4:40.

Boulikas T. Nuclear localization signals (NLS). Crit Rev Eukaryot Gene Expr 1993;3:193.

Boulikas T. A compilation and classification of DNA binding sites for protein transcription factors from vertebrates. Crit Rev Eukaryot Gene Expr 1994;4:117.

Boulikas T. Phosphorylation of transcription factors and control of cell cycle. Crit Rev Eukaryot Gene Expr 1995; 5:1.

Ciechanover A, Schwartz AL. The ubiquitin-mediated proteolytic pathway: mechanisms of recognition of the proteolytic substrate and involvement in the degradation of native cellular proteins. FASEB J 1994;8:182.

Eden S, Cedar H. Role of DNA methylation in the regulation of transcription. Curr Opin Genet Dev 1994;4:255.

Ellenberger TE, Brandl CJ, Struhl K, Harrison SC. The GCN4 basic region leucine zipper binds DNA as a dimer of uninterrupted a helices: crystal structure of the protein-DNA complex. Cell 1992;71:1223.

Ferré-D'Amaré AR, Prendergast GC, Zif EB, Burley SK. Recognition by Max of its cognate DNA through a dimeric b/HLH/Z domain. Nature 1993;363:38.

Ffrench-Constant C. Alternative splicing of fibronectin— Many different proteins but few different functions. Exp Cell Res 1995;221:261.

Geballe AP, Morris DR. Initiation codons within 5′-leaders of mRNAs as regulators of transcription. Trends Biochem Sci 1994;19:159.

Glick BS, Beasley EM, Schatz G. Protein sorting in mitochondria. Trends Biochem Sci 1992;17:453.

Gossen M, Bonin AL, Bujard H. Control of gene activity in higher eukaryotic cells by prokaryotic regulatory elements. Trends Biochem Sci 1993;18:471.

Harrison SC. A structural taxonomy of DNA-binding domains. Nature 1991;353:715.

Hartl FU. Molecular chaperones in cellular protein folding. Nature 1996;381:571.

Hayes SA, Dice JF. Molecular chaperones in protein degradation. J Cell Biol 1996;132:255.

Hendrick JP, Hartl FU. The role of molecular chaperones in protein folding. FASEB J 1995;9:1559.

Hershey JWB, Mathews MB, Sonenberg N. Translational Control. Cold Spring Harbor, NY: Laboratory Press, 1996.

Hesketh JE. Sorting of messenger RNAs in the cytoplasm: mRNA localization and the cytoskeleton. Exp Cell Res 1996;225:219.

Johnson PF, McKnight SL. Eukaryotic transcriptional regulatory proteins. Annu Rev Biochem 1989;58:799.

Klug A. Gene regulatory proteins and their interaction with DNA. Ann NY Acad Sci 1995;758:143.

Lee HK, Marzella L. Regulation of intracellular protein degradation with special reference to lysosomes: role in cell physiology and pathology. Int Rev Exp Pathol 1994;35:39.

Lewin B. Genes V. New York: Oxford University Press; 1994.

Lodish H, Baltimore D, Berd A, Witkowski AL, Matsudiara P, Darnell J. Molecular Cell Biology. 3rd ed. New York: Freeman; 1995.

Maniatis T, Goodbourn S, Ficher J. Regulation of inducible and tissue-specific gene expression. Science 1987;236:1237.

Martienssen RA, Richards EJ. DNA methylation in eukaryotes. Curr Opin Genet Dev 1995;5:234.

McKeown M. Alternative mRNA splicing. Annu Rev Cell Biol 1992;8:155.

Melcher T, Maas S, Herb A, Sprengel R, Seeburg PH, Higuchi M. A mammalian RNA editing enzyme. Nature 1996;379:460.

Monk M. Epigenetic programming of differential gene expression in development and evolution. Dev Genet 1995;17:188.

Nadal-Ginard B, Smith CWJ, Patton JG, Breitbart RE. Alternative splicing is an efficient mechanism for the generation of protein diversity: contractile protein genes as a model system. Adv Enzyme Regul 1990;31:261.

Orkin SH. Regulation of globin gene expression in erythroid cells. Eur J Biochem 1995;231:271.

Pain VM. Initiation of protein synthesis in eukaryotic cells. Eur J Biochem 1996;236:747.

Papavassiliou AG. Transcription factors: structure, function, and implication in malignant growth. Anticancer Res 1995;15:891.

Peltz SW, Brewer G, Bernstein P, Hart PA, Ross J. Regulation of mRNA turnover in eukaryotic cells. Crit Rev Eukaryot Gene Expr 1991;1:99.

Razin A, Shemer R. DNA methylation in early development. Hum Mol Genet 1995;4:1751.

Rechsteiner M, Rogers SW. PEST sequences and regulation by proteolysis. Trends Biochem Sci 1996;21:267.

Rigby PW. Three in one and one in three: it all depends on TBP. Cell 1993;72:7.

Rings EHHM, Büller HA, Neele AM, Dekker J. Protein sorting versus messenger RNA sorting? Eur J Cell Biol 1994;63:161.

Ross J. Control of messenger RNA stability in higher eukaryotes. Trends Genet 1996;12:171.

Rothman JE. Mechanisms of intracellular protein transport. Nature 1994;372:55.

Rudnicki MA, Jaenisch R. The myoD family of transcription factors and skeletal myogenesis. Bioessays 1995;17:203.

Sachs AB. Messenger RNA degradation in eukaryotes. Cell 1993;74:413.

Scott J. A place in the world for RNA editing. Cell 1995; 81:833.

Sharp PA. Split genes and RNA splicing. Cell 1994; 77:805.

Staudt LM, Lenardo MJ. Immunoglobulin gene transcription. Annu Rev Immunol 1991;9:373.

Tarun SZJ, Sachs AB. A common function for mRNA 5′ and 3′ ends in translation initiation in yeast. Genes Dev 1995;9:2997.

Theil EC. The IRE (iron regulatory element) family: structures which regulate mRNA translation or stability. Biofactors 1993;4:87.

Truss M, Beato M. Steroid hormone receptors: interaction with deoxyribonucleic acid and transcription factors. Endocr Rev 1993;14:459.

Vellanoweth RL, Supakar PC, Roy AK. Biology of disease. Transcription factors in development, growth and aging. Lab Invest 1994;70:784.

von Heijne G. Protein targeting signals. Curr Opin Cell Biol 1990;2:604.

Wahle E, Keller W. The biochemistry of polyadenylation. Trends Biochem Sci 1996;21:247.

Walter P, Johnson AE. Signal sequence recognition and protein targeting to the endoplasmic reticulum membrane. Annu Rev Cell Biol 1994;10:87.

Watson JD, Gilman M, Witkowski J, Zollen M. Recombinant DNA. 2nd ed. New York: Freeman; 1992.

Wedel A, Ziegler-Heitbrock HWL. The C/EBP family of transcription factors. Immunobiol 1995;193:171.

Wilkinson DD. Roles of ubiquitinylation in proteolysis and cellular regulation. Annu Rev Nutr 1995;15:161.

Wolberger C, Vershon AK, Liu B, Johnson AD, Pabo CO. Crystal structure of a MAT α2 homeodomain-operator complex suggests a general model for homeodomain-DNA interactions. Cell 1991;67:517.

Mammalian Cell Cycle and Growth Regulation

Introduction

The ability to divide and multiply are fundamental properties of all cells. These properties are essential for the development and growth of living organisms, and for the replacement of cells destroyed by injury or during wound healing. The objectives of cell division are to duplicate the chromosomes and distribute them equally to daughter cells. In higher animals and plants, this is achieved by two processes referred to as mitosis and meiosis. Most somatic cells divide by mitosis, producing two daughter cells with one set of identical complementary diploid chromosomes each. In contrast, meiosis, by which sperm and eggs are produced, generates progeny containing half the number of respective parental chromosomes characteristic of the somatic cells of the species.

In unicellular organisms, each cell is committed to grow and divide continually, as rapidly as the availability of nutrients and the cell's environment will allow. In contrast, most somatic cells of higher organisms are not programmed to divide continually. These cells remain growth arrested in a quiescent state until signals are received to induce them to divide. In this state, the cells grow in neither size nor in number, and their metabolism is at an equilibrium. In these cells, cell division is controlled by several intracellular checkpoints. When the need to multiply arises, the cells are induced by extracellular signals, such as growth factors and nutrients, to overcome the checkpoints and complete the cell division. The mechanisms by which cells overcome growth arrest and divide are similar in all eukaryotic cells from yeasts to mammals. The ordered sequence of events by which cells divide is called the cell cycle.

Stages of the Somatic Cell Cycle

The events involved in the cell cycle process can be divided into four distinct phases. Actual cell division during which daughter cells separate takes place during a brief mitotic (M) phase. The interval between mitotic phases is called the interphase, and nondividing cells spend most of their lifetime in this phase. Preparations for cell division are made during the interphase, which consists initially of the first gap phase (G_1), followed by synthesis of DNA (S phase), and then a second gap phase (G_2) (Fig 2-1a). Cells that are growth arrested remain at G_1 or at a nondividing quiescent G_0 phase. In the presence of mitogenic factors that provide division signals, the cells respond with a cascade of biochemical reactions that overcome the growth-arresting checkpoints and commit them to divide (Norbury and Nurse 1992; Pardee 1989; Pardee et al 1978). The commitment of cells to divide occurs somewhere during the mid-to-late G_1 phase at a restriction point (R point, called START in yeast), after which they no longer require mitogenic factors. The cells then transit to the S phase, at which point the DNA is replicated completely, but only once, so that cells will have exactly twice

the normal DNA content. Preparations for the M phase events are made during the ensuing G_2 phase. During M phase, virtually all cellular synthetic activities are stopped and the entire efforts of the cell are directed toward cell division. At the end of mitosis, one diploid set of chromosomes each is transferred to each of the daughter cells.

Mitosis involves a series of brief and well-defined events (see Fig 2-1b). At prophase, chromatin in the nucleus condenses into visible chromosome fibers, and the nuclear membrane begins to breakdown. Microtubules of the spindle nucleate around the pole bodies and move to opposite poles of the cell. During the ensuing prometaphase, the microtubules enter the nucleus, and sister chromatids (duplicate set of chromosomes each attached at their centromere) move toward the equator of the cell. This is followed by metaphase, when all chromosomes line up equally along the metaphase plate. Then follows anaphase, when the sister chromatids separate and chromosomes move to opposite poles along the microtubules. The poles then separate along with the chromosomes during telophase; at this time the nuclear envelope re-forms around the chromosomes. The final mitotic event is cytokinesis, when the cytoplasm segregates into two daughter cells (for a general treatise on this and other aspects of cells, see Alberts et al 1994). These same events are also involved in meiosis, however, in this case the cells undergo two successive divisions, but only one S phase. During the first meiotic division, centromeres do not divide, and one homologue of each of the sister chromatids is distributed randomly to the daughters. The centromeres separate during the second meiotic division, and one chromosome is dispensed to each of the four haploid daughters.

The time taken to complete each cell division varies in different species, and even among different cell types within the same organism. Cell division is much more rapid during embryogenesis; for example, the first

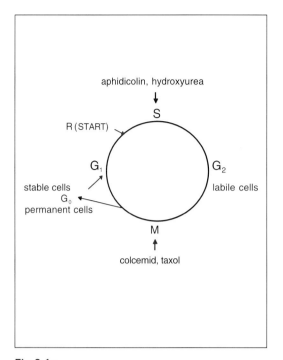

Fig 2-1a

Fig 2-1 A schematic representation of cell division cycle. **(a)** The cell cycle is divided into four phases: gap 1 (G_1), S (DNA synthesis), gap 2 (G_2) and mitosis (M). Mammalian cells normally are arrested in G_1 or G_0 (quiescent) phase until they come across a proliferation stimulus such as a growth factor. Then they proceed through the cell cycle, but division can proceed only if they cross the commitment point (R point; START in the yeast) in mid-to-late G_1. Once the R point is overcome, the cells are committed to divide and no further mitogenic signal is needed. The cells replicate DNA during the S phase, pass through the G_2 phase, and divide during the M phase. The stages at which some inhibitors arrest the cell cycle are indicated. Aphidicolin and hydroxyurea arrest cells in the S phase, whereas colcemid, which depolymerizes microtubules, blocks the cells in metaphase. Differentiated cells have exited the cell cycle and are permanently arrested in G_0. Stable cells have limited division capacity, and they remain dormant at G_0 or G_1. In contrast, labile cells can divide continually. The major mitotic events that lead to cytokinesis are summarized in **(b)**.

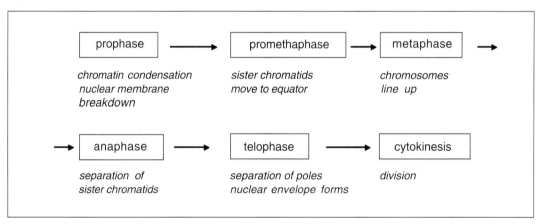

Fig 2-1b

cell division in *Xenopus* occurs in 90 minutes, and 11 subsequent divisions are completed within 7 hours. Exponentially growing human diploid fibroblasts may complete one cycle of division every 24 hours. The length of the G_1 phase in somatic cells is highly variable because cells remain in this phase until the division-promoting signal becomes avail-able. The length of the G_2 phase may also vary to some extent depending upon conditions (eg, due to DNA damage), however the duration of the S and M phases is invariant.

Not all of the cell populations constituting an adult organism divide. Based on their division potential, these cells have been classified into three types. Specialized cells such as nerve cells, cardiac myocytes, and skeletal muscle cells have exited the cell cycle and are differentiated, and they do not divide. These cells are called permanent, or nondividing, cells and they remain in the G_0 state. Parenchymal cells of glandular organs, liver, and kidney, and mesenchymal cells such as fibroblasts, osteoblasts, and glial cells have limited division potential, and these are referred to as stable (or quiescent) cells. Stable cells normally remain quiescent in tissues in G_0-G_1 phase waiting for an appropriate signal to divide. During wound healing, these signals are provided by growth factors and cytokines released during inflammation. The stable cells provide the machinery for wound repair, and they are largely responsible for synthesizing the extracellular matrix components. In contrast to the above two cell types, cells that continually divide and have considerable division potential are called labile cells. Stem cells, which are undifferentiated precursor cells, and basal epithelial cells are labile cells. The labile cells may be pluripotent, with the ability to differentiate into several cell lineages, or unipotent. Splenic, lymphoid, hematopoietic, and bone marrow cells are pluripotent, as they give rise to inflammatory and other cell types. Epithelial cells, on the other hand, are unipotent. This cell type includes those present in the stratified squamous surfaces of the skin, oral cavity, vagina, and cervix; the cells lining the mucosa of gland excretory ducts such as the pancreatic and biliary ducts; the columnar epithelial cells of the gastrointestinal tract, uterus, and fallopian tubes; and cells of the transitional epithelium of the urinary tract.

Biochemical Events Associated with the Cell Cycle

The various activities of a cell, including its division, are influenced by growth factors, hormones, cytokines, and a broad range of other molecules that are collectively known as mitogenic factors. The actions of these substances are initiated when they bind to specific receptors on the cell membrane, initiating a cascade of biochemical reactions within the cell that generate second messengers and amplify the original signal. A number of cellular proteins are involved in these processes, and the final outcome is cell division, differentiation, or other cellular function.

Mitogenic Factors

The mitogenic factors include polypeptide growth factors, cytokines, and many other substances named based on their cellular origin, target cells, and effect (Cantley et al 1991; Nathan and Sporn 1991; Sporn and Roberts 1990). Among these substances, growth factors form an important group. This family includes platelet-derived growth factors (PDGF), epidermal growth factor (EGF), fibroblast growth factors (FGF), insulinlike growth factors I and II (IGF-I and IGF-II), transforming growth factors α and β (TGF-α and β), and nerve growth factor (NGF), insulin, and other hormones (Table 2-1). Target cells for these molecules are mesenchymal, epithelial, and endothelial cells, whereas the action of cytokines, interferons, and colony stimulating factors is largely, but not exclusively, on inflammatory cells. These substances have many properties in common. They are pleiotropic and stimulate similar signaling events in many target cells (Chao 1992; Nathan and Sporn 1991); however, the final outcome of their effect depends upon many factors, especially the type of target cell. Their action may even be opposite in different cell types. Often, several molecules act together in concert, and their overall effect may be additive, synergistic, or contradictory. These substances may be present constitutively in the environment, or derived from an effector cell that secretes mitogenic factors either from storage or after new synthesis. Most

Table 2-1. Some Important Growth Factors, Cytokines, and Lymphokines

Molecule	Structure	Target Cell	Major Effect on Cells
Growth Factors			
PDGF	Homo/hetero dimer of A and B chains	Mesenchymal cells	Growth promotion
FGF1-9	16–18-kd polypeptide	Mesenchymal cells	Growth promotion, angiogenesis
EGF	6-kd polypeptide	Epithelial cells, epidermal cells	Proliferation, differentiation
TGF-α	6-kd polypeptide	Epithelial cells, epidermal cells	Proliferation, differentiation
TGF-β family	~25-kd polypeptide	Epithelial cells, mesenchymal cells	Growth inhibition, matrix synthesis, angiogenesis
BMP2-8	...	Osteoblasts	Bone formation
Cytokines/Lymphokines			
IL-1	17 kd	Many cells, inflammatory cells	Growth promotion, matrix degradation
TNF-α	17-kd polypeptide	Many cells	Growth promotion, matrix degradation
IL-8	10 kd	PMN	Chemotaxis
IFN-γ	20–25 kd	Fibroblasts, monocytes, lymphocytes	Growth inhibition, matrix inhibition

cells require more than one stimulus (mitogenic factor) to traverse past the restriction point and enter from the G_1 phase into the S phase (Pardee 1989).

Although the mitogenic factors fall into several families, they all induce a series of common events that are necessary for cell division. Many of these events are also induced during other cellular functions such as metabolism, neurotransmission, cell migration, and phagocytosis (Ben-Baruch et al 1995; Ihle 1995; Juliano and Haskill 1993). The major events induced by growth factors are described in the following sections.

Growth Factor Receptors

The first event of growth factor action is the binding to specific receptors on the cell surface. Growth factor receptors comprise a large family of transmembrane proteins with more than 50 members. Based on the location of N- and C-terminal domains, receptors are classified as type I (N-terminal side outside the cell, C-terminal end in the cytoplasmic side; or type II (N-terminal end on the cytoplasmic side). Virtually all growth factor receptors are type I. Growth factors bind to the extracellular N-terminal domain, and the C-terminal cytoplasmic end of the receptors usually contains kinase domains. The kinase domain may have tyrosine, or serine and threonine kinase activity, or no kinase activity at all (Fig 2-2a). Receptors with tyrosine kinase activity have been divided into more than 10 classes, based on structural features (Fantl et al 1993). One of these classes is the EGF receptor family; these are monomeric molecules that contain two cysteine-rich clusters at the extracellular domain and src-like (src is a protein kinase and a product of the v-*src* onco-

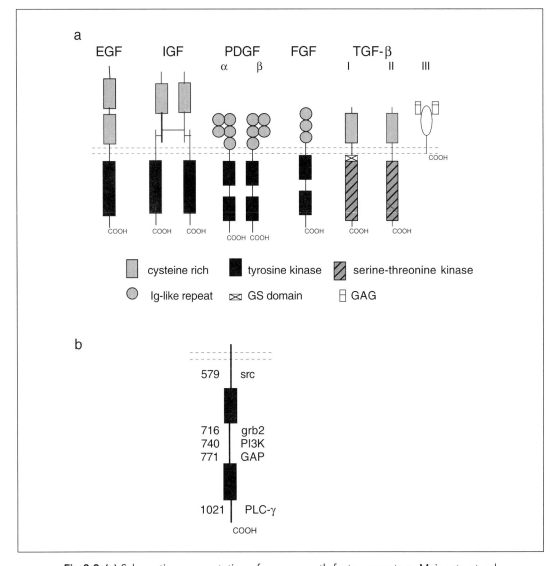

Fig 2-2 (a) Schematic representation of some growth factor receptors. Major structural and functional domains in these molecules are indicated. Growth factors bind to the extracellular N-terminal domain. EGF, IGF, FGF, and PDGF receptors have intrinsic tyrosine kinase activity at the cytoplasmic domain. Type I, II, and III receptors for TGF-β are shown; types I and II have a serine-threonine kinase domain. The GS domain in the type I receptor is rich in Gly-Ser. The type III receptor, also called betaglycan, contains covalently attached heparan sulfate and chondroitin sulfate glycosaminoglycan chains (Reprinted with permission from Attisano et al 1994; Fantl et al 1993). These figures are not drawn to scale. (b) Cytoplasmic tyrosine kinase domains of the PDGF β receptor showing the sites where SH2 proteins bind. The tyrosine residues that bind to src, grb2, PI3K, GTP-ase activating protein (GAP), and PLC-γ are indicated (Reprinted with permission from Claesson-Welsh 1994).

gene originally identified in Rous sarcoma virus) cytoplasmic domains (see Fig 2-2a). The insulin receptor and the IGF-I receptor represent a second family; these are heterodimers made up of one α and β subunit each, linked by disulfide bonds. The α subunit contains a cysteine-rich cluster that binds to the ligand, while the β subunit has the tyrosine kinase activity. The receptor for PDGF is also a dimer of α and β subunits, however the dimer may be composed of either or both subunits. Each subunit has its own extracellular ligand binding domain that contains immunoglobulinlike repeats, and a cytoplasmic tyrosine kinase domain. The latter is interrupted by a kinase insertion domain (see Fig 2-2b). Unlike the PDGF and EGF receptors, TGF-β binds to three receptors, designated as types I, II, and III. Among these, types I and II consist of an extracellular cysteine-rich ligand-binding domain, a transmembrane domain, and a cytoplasmic serine-threonine kinase domain. These two receptors mediate signaling events as a heterodimeric complex (Attisano et al 1994). The type III receptor, also called betaglycan (see Chapter 6), does not have kinase activity, and it contains an extracellular domain to which the heparan sulfate and chondroitin sulfate glycosaminoglycans are attached.

These receptors are responsible for mediating their targeted functions, and they bind to their ligands with high affinity. In addition, some growth factors such as FGF and TGF-β also bind to other cell surface components with lower affinity. The latter are normally hybrid molecules consisting of proteins and polysaccharides (eg, TGF-β receptor betaglycan). They do not directly mediate mitogenic action, but they appear to possess accessory functions such as sequestering growth factors and presenting the ligands to their primary receptors (Schlessinger et al 1995).

The first reaction that occurs immediately following the binding of a growth factor to its receptor is the dimerization of the receptor. This is accompanied by tyrosine autophosphorylation of its cytoplasmic domain, if the receptor is a tyrosine kinase (Lemmon and Schlessinger 1994; Seedorf 1995). Autophosphorylation may occur at one or more of the tyrosines and leads to the activation of its tyrosine kinase activity located on the cytoplasmic side. The tyrosine autophosphorylation makes it possible to bind to other proteins containing one or more amino acid sequences homologous to the src protein kinase (these domains are called SH2 and SH3 domains for src homology 2 and 3) (see Fig 2-2b). The latter are signaling proteins such as phospholipase C_γ (PLC-γ), phosphatidylinositol-3′ kinase (PI3 kinase), Grb2, and src. These molecules become phosphorylated and activated by their binding to growth factor receptors, and generate second messengers in turn. An exception to this scheme is the insulin receptor; this receptor does not bind to SH2 proteins directly, but it activates a docking protein, referred to as IRS-1 (insulin receptor substrate-1), to which the SH2 proteins bind (White and Kahn 1994).

Induction of Second Messengers

Each of the activated SH2/SH3 proteins initiates another series of reactions in parallel. The adapter molecule Grb2 binds to another protein, sos, and together they replace guanosine 5′-diphosphate (GDP) from the ras-GDP complex with GTP. GDP-bound ras is inactive and replacement with guanosine 5′-triphosphate (GTP) activates ras, which is a serine-threonine kinase. The activation of ras occurs at close proximity to the membrane. The activated ras in turn activates another serine-threonine kinase, raf-1. Activation of raf-1 is the first step in the mitogen activated protein kinase (MAPK) cascade. The MAPK cascade is a major mediator of several cellular functions (see page 35). The enzyme PLC-γ hydrolyzes the membrane-bound phospholipid, phosphatidylinositol 4,5-bisphosphate (PIP_2) to inositol-1,4,5-triphosphate (IP_3) and diacylglyc-

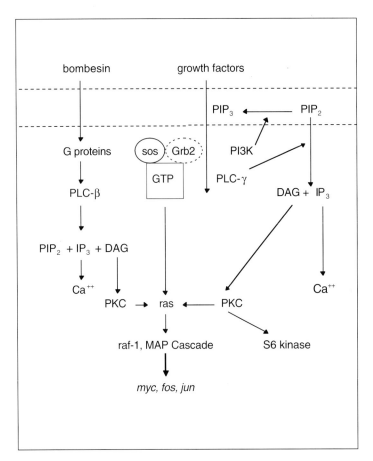

Fig 2-3 Summary of major mitogenic signal transduction events. Binding to a ligand induces receptor dimerization and autophosphorylation in receptors with tyrosine kinase activity. The autophosphorylated receptor binds to Grb2, PI3K, PLC-γ, and other proteins containing SH2 and SH3 domains, and activates them. The IGF-1 receptor, however, does not bind to SH2 proteins directly, but through a docking protein called IRS-1. Activation of the adapter molecule Grb2 results in activation of ras, which in turn activates raf-1 and the MAPK cascade. The PLC-γ hydrolyzes membrane phospholipids to IP_3 and DAG, which cause Ca^{++} mobilization and PKC activation, respectively. PKC phosphorylates and activates raf-1 and S6 kinase. The ras is also activated by receptors without tyrosine kinase activity through a different mechanism involving cAMP/cGMP and G proteins (not shown). Ca^{++}, DAG, PKC, ras, cAMP, and cGMP are second messengers.

erol (DAG); these two molecules are called second messengers, and cause the movement of Ca^{++} from endoplasmic reticulum reserves and activation of protein kinase C (PKC), respectively (Fig 2-3) (Berridge 1993; Clapham 1995; Divecha and Fine 1995; Means 1994). PKC, among its many activities, also activates raf-1 directly. The PI3-kinase phosphorylates PIP_2 to phosphatidylinositol-3,4,5-triphosphate (IP_3). This enzyme also associates with focal adhesion kinase (FAK), which assembles with paxillin, talin, and other cytoskeletal proteins for cytoskeletal organization.

While the receptors for PDGF and EGF induce growth signals in the above manner, other growth factor receptors interact with a transmembrane protein, G protein (guanine nucleotide binding protein). This protein consists of α, β, and γ subunits; the α subunit binds to guanine nucleotides. Like ras, the G protein is inactive when bound to GDP, and it remains in this state as a complex of the α and β subunits. Binding of the ligand to its receptor results in replacement of GDP with GTP, and this leads to the activation of the α subunit and its dissociation from the other subunits. The GTP-bound α subunit activates adenyl cyclase, an enzyme that catalyzes the synthesis of cyclic adenosine monophosphate (cAMP). During this process, GTP is hydrolyzed to GDP and the α subunit–GDP complex reassociates with the β and γ subunits to become inactive again. Adenyl cyclase activates protein kinase A, an important enzyme that phosphorylates several cellular proteins. The G proteins can also activate another enzyme, PLC-β, which, like PLC-γ, generates DAG (Berridge 1993).

The G protein–mediated pathway is triggered by neuropeptide mitogens such as bombesin, and it is sensitive to pertussis toxin (see Fig 2-3).

Binding of cytokines such as IFN-γ and interleukin-2 to cells activates a family of transcription factors called signal transducers and activators of transcription (STAT). These transcription factors are involved in functional, not mitogenic, responses of cytokines, and their regulatory function on lymphoid and myeloid cells is mediated through the JAK family of tyrosine kinases.

Protein Kinases and the MAPK Cascade

Phosphorylation-dephosphorylation of signal peptides is a reversible mechanism for the activation-deactivation cycle of many regulatory proteins. These reactions are catalyzed by protein kinases and phosphatases, respectively. Phosphorylation can occur either at tyrosine residues, catalyzed by protein tyrosine kinases, or at serine and threonine residues, catalyzed by PKC. The PKCs are a family of at least 12 isoenzymes activated by DAG, or by DAG plus Ca^{++}, or by other factors (Newton 1995). One target for PKC is the MAPK cascade. Proteins are also phosphorylated by another family of kinases called protein kinase A; these enzymes (also called cAMP-dependent protein kinases) are primarily involved in mediating the biologic actions of cAMP (Cohen 1988).

The enzymes associated with the MAPK cascade are threonine-serine kinases. Their activation represents a major step toward translating extracellular signals into various cellular functions. Up to six tiers have been described, and the outcome of MAPK activation may be cell proliferation, differentiation, or other cellular functions. The MAPK activation induces the expression of the c-*fos* gene and phosphorylation of c-*jun;* these two molecules combine to form active AP1 transcription factor. The MAPK cascade is initiated when ras and PKC activate raf-1. Raf-1 in turn activates the mitogen-activated protein kinase kinase (MAPKK), and other enzymes are activated in sequence. Different cellular functions use the above basic scheme of activation; however, they utilize different isoforms of enzymes, but with no cross-reactivity among pathways (Seger and Krebs 1995). Two such pathways are shown in Fig 2-4. These parallel systems are triggered during growth and stress responses, and involve different enzymes. For example, the stress response utilizes another enzyme, MEKK, instead of raf-1, and it activates JNK, the equivalent to extracellular-signal-regulated kinases (ERKs) (Cobb and Goldsmith 1995) (see Fig 2-4).

The different MAP cascades may be redundant, generating different functions in different cell types (Seger and Krebs 1995). For example, FGF causes cell proliferation in fibroblasts, but differentiation in other cell types. The kinetics of MAP activation may also vary during different cellular responses. For example, mitogenic stimulation involves a transient activation of the MAP cascade, whereas sustained stimulation is needed for differentiation.

Late Mitogenic Events

The reactions described above occur from the first seconds to the first hour after growth factor binding. These are followed by later events. One of these is the activation of immediate early genes (eg, AP1 components) that do not require de novo protein synthesis. The outcome of these reactions is induction of new protein synthesis or activation of existing proteins involved in the progression of cells through the G_1, S, and M phases of the cell cycle. Molecules participating in these reactions include cyclins and tumor suppressor gene products; these are described in the next section.

The signaling events induced by growth factors have several features in common. The various reactions are interconnected and re-

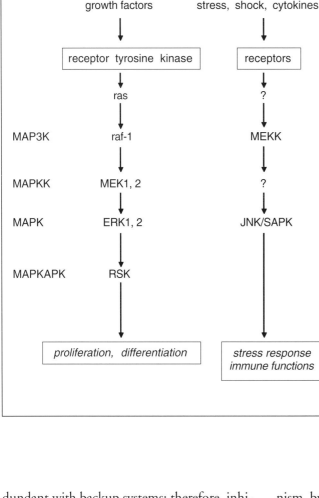

Fig 2-4 Two pathways of the MAPK cascade. The left and right panels show the reactions induced in response to growth factors, and to stress, shock, and cytokines, respectively. Both cascades involve isoforms of the same enzymes with similar mechanisms of action, but with different outcomes. Growth factor binding to the receptor leads to activation of ras, which activates raf-1. The latter activates MAP kinase kinase (MAPKK, also called MEK), which in turn activates ERK1 and ERK2 (extracellular-signal-regulated kinases); RSK (ribosomal S6 kinase) is then activated. Stress response such as heat shock, and cytokines such as IL-2 and IFN-γ induce the enzymes indicated on the right panel, activating JNK/SAPK (Jun-N-terminal kinase/stress activated protein kinase) protein kinases. For terminology and more details, see Seger and Krebs (1995) and Cobb and Goldsmith (1995). A question mark (?) indicates enzymes that have not yet been characterized.

dundant with backup systems; therefore, inhibition of one or a few of the individual reactions does not usually block the biological activity. The signals produced enable the cell to judge its relationship with neighboring cells and its environment, and to respond accordingly; however, how the cells respond depends upon several factors including the type of effector molecules, cell type, and the presence of a matrix. The activation may be transient or sustained, and the kinetics of activation often depends upon the activator as well as its function. Finally, the signaling reactions induced are always kept in check, otherwise, cell function may be adversely affected, leading to abnormalities and oncogenesis. One mecha-

nism by which a growth factor response is regulated is degradation of the ligand and its receptor. Ligand binding to receptors usually leads to internalization of the receptor-ligand complex by endocytosis, followed by either degradation or recycling of the ligand and the receptor. The internalization is mediated by the specific amino acid sequence Asn-Pro-x-Tyr. Alternatively, phosphatases may hydrolyze, and thereby inactivate, phosphorylated proteins. Although phosphorylation activates many enzymes, it may also decrease their activity. Examples of inactivation by phosphorylation are the initiation factor eIF2; the retinoblastoma protein, pRB; and the cyclin-dependent kinase, cdc2.

Regulation of Cell Proliferation

As discussed previously, the ability of eukaryotic cells to divide is regulated by the presence or absence of division-inducing signals. In many cell types, differentiation and division are mutually exclusive processes, and terminally differentiated cells do not divide. In contrast, labile cells retain the capacity to divide continually. In all these cases, growth regulation is mediated through many molecules. Among these, two families of proteins called cyclins and tumor suppressors regulate cell cycle events such that the cells replicate DNA and complete division in a precisely programmed manner through temporally ordered sequence of events, and they arrest cell growth as and when needed.

How some environmental factors regulate cell division is discussed in this section, and this is followed by a description of cyclins, tumor suppressor gene products, and other molecules.

Regulation by Extracellular Matrix and Cell-Cell Interactions

The extracellular matrix is a major environmental determinant of cell division and differentiation. Apart from the availability of mitogenic signals, the cells need to remain attached to a substratum through focal contacts in order to be able to divide. This is referred to as anchorage dependence. Most normal cells kept in suspension, with the exception of hematopoietic cells, do not divide. Cultures of anchorage dependent cells, especially fibroblasts, must first attach to, and spread on, a substrate before they can progress through the G_1 phase into S phase. However, once they cross the restriction point they no longer require anchorage. The property of anchorage dependence is lost in cancer cells. The extracellular matrix serves as the substrate for anchorage, and the cells are embedded in the matrix in a three-dimensional setting. The matrix affects the geometry and polarity of cells, and regulates the spatial organization of cell surface receptors. It often determines the outcome of cellular response to agonists, and the effects in the presence and absence of the matrix may even be opposite. For example, the extracellular matrix facilitates the differentiation of cells in response to growth factors, but it suppresses division.

The actions of the matrix are dependent upon adhesive interactions between the matrix macromolecules and cells, and these interactions play a crucial role in cell differentiation and during embryogenesis (Adams and Watt 1993; Schuppan et al 1994; Gumbiner 1996; Hay 1993; Ingber 1991). For example, mammary epithelial cells require a matrix to differentiate and express β-casein (Roskelley et al 1995). Adhesion to a matrix induces the expression of c-*fos* and proα1[I] genes, and adhesion to fibronectin and laminin enhances cellular activation. The matrix, however, only activates, but does not significantly change, predetermined developmental patterns of gene expression. In addition to serving as a substratum, the matrix also serves as a reservoir for growth factors and cytokines, and presents these molecules to high-affinity cell surface receptors (Ruoslahati and Yamaguchi 1991; Schlessinger et al 1995).

The extracellular matrix consists of fibrous proteins (collagens and elastin), adhesion molecules (fibronectin and laminin), other proteins and proteoglycans (see Chapters 4–6). Mesenchymal cells reside in a matrix composed of primarily type I collagen, whereas endothelial and epithelial cells are in contact with a basement membrane made up of type IV collagen, laminin, and nidogen. Contact of cells to the matrix is through a family of receptors called integrins. The integrins comprise a family of heterodimeric receptors made up of one α and one β subunit each, and consist of a large extracellular domain, a transmembrane domain, and a short cytoplasmic domain (see Chapter 5). They do not have tyrosine kinase domains as do growth factor receptors, nevertheless, binding of ligands to these receptors mimics growth factor binding and generates many of the same signaling events such as Ca^{++} mobilization, activation of PI3-kinase, PLC-γ, and the MAPK cascade, and tyrosine phosphorylation of p125[FAK]. These events, especially the activation of p125[FAK], lead to cytoskeletal reorganization and other cellular functions (Juliano and Haskill 1993). The matrix-mediated signaling reactions constitute a major determinant of tissue-specific gene expression (Roskelley et al 1995).

The activities of a cell are also regulated by its interactions with other cells. Within a small group, cells communicate with each other by direct contact through specialized junctions in plasma membranes; this type of interaction is especially important in developing tissues. Interactions with other cells and organs are mediated by soluble paracrine and endocrine molecules (these terms refer to substances that act on neighboring cells, and those that are carried by circulation to different organs, respectively) such as growth factors and hormones. Normal cells in culture do not divide when they remain in contact on all sides with other cells. This contact or density-dependent inhibition of growth is also a property of normal cells that is lost in cancer cells.

Cyclins and Cyclin-Dependent Kinases

The cyclins and cyclin-dependent kinases (Cdks) are active enzyme complexes in which the cyclins are the activating units, and Cdks are the catalytic units. Together they regulate eukaryotic cell cycle events (Draetta 1994; Nasmyth 1993; Pines 1995). Originally the cyclins were defined as proteins that are specifically degraded at every mitosis (hence the name cyclins), but now the definition has been enlarged to include those proteins containing a cyclin box domain of approximately

100 amino acids that can bind to Cdks (Pines 1995). In eukaryotic cells, several families of cyclins have been identified and designated as A, B, C, D, E, F, G, and H (Table 2-2). Many, but not all, of these molecules are periodically synthesized or activated during specific periods during the cell cycle. The Cdks also share common structural features among themselves, the most important of which is a canonical EGVPSTAIRISLLKE amino acid–sequence motif (for one-letter codes for amino acids, see Table 1-2). Cyclins and their role in the cell cycle have been studied extensively in the budding *(Saccharomyces cerevisiae)* and fission *(S pombe)* yeasts. Cyclins and Cdks are highly homologous between yeasts and humans, and have identical functions; this high degree of conservation indicates their importance in eukaryotic systems (Pines 1995; Nasmyth 1993).

Both the D and E cyclin families regulate the G_1 phase of the eukaryotic cell cycle. The catalytic units for these cyclins are Cdk2, Cdk4, Cdk5 and Cdk6, and Cdk2, respectively (see Table 2-2). The D cyclins are short-lived, with a half-life of approximately 25 minutes. The genes encoding the D_1, D_2, and D_3 cyclins are progressively induced in response to mitogenic stimulation by extracellular signals. Thus, in the absence of growth factors, the D_1 cyclins are rapidly degraded and their accumulation prevented; therefore, the cells do not have active Cdks to traverse past the R point in the G_1 phase. The presence of mitogenic stimulation makes it possible to accumulate sufficient D cyclins and cross the restriction point. In contrast to the D species, expression of E, A, and B cyclins does not seem to be dependent on extracellular signals, although they are also synthesized at specific periods during the cell cycle. The D cyclins appear first during G_1 phase, and their levels subsequently peak during the latter half of the G_1 phase. Cyclin E appears later and its level reaches maximum during the late G_1 or early S phase.

Cyclin D_1–Cdk4 and cyclin E–Cdk2 form enzymatically active complexes for a short

Table 2-2. Some Mammalian Cyclins

Cyclin Type	Cyclin-Dependent Kinase	Inhibitor	Active Cell Cycle Phase
A_1, A_2	cdc2, Cdk2	p21[†]	S, G_2, M
B_1, B_2, B_3	cdc2*	p21[†], p24	Mitosis
C	...[†]	...[†]	G_1
D_1, D_2, D_3	Cdk 2, 4, 5, 6	p15, p16, p21, p27	R point
E	Cdk 2	p15, p21, p27	G_1/S
H	Cdk7	...[†]	G_1-G_2

*cdc28 in *S Cerevisiae*.
†? Currently unknown.

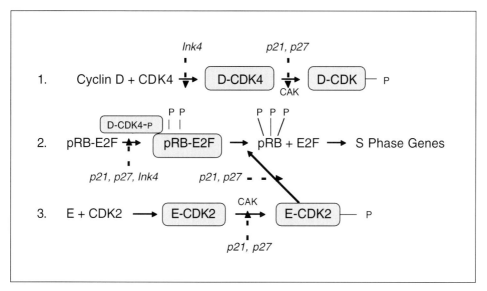

Fig 2-5 A summary of the action of the D and E cyclins and their associated kinases. Early in G_1 phase, mitogenic factors activate the synthesis of cyclin D so that it accumulates and assembles with Cdk4 (and Cdk2 and Cdk6) (Reaction 1). Cyclin E is expressed slightly later, and it assembles with Cdk2 (Reaction 3). Cyclin D–Cdk and cyclin E–Cdk are activated by cyclin H–Cdk7, called CAK. Both cyclin D–Cdk4 and cyclin E–Cdk2 phosphorylate pRB, thereby releasing E2F, and the transcription of S-phase proteins begins (Reaction 2). Cdk activity is regulated by at least three mechanisms: by synthesis and accumulation of cyclins; phosphorylation-dephosphorylation of Cdk, and by the levels of cdk inhibitors p21, p27, p16, and the Ink family proteins. The inhibition points of some of these inhibitors (in italics) are indicated.

period at the R point, and between the R point and the S phase; these complexes phosphorylate and activate a group of proteins necessary for the G_1 to S transition (Fig 2-5). One of these is the retinoblastoma protein, pRB, which is the product of retinoblastoma *(rb)* tumor suppressor gene. Un- and hypophosphorylated pRB exist as a complex with E2F. The E2F is a transcription factor for DNA polymerase α, ribonucleotide reductase, thimidylate synthetase, PCNA (proliferating-cell nuclear antigen, a protein subunit of

DNA polymerase δ), dihydrofolate reductase, thymidine kinase, and other S-phase proteins required for DNA replication.

Normally, the E2F proteins sequestered by unphosphorylated pRB are inactive. At the R point during mid-G_1 phase, the pRB is phosphorylated by the cyclin D/E–Cdks, consequently E2F is released from the pRB. The liberated E2F then induces transcription of S-phase proteins. The pRB remains phosphorylated during the remaining G_1/S phase and until the end of mitosis; it is then dephosphorylated by a phosphatase, PP1. The dephosphorylated pRB again combines with E2F and inactivates it to arrest cells in the G_1 phase. D cyclins bind to pRB through the amino acid sequence LXCXE (X = any amino acid) present at the N-terminus. The cyclin D–Cdks also phosphorylate E2F transcription factors. Cyclin E–Cdk2 is an important regulator of pRB, and the cyclin E–Cdk2 complex must be active for the cells to initiate DNA synthesis (Roberts et al 1994; Solomon 1993) (see Fig 2-5). Another cyclin active during this time is the A cyclin, appearing later than the D cyclin. The synthesis of this cyclin is also induced when cells adhere to matrix substrates. Overexpression of cyclin A overcomes anchorage dependence (Hunter and Pines 1991).

The B and A (A_1, A_2, and A_3) cyclins function during the G_2 phase of the cell cycle. They are stable throughout the interphase, but are destroyed at mitosis. These cyclins combine with the cyclin-dependent kinases cdc2 (the cdc2 is called cdc28 in *S cerevisiae*). The cyclin B cdc2 was originally identified from *Xenopus* eggs and referred to as mitosis promoting factor (MPF). This molecule has also been called maturation promoting factor since microinjection of the MPF into G_2-arrested oocytes induces them to mature into eggs in the absence of progesterone. The activity of cdc2 is regulated by phosphorylation-dephosphorylation cycle. During the G_2 phase of the cell cycle, the activity of *S pombe* cdc2 remains inhibited due to phosphorylation at Tyr_{15} (Thr_{14} in mammals) by the Wee 1 family of kinases. At the onset of M phase, cdc2 is dephosphorylated by the phosphatase cdc25 and becomes activated. The cdc2 is also activated by phosphorylation of $thr_{160,161}$ by the enzyme CAK (the CAK is a complex of cyclin H and Cdk7). Cyclin B-cdc2 kinase is a serine-threonine kinase, and its substrates include nuclear lamins (lamins are intermediate filament components associated with the inner nuclear envelope), vimentin, caldesmon, and H1 histone. Phosphorylation of lamins and other cytoskeletal proteins leads to cytoskeletal reorganization at M phase and causes nuclear envelope breakdown (Draetta 1994; Pines 1995).

The activities of cyclin-Cdks are regulated by at least three mechanisms. The first is proteolysis; proteolysis occurs either through the specific PEST (Pro-Glu-Ser-Thr) recognition sequence or by the ubiquitin degradation pathway (see Chapter 1). The second mechanism of regulation is through a phosphorylation-dephosphorylation cycle to activate or deactivate the protein. One example of this type of regulation is the inactivation of cdc2 by phosphorylation at Tyr_{15} or Thr_{14} and its activation by dephosphorylation of Tyr_{15} or Thr_{14} described above. Finally, the activities of cyclins-Cdks are controlled by several highly specific polypeptide inhibitors. Two such inhibitors are p21[cip1,waf1] and p27[kip1] (abbreviated p21 and p27, respectively). These proteins bind with cyclin-Cdk complexes stoichiometrically and inactivate them (see Fig 2-5). In cells, p21 forms complexes with Cdk2 and Cdk4, cdc2, and PCNA, and can act as a universal inhibitor of the Cdks. The levels of p21 are greater in differentiated and senescent cells, therefore the Cdk remains inactive and cells cannot divide. Cells in which DNA is damaged also accumulate p21. Like p21, the inhibitor p27 binds to cyclin-Cdks and inhibits the activity of cyclins D and E (see Fig 2-5) and cyclin A– and cyclin B–dependent Cdks (Roberts et al 1994; Sherr and Roberts 1995). The p27 levels are high in quiescent fibroblasts, and in some cells TGF-β induces cell cycle arrest through this inhibitor. The p27 levels are also increased by cyclic AMP, and it is down-regulated by IL-2 in T-lymphocytes. TGF-β also up-regulates another inhibitor p15^{Ink4A} (Alexandrow and Moses 1995).

Most cells require more than one mitogenic stimulus to coordinate the production and activation of cyclins, allowing completion of the G$_1$ and S phases of the cell cycle. For example, in T lymphocytes, the first signal is the antigen receptor, which induces the expression of cyclin E, cyclin A, and Cdks; but cyclin A–Cdk2 and cyclin E–Cdk2 are not active because of inhibition by p27. A second signal, IL-2, removes this inhibition.

Oncogenes and Regulation of Cell Growth by Tumor Suppressor Genes

The number of cells in each tissue and organ is regulated to precisely suit its functional requirements. As mentioned previously, the division potential of different cell types varies with their differentiation status, but, for the most part, normal eukaryotic cells remain growth arrested unless there is demand for cell division. Growth-arrested cells remain flat and in extended shapes, retain diploid constitution of their chromosomes, and manifest anchorage dependence and contact inhibition of growth. These features are lost when a cell is transformed, and the transformed cell may expand indefinitely and become a tumor (Hartwell and Kastan 1994). A tumor consisting of cells that closely resemble normal cells in properties is considered to be benign. In contrast, an invasive tumor or cancer consists of malignant cells, which are usually less well differentiated. They have abnormal numbers of chromosomes that are unstable, and the chromosomes have abnormalities. Cancer cells are also characterized by high nucleus-to-cytoplasm ratios, prominent nucleoli, and many mitoses. They lose differentiation and become less drug sensitive.

Although the mechanisms that cause aberrant growth properties in cancer cells are not precisely known, at least two factors are associated with the interference of their growth regulation. These are the overproduction of cellular proteins called oncogene proteins, and mutations in tumor suppressor genes.

Oncogenes. Oncogenes are discrete genetic elements carried by DNA and RNA tumor viruses. The oncogenes of DNA tumor viruses code for specialized proteins that have complex and multiple actions. Examples are the T-antigen of SV40 and polyoma virus, the adenoviral E1A and E1B, and E6 and E7 of the papilloma virus. The major in vivo effect of these proteins is to activate host cell DNA replication machinery so that viral DNA can be replicated. Activation of host replicative machinery uncouples the host cells from their cell cycle regulatory controls, and the host cells become tumor cells. In contrast, RNA retroviral oncogenes are counterparts of normal cellular genes called proto-oncogenes or c-oncogenes, which are involved in the regulation of cell growth. The cellular and viral counterparts are designated with the prefixes c- and v-, respectively (eg, c-*sis* and v-*sis* refer to cellular and viral genes coding for a PDGF-like growth factor). The gene suffixes and their protein products are designated in italic and nonitalic characters, respectively. More than 25 such genes have been characterized, and, based on the action of their products, they are classified roughly into the following four groups: (1) growth factors (*sis* coding for PDGF, *int-2* which codes for FGF), (2) growth factor receptors (CSF-1 receptor *fms*, EGF receptor *erbB*, and NGF receptor *trk*), (3) signaling molecules (protein tyrosine kinases *src, abl*, and *met*; serine-threonine kinases *raf* and *ras*, adaptor protein *crk*, and transcription factors *jun, fos, myc*, and *myb*), and (4) tumor suppressor genes *p53* and *pRB* (Bishop 1991; Cantley et al 1991; Hunter 1991; Marshall 1991).

Oncogenes representing signal transduction enzymes appear to be the most common. This family of oncogenes encodes enzymes such as tyrosine kinase and serine-threonine kinases, as well as the G protein. These molecules may evade normal cell regulatory processes by novel mechanisms. For example, the product of the Rous sarcoma viral (RSV) oncogene *src* is a 60-kd protein tyrosine kinase, which, like its normal counterpart, contains SH2 and SH3 domains, and N-terminal sequences for myristylation for attaching to a membrane; but, unlike the normal molecule, it does not have a C-terminal tyrosine$_{527}$, which, when phosphorylated, represses kinase activity. Therefore, the src is not subjected to regulation and it remains continuously active. Another example is the *ras* family of oncogenes involved in several bladder carcinomas. These genes encode proteins without their intrinsic GTP-ase activity; therefore, the protein cannot convert GTP to GDP to become inactive. Thus, the oncogenic *ras* always remains in its active conformational state.

Tumor suppressor genes. Recent studies have shown that the transformation of a normal cell into a cancer cell may involve alterations in certain genes that negatively regulate cell proliferation (Marshall 1991). Most studied among this group are the tumor suppressor genes *rb* and *p53*. A number of tumors are associated with mutations in these genes.

Retinoblastoma protein. The product of the *rb* gene is the retinoblastoma protein (p110^{RB} or pRB), a 110-kd protein localized in the nucleus. It consists of discrete domains for oligomerization, phosphorylation, and binding to DNA. The pRB exerts its effect in the G$_1$ phase of the cell cycle, regulating the activities of the E2F family of transcription factors as described in the previous section (see Fig 2-5) (Kranenburg et al 1995; Riley et al 1994; Weinberg 1995). Besides the E2F, the pRB also interacts with protein kinases, growth regulators such as c-*myc*, N-*myc*, protein phos-

phatases, and nuclear matrix proteins. DNA viral oncoproteins such as SV40 large T antigen, adenoviral E1A, and papilloma virus E6/E7 bind to pRB; the binding mimics phosphorylation and dissociates hypophosphorylated pRB from E2F; therefore the host cells enter into S phase. The pRB is also a target for other growth inhibitory signals such as cAMP and TGF-β. TGF-β exerts its effect by inducing the synthesis of the Cdk inhibitors p27 and p15. Radiation and other agents that damage DNA block pRB phosphorylation through p21 (see later; Fig 2-6) (Hainaut 1995).

Retinoblastoma protein appears to play a key role in cellular differentiation and development as well. For example, pRB binds to MyoD, and when pRB is inactivated, myoblast differentiation is inhibited and myotubes reenter the cell cycle. In terminally differentiated myotubes and senescent fibroblasts, the pRB remains underphosphorylated and it cannot be phosphorylated by growth factors. Unphosphorylated pRb accumulates in terminally differentiated neurons, and traps C-*Abl*, E2F, and myoD. Cells without functional pRB may be predisposed to apoptosis (apoptosis refers to genetically programmed cell death).

p53 Tumor suppressor gene. The product of the p53 tumor suppressor gene is a multifunctional nuclear phosphoprotein associated with tumor suppression function. Sixty percent of human cancers are associated with mutations in this protein. This gene is a transcription factor that contains an N-terminal transactivation domain, a middle DNA binding domain, an oligomerization domain that helps formation of p53 tetramers, a nuclear localization signal, and a C-terminal negative regulation domain. It binds to several transcription factors and affects the expression of many genes. Most notably, it binds to the TATA-box binding protein (TBP) subunit of transcription factor TFIID and represses general transcription. Other transcription factors that bind to p53 include SP-1, WT-1, and

Fig 2-6 Interaction between p53, pRB, cyclin-cdk inhibitors, and apoptosis. The p53 pathway is activated by DNA damage due to radiation, chemicals, or stress. Accumulation of the p53 gene product induces the synthesis Gadd45 gene product, and this causes G_1 arrest. The p53 also induces p21 synthesis. This protein inhibits cyclin-Cdks; therefore pRB is not phosphorylated and cells are arrested in the G_1 phase. The p21 also inactivates PCNA by binding to it (not shown); this is another mechanism of G_1 arrest. Another action of the p53 is promotion of apoptosis; this is achieved by up-regulation of the *Bax* gene that promotes apoptosis and down-regulation of *bcl-2*, which protects cells from apoptosis.

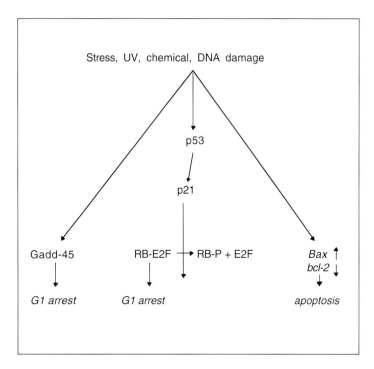

CCAAT binding factor. The p53 also binds to single-stranded DNA and to the oncoproteins SV40 large T antigen, E1B, and E6 (Hainaut 1995). The p53 activates the genes for p21 and Gadd45 (growth arrest and DNA damage 45, a protein involved in G_1 arrest) and arrests cells in G_1 (Fig 2-6). In addition, the *Bax* gene is up-regulated, and *bcl*-2 is reciprocally down-regulated to promote apoptosis by the p53.

The p53 tumor suppressor gene is believed to play a prominent role in DNA repair. When DNA is damaged by UV, γ radiation, chemicals, or by other stress, p53 senses the damage and activates two types of cellular responses. It induces G_1 (or G_2) arrest transiently by any of the mechanisms mentioned above to provide adequate time for the cells to repair DNA damage. In some cells, proliferation may even be arrested permanently. Alternatively, p53 may induce cells such as thymocytes to undergo apoptosis. The interrelationship among p53, pRB, and apoptosis is summarized in Fig 2-6.

Telomerase. The ends of eukaryotic chromosomes contain protein-DNA structures called telomeres that are believed to protect the ends of chromosomes from damage and from illegitimate recombination. The telomeres in most organisms consist of tandem arrays of short repeats. The telomeric DNA is not replicated by conventional DNA polymerases, thus, with every cell division, telomeres in somatic cells become shortened. Replication of telomeres is carried out by telomerase, and this enzyme is regulated developmentally and by the cell cycle. In most somatic cells, the activity of the telomerase is repressed and lost during replicate aging. However, cells that divide repeatedly, such as cancer cells, germ line cells, and immortalized cells, and microorganisms like yeast contain the active enzyme; these cells retain a stable telomere length. While this indicates that the telomerase plays a role in regulation of cell division, the actual mechanisms involved are currently unclear (Shay and Wright 1996; Zakian 1995).

Cell Death and Apoptosis

Other than accidental or incidental death during inflammation, cells can also be induced to die due to developmental instructions in a mechanism resembling suicide. This type of cell death occurs under a variety of physiologic conditions, and it is known by two interchangeable terms, apoptosis and programmed cell death. Apoptosis is distinguished from necrosis, a process that represents morphologic changes caused by cell death due to progressive degradative action of enzymes. Apoptosis, on the other hand, may be a normal feature of differentiation and maturation of organisms; it is induced when cells are damaged or no longer needed. Apoptosis is particularly important in the development of nervous and immune systems, and it plays a prominent role in elimination of self-reactive T lymphocytes that cause autoimmunity. It is increasingly becoming clear that apoptosis is a key component of the repertoire of cellular responses, and that aberrations in apoptosis may be associated with the development of cancer and autoimmune diseases, including AIDS.

Several changes occur in cellular organelles during apoptosis. The chromatin becomes fragmented and condensed, and cell organelles shrink. One characteristic feature is fragmentation of DNA into 180 to 200-bp ladders (fragments) due to nuclease cleavage between nucleosomes; this is associated with the breakdown of the nuclear envelope caused by irreversible disassembly of lamins. The breakdown of DNA is believed to be caused by the enzyme DNase-1. During apoptosis, several changes occur in the cytoplasm independently of the DNA fragmentation; these include the breaking down of cells into apoptotic bodies formed by budding of membranes by cell surface blebbing. There are extensive cell-membrane alterations, and cells detach from neighboring cells and substratum (Hale et al 1996).

Apoptosis involves several gene products; many have been identified in the nematode *Caenorhabditis elegans.* This organism consists of 1090 somatic cells in the adult hermaphrodite, of which 131 cells undergo programmed cell death in a predictable fashion. Death of these cells involves fourteen genes that specify which cells die, and those cells that carry out cell death, engulf dead cells, and digest the corpse (Hale et al 1996). Cell death is induced by the *ced-3* gene, which is activated by the product of gene *ced-4.* The *ced-3* gene codes for an enzyme similar to mammalian interleukin-1$_\beta$ converting enzyme (ICE); this is a cysteine protease that converts the proIL-1$_\beta$ precursor to IL-1$_\beta$. Death is inhibited by the product of another gene, *ced-9*, that protects cells from death. The cascade of apoptotic cell death appears to involve three major stages: receipt of death signals, execution of death through activation of *ced-3*, and cellular alterations that follow death.

The mammalian equivalent of *ced-3* is a family of at least 10 ICEs now referred to as caspases. These enzymes have several substrates. One of these is the product of a gene called CPP32$_\beta$ (*Yama*), which is activated by proteolytic cleavage, and it in turn cleaves poly(ADP-ribose) polymerase (PARP; this is an enzyme involved in DNA repair). The caspases appear to play a role in apoptosis in human cells mediated by tumor necrosis factor, in neuronal cell death induced by withdrawal of nerve growth factor, in epithelial cell death caused by growth factor withdrawal, and in cytotoxic T-lymphocyte–induced macrophage apoptosis. Other proteases such as cathepsins B and D and collagenase are also expressed during apoptosis (Hale et al 1996).

The mammalian genes corresponding to *C elegans ced-9* are the members of *bcl-2* (B-cell lymphoma/leukemia-2 family), *bcl-x, Bax, mcl-1,* and *bak-2.* The *bcl-2* gene, like *ced-9*, is a negative regulator and it protects cells from death. Its overexpression prolongs cell survival and blocks cell death from drugs, heat shock, ionizing radiation, and other forms of cell injury (Reed 1994), but not by TNF. Overexpression of *bcl-2* can prolong cell survival without concomitant cell proliferation. The product of the *bcl-2* gene is a 25 to 26-kd protein that has a stretch of 19 hydrophobic amino acids near the carboxy terminus, followed by two charged residues for anchoring the protein membranes. This protein resides in the outer mitochondrial membrane, nuclear envelope, and in parts of ER. It is believed that the bcl-2 family of proteins (BAX, BAD, bcl-x$_L$, bcl-2) interact with each other and with ced-4. The ced-4 activates caspases and brings forth cell death. BAD is proapoptotic when it heterodimerizes with bcl-2/bcl-x$_L$; when it is phosphorylated by Raf-1, it releases bcl-2 and the released bcl-2 protects cells from death. The activities of bcl-2 include blocking CPP32 activation, prevention of mitochondrial membrane depolarization, and inhibiting the release of mitochondrial cytochrome *c* into the cytoplasm (Yang et al 1997). Other components that participate in apoptosis include cell surface receptors Fas/Apo-1, tumor necrosis factor receptor-R1 (TNF-R1), and c-*myc* proto-oncogene. The TNF-R1 receptor contains a cytotoxic signal in an 80–amino acid death domain. Several tumor promoting genes, such as those coding for GTP-binding proteins (ras, raf), transcription factors (AP-1, *R*-myc, myb, E2F), and viral proteins also influence cell death.

Summary

The ability to regulate cell division and growth is an essential part of development and growth of all organisms. Differentiated cells of higher eukaryotes are usually permanently arrested from division. In cells capable of division, several restrictions are to be overcome if a cell is going to divide. This involves synthesis of new proteins and activation of existing proteins. The activities of these molecules are regulated by several mechanisms, including covalent modification of certain amino acids, inhibition by polypeptide inhibitors, and by proteolysis. The importance of signaling reactions involved in cell growth regulation is apparent by their redundancy and the presence of several backup systems. Aberrations in any of these mechanisms can lead to transformation of cellular properties and to cancer. During wound healing, restrictions for cell growth are overcome in a complex series of signaling reactions. The regulatory mechanisms and the type of cells available presumably determine whether the wound heals by regeneration or by repair. Many of the signaling mechanisms described here have been shown to be involved in the regulation of periodontal cell types, and the generic mediators described above, as well as others that are periodontium-specific, have been demonstrated to be present in the periodontal components. Thus, the mechanisms elaborated in this chapter are highly relevant to the periodontium in which regeneration involves many tissue components. These principles are discussed in Chapter 3 and in Part III.

References

Adams JC, Watt FM. Regulation of development and differentiation by the extracellular matrix. Development 1993;117:1183.

Alberts B, Bray D, Lewis J, Raff M, Roberts K, Watson JD, eds. Molecular Biology of the Cell. 3rd ed. New York: Garland; 1994.

Alexandrow MG, Moses HL. Transforming growth factor β and cell cycle regulation. Cancer Res 1995;55:1452.

Attisano L, Wrana JL, López-Casillas F, Massagué J. TGF-β receptors and actions. Biochem Biophys Acta 1994; 1222:71.

Ben-Baruch A, Michiel DF, Oppenheim JJ. Signals and receptors involved in recruitment of inflammatory cells. J Biol Chem 1995; 270:11703.

Berridge MJ. Inositol trisphosphate and calcium signaling. Nature 1993;361:315.

Bishop JM. Molecular themes in oncogenesis. Cell 1991; 64:235.

Cantley LC, Auger KR, Carpenter C, et al. Oncogenes and signal transduction. Cell 1991;64:281.

Chao MV. Growth factor signaling: where is the specificity. Cell 1992;68:995.

Claesson-Welsh L. Platelet-derived growth factor receptor signals. J Biol Chem 1994;269:32023.

Clapham DE. Calcium signaling. Cell 1995;80:259.

Cobb MH, Goldsmith EJ. How MAP kinases are regulated. J Biol Chem 1995;270:14843.

Cohen P. Protein phosphorylation and hormone action. Proc R Soc Lond B Biol Sci 1988;234:115

Divecha N, Fine RF. Phospholipid signaling. Cell 1995; 80:269.

Draetta GF. Mammalian G_1 cyclins. Curr Opin Cell Biol 1994;6:842.

Fantl WJ, Johnson DE, Williams LT. Signalling by receptor tyrosine kinases. Annu Rev Biochem 1993;62:453.

Gumbiner BM. Cell adhesion: The molecular basis of tissue architecture and morphogenesis. Cell 1996;84:354.

Hainaut P. The tumor suppressor protein p53: a receptor to genotoxic stress that controls cell growth and survival. Curr Opin Oncol 1995;7:76.

Hale AJ, Smith CA, Sutherland LC, et al. Apoptosis: molecular regulation of cell death. Eur J Biochem 1996;236:1.

Hartwell LH, Kastan MB. Cell cycle control and cancer. Science 1994;266:1821.

Hay ED. Extracellular matrix alters epithelial differentiation. Curr Opin Cell Biol 1993;5:1029.

Hunter T. Cooperation between oncogenes. Cell 1991; 64:249.

Hunter T, Pines J. Cyclins and cancer. Cell 1991;66:1071.

Ihle JN. Cytokine receptor signalling. Nature 1995;377: 591.

Ingber D. Extracellular matrix and cell shape: potential control points for inhibition of angiogenesis. J Cell Biochem 1991;47:236.

Juliano RL, Haskill S. Signal transduction from the extracellular matrix. J Cell Biol 1993;120:577.

Kranenburg O, van der Eb AJ, Zantema A. Cyclin-dependent kinases and pRb: regulators of the proliferation-differentiation switch. FEBS Lett 1995;367:103.

Lemmon MA, Schlessinger J. Regulation of signal transduction and signal diversity by receptor oligomerization. Trends Biochem Sci 1994;19:459.

Marshall CJ. Tumor suppressor genes. Cell 1991;64:313.

Means AR. Calcium, calmodulin and cell cycle regulation. FEBS Lett 1994;347:1.

Nasmyth K. Control of the yeast cell cycle by the cdc28 protein kinase. Curr Opin Cell Biol 1993;5:166.

Nathan C, Sporn M. Cytokines in context. J Cell Biol 1991;113:981.

Newton AC. Protein kinase C: structure, function and regulation. J Biol Chem 1995;270:28495.

Norbury C, Nurse P. Animal cell cycles and their control. Annu Rev Biochem 1992;61:441.

Pardee AB. G_1 events and regulation of cell proliferation. Science 1989;246:603.

Pardee AB, Dubrow R, Hamlin JL, Kletzien RF. Animal cell cycle. Annu Rev Biochem 1978;47:715.

Pines J. Cyclins and cyclin-dependent kinases: a biochemical review. Biochem J 1995;308:697.

Reed JC. Bcl-2 and the regulation of programmed cell death. J Cell Biol 1994;124:1.

Riley DJ, Lee EY, Lee WH. The retinoblastoma protein: More than a tumor suppressor. Annu Rev Cell Biol 1994; 10:1.

Roberts JM, Koff A, Polyak K, et al. Cyclins, Cdks, and cyclin kinase inhibitors. Cold Spring Harb Symp Quant Biol 1994;59:31.

Roskelley CD, Srebrow A, Bissell MJ. A hierarchy of ECM-mediated signaling regulates tissue-specific gene expression. Curr Opin Cell Biol 1995;7:736.

Ruoslahti E, Yamaguchi Y. Proteoglycans as modulators of growth factor activities. Cell 1991;64:867.

Schlessinger J, Lax I, Lemmon M. Regulation of growth factor activation by proteoglycans: What is the role of the low affinity receptors? Cell 1995;83:357.

Schuppan D, Somasundaram R, Dieterich W, Ehnis T, Bauer M. The extracellular matrix in cellular proliferation and differentiation. Ann NY Acad Sci 1994;733:87.

Seedorf K. Intracellular signaling by growth factors. Metabolism 1995;44:24.

Seger R, Krebs EG. The MAPK signaling cascade. FASEB J 1995;9:726.

Shay JW, Wright WE. The reactivation of telomerase activity in cancer progression. Trends Genet 1996;12:129.

Sherr CJ, Roberts JM. Inhibitors of mammalian G_1 cyclin-dependent kinases. Genes Dev 1995;9:1149.

Solomon MJ. Activation of the various cyclin/cdc2 protein kinases. Curr Opin Cell Biol 1993;5:180.

Sporn MB, Roberts AB. Peptide Growth Factors and Their Receptors. Berlin: Springer 1990;1–2.

Weinberg RA. The retinoblastoma protein and cell cycle control. Cell 1995;81:323.

White MF, Kahn C. The insulin signaling system. J Biol Chem 1994;269:1.

Yang J, Liu X, Bhalla K, et al. Prevention of apoptosis by Bcl-2: release of cytochrome c from mitochondria blocked. Science 1997;275:1129.

Zakian VA. Telomeres: Beginning to understand the end. Science 1995;270:1601.

3

Inflammation and Wound Healing

Introduction

Following injury to tissues, vertebrates respond by initiating a series of events designed to eliminate the agent causing the injury, contain the damage, and reconstitute the damaged tissues. In unicellular organisms, the injurious agent is first engulfed and disposed of by phagocytosis. While this basic mechanism is retained in vertebrates, the overall response to injury involves additional events requiring the active participation of the vascular system and the specialized cells residing within the affected tissues. This process is called inflammation and may be defined as the response of vascularized living tissues to injury.

Inflammation is characterized by the movement of fluid and white blood cells from the blood stream to the site where the injury has occurred. It is a fundamental response that aims to confine the injury, eliminate the offending agents and their effects, remove dead and damaged tissue and, more importantly, to initiate the reactions necessary for healing the damaged tissue.

The cell types participating in inflammation include polymorphonuclear leukocytes (PMN),

47

Table 3-1. A Comparison of Major Features Associated with Acute and Chronic Inflammation

Feature	Acute Inflammation	Chronic Inflammation
Vascular reaction	Prominent with clinical signs	Less prominent, cold swelling
Inflammatory cell	Polymorphonuclear leukocytes	Monocytes, lymphocytes, plasma cells
Pus	Present	Not characteristic
Pain	Often severe	Often absent
Connective tissue destruction	Prominent	Prominent
Fibroblast proliferation	Absent	Present
New connective tissue	Absent	Present

monocytes, lymphocytes, and platelets. The polymorphonuclear leukocytes are a family of cells that consists of neutrophils, eosinophils, and basophils/mast cells. These three cell types have different functions. The neutrophils are phagocytic cells and are the primary cells responsible for phagocytosis. The eosinophils and basophils are not normally phagocytic, but they release mediators during allergic responses. Eosinophils are often associated with parasitic infections, while basophils are the major inflammatory cells participating in allergic responses. Monocytes/macrophages are also a major source of inflammatory mediators, and these cells, unlike platelets and polymorphonuclear leukocytes, can synthesize mediators de novo and secrete these molecules at the sites of injury. Among the lymphocytes, B cells produce antibodies locally, while T cells participate in cell-mediated host response. Platelets are a rich source of vasoactive amines, growth factors, and several other mediators. During inflammation these inflammatory cells are activated by antigen-antibody complexes, foreign bodies, bacterial endotoxins, chemical mediators, and other molecules to move to the site of the injury, adhere, and release their contents by degranulation.

Inflammation may be acute or chronic, depending on the persistence of injury, the nature of the inflammatory response, and its clinical symptoms. The hallmarks of acute inflammation are short duration, accumulation of fluid and plasma components in the affected tissue, intravascular stimulation of platelets, and infiltration of the affected tissues by inflammatory cells, which are predominantly neutrophils. Chronic inflammation, on the other hand, is of longer duration, and it involves mostly monocytes/macrophages, lymphocytes, and plasma cells. It is often associated with proliferation of blood vessels and connective tissue indicating episodes of healing (Cotran 1994) (Table 3-1).

Events Associated with Acute Inflammation

Vascular Changes

Acute inflammation consists of specific vascular and cellular events. It may last from minutes to days, and its cardinal signs are those described by Celsus in the first century AD: *rubor* (redness), *calor* (heat), *tumor* (swelling), and *dolor* (pain). These signs are associated primarily with vascular changes, and they are caused by chemical mediators (Cotran 1994). The vascular events occur in the microvasculature and usually become apparent within 15 to 30 minutes after injury. During the first minutes following injury, arterioles undergo transient vasoconstriction caused by neurogenic and chemical mediators; this usually resolves in seconds to minutes and is of no consequence. Then follows the vasodilation of arterioles, and almost immediately afterward, vasodilation of venules and capillaries. During this time, blood flow increases, causing localized redness and heat. The intravascular hydrostatic pressure increases both at the arterial and the venous ends, therefore, fluid escapes to the extravascular space. Fluid leakage also occurs through gaps generated between endothelial cells when they contract.

Fluid Exudate

Endothelial cells play a major role in the fluid leakage that occurs in the venules. Chemical mediators released during inflammation cause contraction of these cells and generate gaps at intercellular junctions; this results in increased vascular permeability. The extent and type of injury to the endothelium determine the kinetics of the vascular response. For example, after a mild injury, fluid leakage begins immediately, peaks in 5 to 10 minutes, and then resolves. However, if the endothelial cells are killed, as happens in severe burns, the leakage may persist for days until the damaged vessels are either restored or thrombosed. In certain cases, the leakage may begin after a delay and last for several hours or even days; examples of this type of injury are mild thermal injury, exposure to UV or X-ray radiation, sunburn, certain bacterial toxins, and delayed hypersensitivity reactions.

The escaping fluid from the vessels is rich in proteins such as fibrinogen and immunoglobulins; these proteins are not reabsorbed at the venous end due to high hydrostatic pressure, therefore a protein-rich exudate accumulates within the tissues. With time, the exudate may also contain cells and cellular debris. The continuing accumulation of both the cellular and

fluid exudates eventually causes swelling (edema). Chemical mediators released during these reactions produce pain.

In general, the inflammatory exudate has several beneficial roles. For example, it contains the necessary proteins for activation of the complement cascade, which ultimately leads to cell lysis. In addition, the fluid exudate contains antibodies, which are bactericidal, and opsonins, which coat foreign matter and allow them to be recognized as foreign and permit phagocytosis to occur. The presence of fibrin within the fluid exudate is considered to be beneficial in generating a barrier against infection.

Cellular Exudate

These vascular events are followed by cellular events. Increased permeability in the microvasculature leading to the fluid exudate also results in higher blood viscosity, an increase in the concentration of red blood cells, and subsequent slowing of the circulation (stasis). With the decrease in rate of blood flow, the white blood cells move towards the periphery of the vessels. During this process the cells appear to tumble and roll, and eventually they contact the endothelium lining the vessel walls. This process is referred to as margination. Subsequently, the cells line up on, and adhere to, the endothelium and assume a flattened shape. This phenomenon is called pavementing.

Cell adhesion to endothelium. The adherence of leukocytes to endothelial cells is through specific interactions between complementary adhesion molecules present on the cell surfaces of both cell types. Three groups of adhesion molecules participate in this process—the selectins, integrins, and cell adhesion molecules (CAM) (Albeda et al 1994; Rosen and Bertozzi 1994). During inflammation, the activity of these adhesion molecules is invoked by at least three mechanisms: by

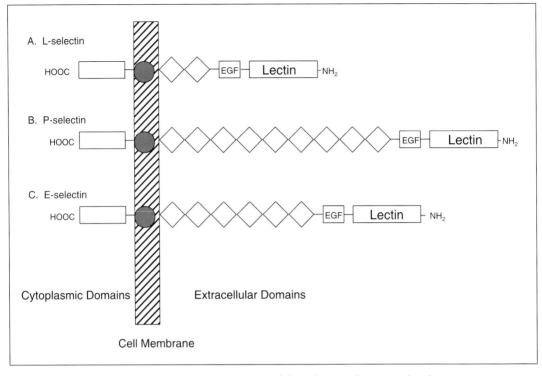

A. L-selectin

HOOC ⬦⬦ EGF Lectin NH₂

B. P-selectin

HOOC ⬦⬦⬦⬦⬦⬦⬦ EGF Lectin NH₂

C. E-selectin

HOOC ⬦⬦⬦⬦ EGF Lectin NH₂

Cytoplasmic Domains   Extracellular Domains

Cell Membrane

Fig 3-1 Schematic representation of the selectin adhesion molecules.

synthesis of adhesion molecules not normally present, by translocation of already existing molecules from cytoplasm to plasma membranes, and by modifying the conformation of adhesion molecules such that their affinity to the ligand is enhanced.

Selectins. The process by which leukocytes slow down in their passage through the blood vessels is known as rolling and is due to the presence of selectins on their cell surface. Selectins are a family of cell adhesion molecules that bind carbohydrates (lectins) and mediate interactions between leukocytes, platelets, and endothelial cells (Bevilacqua et al 1991; Bevilacqua 1993). To date, three selectins have been described, all of which share similar structural features (Lasky 1990; Bevilacqua and Nelson 1993). These are cell surface glycoproteins that contain an extracellular por-

tion located at the amino terminal lectinlike domain followed by an epidermal growth factor–like domain and multiple (ranging from 2 to 9) short domains similar to those found in complement (C3/C4) binding proteins (Fig 3-1). In addition, a transmembrane domain and an intracellular domain have been identified in these molecules. In general terms, the selectins are categorized according to the cell type from which they were first isolated. Thus, they have been termed L-selectin for leukocytes, P-selectin for platelets, and E-selectin for endothelial cells.

L-selectin has been known by a variety of names, including lectin adhesion molecule-1, lectin-EGF-complement adhesion molecule-1 (LECAM-1), TQ1, and Leu 8, and is believed to be intimately associated with lymphocyte binding to endothelium (Tedder et al 1990). This molecule contains only two comple ment-binding proteinlike domains and is found on lymphocytes, polymorphonuclear leukocytes, and monocytes (Stoolman 1989). The expression of this molecule is closely associated with cell activation and adhesion. Following adhesion to endothelial cells, the expression of L-selectin is diminished, with a concomitant increase in the expression of other leukocyte integrins that play important roles in the attachment and transendothelial migration of the cells (Tedder et al 1990).

P-selectin, found mainly on platelets, contains the largest number (nine) of complement-binding protein–like sequences of all the selectins (Bevilacqua and Nelson 1993). This molecule is not constitutively expressed on endothelial cells and requires activation of platelets by thrombin, histamine, or phorbol esters (Larsen et al 1990; Toothill et al 1990). The role of P-selectin in platelet adhesion to endothelial cells is recognized but poorly understood.

E-selectin (also known as endothelial-leukocyte adhesion molecule-1 or ELAM-1) was originally identified as a cytokine-inducible endothelial glycoprotein that bound both neutrophils and monocytes (Pober et al 1986; Cotran et al 1986). This selectin has at least six complement-binding protein–like sequences. This selectin is induced by cytokines and is not normally expressed on endothelial cells of uninflamed tissues. However, it is strongly expressed by endothelial cells at sites of polymorphonuclear leukocyte migration and mononuclear cell accumulation, and it is associated with a wide variety of inflammatory conditions. Because the presence of ELAM-1 requires new synthesis, there is a time lag of a few hours between exposure to a cytokine and the appearance of ELAM-1 on the endothelial cell surface; during this lag period, other cell adhesion molecules presumably carry out the leukocyte adherence.

Integrins. The second group of molecules involved in leukocyte adhesion to the endothelial cells are the integrins, which are a family

Table 3-2. Nomenclature of Leukocyte Integrins

Name Used	Other Names
$\alpha1\beta2$	LFA-1, CD11a/CD18, alb2
$\alpha2\beta2$	Mac-1, Mo-1, CR3, amb2, CD11b/CD18
$\alpha3\beta2$	p150, 95, CR4, axb2, CD11c/CD18

of cell surface receptors composed of one α and one β subunit each. At present, eight β chains and 16 α chains have been identified. Thus, the number of different combinations of α and β chains is very large. Within this family of molecules, those containing the $\beta2$ chain are considered to be most important in leukocyte adhesion. Examples of leukocyte integrins, together with their alternative names, are shown in Table 3-2. A more detailed description of the structure and properties of integrins is presented in Chapter 5.

Immunoglobulin superfamily cell adhesion molecules. The third family of molecules involved in leukocyte adhesion to endothelial cells is called cell adhesion molecules (CAM) (Albeda et al 1994; Rosen and Bertozzi 1994). These molecules, which belong to the immunoglobulin superfamily of proteins, are present on endothelial cell surfaces and are characterized by the presence of multiple repeat domains containing immunoglobulin-like sequences (Fig 3-2). Members of the CAM family of molecules have been named according to their location and function in mediating cell attachment.

Intercellular adhesion molecule-1 (ICAM-1) is a transmembrane protein of approximately 55 kd. It contains five immunoglobulin-like domains of varying glycosylation, and was first described as a lymphocyte activation marker that could bind the leukocyte integrin, lymphocyte function–associated antigen, LFA-1 ($\alpha1\beta2$). In addition to the membrane-bound form, ICAM-1 can also be shed from the cell surface and enter the circulation,

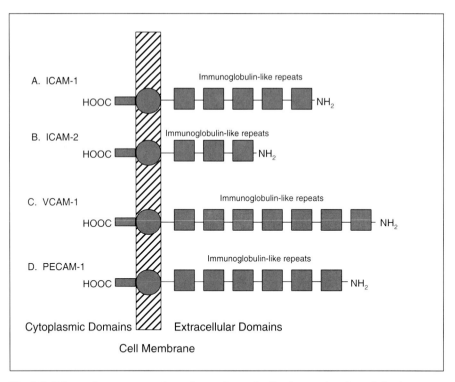

Fig 3-2 Schematic representation of a variety of adhesion molecules of the immunoglobulin gene superfamily.

where it retains its ability to bind several of the leukocyte integrins. ICAM-1 is constitutively expressed, in low levels, on some hematopoietic cells, endothelial cells, fibroblasts, and keratinocytes. The expression of ICAM-1 on these cells is significantly increased at sites of inflammation; this is most likely due to a response to various cytokines such as interferon gamma and tumor necrosis factor-α. Recent studies have demonstrated that both the membrane-bound and the shed forms of ICAM-1 exist in a noncovalent-dimer relationship, and that such dimerization is related to enhanced binding capacity.

ICAM-1 was originally identified as the counter receptor for the leukocyte integrin LFA-1 (α1β2). Recently it has been demon-strated to interact with other leukocyte integrins including α2β2 and α3β2 (de Fourg-erolles 1993). In addition, ICAM-1 can serve as a receptor for rhinoviruses and *Plasmodium falciparum*. Interestingly, all three binding reactions appear to be mediated via different portions of the extracellular domain of the ICAM-1 molecule. The intracellular portion of ICAM-1 appears to bind to actin, and thus provides a mechanism for linking the external environment of leukocytes to the cytoskeleton.

Intercellular adhesion molecule-2 (ICAM-2), which shares some homology with ICAM-1, is comprised of a 33-kd protein containing two extracellular immunoglobulinlike domains that show the highest homology to the two amino terminal domains of ICAM-1. As for ICAM-1, ICAM-2 binds selectively to the leukocyte integrin α1β2 (Diamond et al 1990). In addition, recent evidence indicates that a 22–amino acid binding peptide, P1, located in the first domain of ICAM-2 interacts with the α2β2 integrin (Xie et al 1995). ICAM-2 is expressed predominantly on endothelial cells and may be expressed, to varying levels, on hematopoietic cells. While the biologic significance of ICAM-1 is largely unclear, it has been suggested that it may act on endothelium to aid in triggering the migration of adherent leukocytes (Somersalo et al 1995).

Intercellular adhesion molecule-3 (ICAM-3) is the third member of the group of intercellular adhesion molecules that has been identified as counter receptors for the LFA-1 (α1β2) integrin. The core protein of ICAM-3, which is highly glycosylated and has a molecular mass of 87 kd, contains five immunoglobulin-like domains. Electron-microscopic studies show that ICAM-3 has a head-to-tail arrangement of the immunoglobulin-like domains, forming a straight rod-shaped structure approximately 15 nm long (Sandhu et al 1994). Cloning and expression studies (de Fourgerolles et al 1993) have revealed that the five immunoglobulin-like domains of ICAM-3 have significant homology to both ICAM-1 (52%) and ICAM-2 (37%). Although ICAM-1 and ICAM-3 are highly homologous, ICAM-3 does not possess the same affinity that ICAM-1 has for other leukocyte integrins such as α2β2 and α3β2. ICAM-3 is expressed on hematopoietic cells and Langerhans' cells, but not on endothelial cells (Vaseaux et al 1992; Teunissen et al 1995) and may be involved in the initiation of antigen-specific activation of T lymphocytes.

Vascular cell adhesion molecule-1 (VCAM-1), originally identified as a membrane-associated glycoprotein found on endothelial cells involved in aiding adhesion of melanoma cells and lymphocytes, belongs to the same structural group of the immunoglobulin superfamily that includes the ICAM molecules. Structurally, VCAM-1 contains seven immunoglobulin-like domains, of which the first and fourth can bind the ligand α4β1. Although the bivalent form has increased binding capacity, ligand binding may occur with the presence of only one of these domains (Osborn et al 1992). Unlike other members of the ICAM family of molecules, VCAM-1 is not constitutively expressed by endothelial cells. However, VCAM-1 is induced on endothelial cells by several inflammatory cytokines, including interleukin-1 (IL-1) and tumor necrosis factor-α (TNF-α) or IL-4. The natural ligand for VCAM-1 is the integrin β1α4, which is expressed on lymphocytes, monocytes, eosinophils, and basophils (but not on polymorphonuclear leukocytes), and provides a means by which these cells may bind to endothelial cells expressing VCAM-1. Through these interactions, VCAM-1 may play a role in a variety of functions such as B-cell development, leukocyte activation and recruitment to sites of inflammation, atherosclerosis, and tumor cell metastasis.

Platelet endothelial cell adhesion molecule-1 (PECAM-1) is a cell surface glycoprotein of 130 kd found on platelets, endothelial cells, monocytes, neutrophils, and some T-cell subsets. With six extracellular immunoglobulin-like domains, PECAM-1 is a member of the immunoglobulin gene superfamily. PECAM-1 also has a short, 19–amino acid transmembrane domain and a 118–amino acid cytoplasmic portion. The cytoplasmic portion has sites with potential for phosphorylation or lipid modification, which could play roles in cell adhesion or motility. Within the N-terminal immunoglobulin-like domains, there are numerous functional domains that appear to be required for migration and possibly for cell aggregation (Yan et al 1995). Multiple isoforms of PECAM-1 have been noted; these result from significant alternate splicing of exons that code for the cytoplasmic domain. These isoforms may be related to cell function through modulating ligand specificity and cell adhesion properties. Recently, a soluble form of PECAM-1 has been identified in both cell culture and human plasma; it is slightly smaller than the cell-associated form, but still retains the cytoplasmic tail and may be involved in modulating inflammatory reactions (Goldberger et al 1994). In blood vessels, PECAM-1 is localized at the intercellular junctions of endothelial cells and probably plays an important role in maintaining endothelial cell-cell relations. It has been suggested that alterations in the distribution of PECAM-1 on endothelial cells may provide a means by which endothelial cells may lose their adhesiveness and permit migration of leukocytes across the vessel wall. The ligand for PECAM-1 may be the leukocyte $\alpha V\beta 3$ integrin.

macrophage products MCP-1 (monocyte chemotactic protein-1), MCP-2, MCP-3, IL-8, and RANTES (regulated upon activation normal T cells expressed and presumably secreted) (Sozzani et al 1996; Ward 1996). Although the majority of chemokines are effective toward several inflammatory cell types, some are highly selective; for example, eotaxin is highly specific toward the eosinophils and IL-8 for polymorphonuclear leukocytes. Bacterial products with amino terminal N-formylmethionyl groups are potent chemotactic agents to neutrophils. Chemotactic agents, which are produced as byproducts of inflammation and tissue destruction, are discussed in the next section, which concerns chemical mediators of inflammation.

Cell Migration

Migration of inflammatory cells to the site of injury is the step that follows margination and pavementing. This process appears to be confined to the venules. In the first 6 to 24 hours of an acute inflammatory reaction, the migrating cells are predominantly neutrophils. Later, monocytes become the majority of cells. However, this pattern may vary in specific instances. For example, in some hypersensitivity reactions, eosinophils are the main type of migrating cell.

The inflammatory cells are attracted to the site of injury by chemotaxis, which is defined as the unidirectional migration of cells toward an increasing concentration gradient of a compound called a chemotactic agent. Chemotaxis involves interactions between cell surface receptors and the chemotactic agent, and many of the signaling events described in Chapter 2 are necessary for cell migration (Ben-Baruch et al 1995; Ihle 1995). A family of chemotactic agents called chemokines are secreted by monocytes and other cells. These cysteine-containing proteins play an important role in the recruitment of leukocytes to the site of inflammation, and include the

Phagocytosis

The final step in the cellular events of acute inflammation is phagocytosis, by which bacteria, other foreign agents, and dead tissue are removed. This is an energy-dependent process that requires three distinct but interrelated steps: (1) recognition and attachment to the material to be phagocytosed, (2) their engulfment, and (3) killing and degradation. Recognition and attachment are facilitated by coating target objects with opsonins; this class of agents includes the C3b complement fragment and plasma fibronectin. The opsonized objects are then engulfed by phagocytic cells, which extend their membranes to surround the object and enclose it. The resulting phagosomes fuse with cytoplasmic lysosomal granules, which degranulate and discharge their contents into the phagosomes.

Killing and degradation are accomplished by oxygen-dependent and oxygen-independent mechanisms. Oxygen-dependent cell killing is a very efficient, and highly potent, mechanism of cell killing that involves oxygen-derived metabolites and free radicals. Phagocytosis activates the enzyme NADPH oxidase and the hexose monophosphate shunt; this leads to increased oxygen consumption referred to as the respiratory burst. Oxygen is metabolized producing superoxide ion (O_2^-), which, by spontaneous dismutation, forms hydrogen peroxide (H_2O_2). In the presence of chloride ions, the H_2O_2 is converted to hypochlorous acid (HOCl). The conversion is catalyzed by myeloperoxidase, an enzyme present in azurophilic granules of the neutrophils. The HOCl is a powerful oxidant and antimicrobial agent. Hydrogen peroxide, superoxide ion, singlet oxygen, and hydroxyl radicals formed during the oxidative metabolism are also effective at killing bacteria. Once bacteria are killed, they are digested by the lysosomal enzymes. The myeloperoxidase system is the most efficient bactericidal system in neutrophils, but it is not present in the macrophage. In chronic granulomatous disease, H_2O_2 production in neutrophils is deficient, and individuals with this disease are predisposed to recurrent infections.

Oxygen-independent mechanisms of cell killing utilize acidic pH, lysosomal enzymes, and complement. Cationic proteins present in neutrophil granules and lactoferrin (an iron-binding protein) enhance the bactericidal activity by the oxygen-independent mechanism.

After killing phagocytosed organisms, neutrophils themselves are killed by their own destructive enzymes. The monocytes/macrophages, however, are not killed, and they continue to produce inflammatory mediators. Eosinophils and basophils do not take an active part in phagocytosis.

Chemical Mediators of Inflammation

During inflammation, numerous molecules are produced, either as byproducts of proteolytic action or by secretion from inflammatory cells. These substances, which participate in and mediate the inflammatory response, can be classified into several families.

Vasoactive Amines and Peptides

These molecules increase vascular permeability by dilating small blood vessels. Histamine and serotonin (5-hydroxytryptamine) are the most potent and important members of this family. They are stored in the granules of mast cells, basophils, and platelets, and are released by anaphylatoxins C5a and C3a (anaphylatoxins are substances that increase vascular permeability by releasing histamine from mast cells and platelets), or by physical agents such as heat and cold. Apart from the amines, other mediators derived from the plasma, including bradykinin, lysyl bradykinin, and peptides derived from fibrin degradation are also vasoactive.

Plasma Proteases

Inflammation activates a group of three inter-related proteolytic systems that are present as inactive zymogens in the blood. These are the complement cascade, kallikrein-kinin, and the fibrinolytic clotting system. The interrelationships among these three proteinase cascades are summarized in Fig 3-3.

Complement. The complement cascade consists of a group of 20 plasma proteins that are activated by two different pathways. The first pathway is the classic pathway; this is initiated primarily by immunologic stimuli (ie, antigen-antibody complexes), bacterial products, and viruses. These substances bind to the C1q subunit of C1 complement, which self-activates and then triggers the cascade of proteinases in the order C4, C2, C3, C5, C6, C7, C8, and C9. The second pathway is termed the alternative pathway. This is a relatively slower process, and it is activated by nonimmune stimuli such as foreign bodies (eg, cobra venom) and aggregated immunoglobulins. This pathway utilizes two plasma proteins (B and D) instead of C1, C2, and C4 complements; however, other reac-

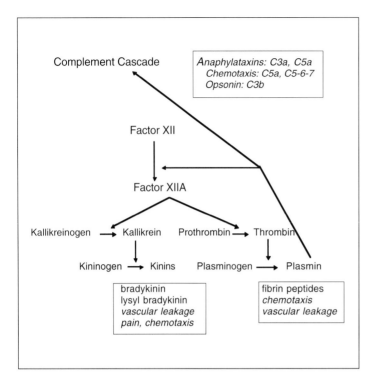

Complement Cascade

Anaphylataxins: C3a, C5a
Chemotaxis: C5a, C5-6-7
Opsonin: C3b

Factor XII

Factor XIIA

Kallikreinogen → Kallikrein   Prothrombin → Thrombin

Kininogen → Kinins   Plasminogen → Plasmin

bradykinin
lysyl bradykinin
vascular leakage
pain, chemotaxis

fibrin peptides
chemotaxis
vascular leakage

Fig 3-3 Generation of inflammatory mediators through the complement, kallikrein-kinin, and clotting systems. Although the major role of the complement cascade is cell lysis, during its activation, peptides that affect inflammatory events are generated. Activated Hageman factor XIIA generates kallikrein and kinins, and it also activates prothrombin and plasminogen to thrombin and plasmin, respectively. Plasmin produces fibrin peptides and can also activate the complement cascade. The mediators generated, and their biologic actions, are enclosed in boxes. Both pathways generate several metabolites, and only those discussed in the text are shown. Their biologic actions are indicated in italics.

tions are the same as the classic pathway. The outcome of both pathways is the formation of a membrane attack complex, C5b-C6-C7-C8-C9, which causes cell lysis. During these reactions, peptide fragments are generated and some of the peptides serve as anaphylatoxins (C3a and C5a), chemotactic factors (C5a, and C5-C6-C7), and opsonins (C3b, C5b) (Table 3-3).

Kallikrein-kinin system. The kallikrein-kinin system is activated when factor XII (Hageman factor) is converted to active XIIA by contact with negatively charged surfaces such as basement membrane, collagen, endotoxins, and foreign materials. Activated XIIA converts plasma prekallikrein to enzymatically active kallikrein, which in turn cleaves high molecular weight kininogen to bradykinin and lysyl bradykinin. Bradykinin, a nonapeptide, increases vascular permeability by vasodilation, contracts smooth muscle, and produces pain. Kallikrein is chemotactic to, and promotes, aggregation of neutrophils.

Fibrinolytic clotting system. The clotting system is the third protease cascade that results in the formation of fibrin. The fibrin is degraded by plasmin, which is activated from its precursor, plasminogen, by factor XIIA. Peptides formed from fibrin induce vascular permeability and are chemotactic for leukocytes. The plasmin also catalyzes the conversion of factor XII to XIIA. In addition, it can activate C3 complement, thus triggering the complement cascade. Thus, these three enzyme systems, although targeted individually for different functions, form an integrated network by which numerous inflammatory mediators are generated.

Arachidonic Acid Metabolites

Arachidonic acid (AA; 5,8,11,14-eicosatetraenoic acid) is a 20-carbon polyunsaturated fatty acid present in cell-membrane phospholipids. It is released from phosphatidylcholine by the enzyme phospholipase A_2, and from

Table 3-3. Common Mediators of Inflammation

Mediator	Source	Action
Histamine and serotonin	Platelets, mast cells, and basophils	Vascular leakage
Bradykinin	Plasma	Vascular leakage, pain
Kallikrein	Plasma	Chemotaxis to PMN
C3a	Complement C3	Vascular leakage
C3b	Complement C3	Opsonin
C5a	Complement C5	Vascular leakage, chemotaxis
PGD_2, PGE_2	Membranes, mast cells	Vasodilation, bronchodilation
PGI_2	Membranes, mast cells	Inhibits platelet aggregation
PGE_2	Membranes, mast cells	Vasodilation, fever, bronchoconstriction
TXA_2	Membranes, mast cells	Vasoconstriction, bronchoconstriction
LTB_4	Membranes, leukocytes	Chemotaxis to PMN, monocytes
LTC_4, D_4, E_4 (SRS-A)	Leukocytes, mast cells	Vascular leakage, bronchoconstriction, vasoconstriction
Cationic proteins	Leukocytes	Vascular leakage, immobilization of neutrophils
PAF	Leukocytes	Vascular leakage, chemotaxis, bronchoconstriction
IL-1 and TNF-α	Monocytes	Pain, fever, acute-phase reactions, chemotaxis
IL-8	Monocytes	Chemotaxis to PMN
Chemokines	Monocytes, other cells	Chemotaxis
(MCP-1, -2, -3, RANTES) eotaxin	Monocytes	Chemotaxis (eosinophils)

diacylglycerol by diacylglycerol lipase. Arachidonic acid released from these two phospholipids is metabolized through two pathways (Fig 3-4). The first is the prostanoid pathway, mediated by the enzyme cyclooxygenase. This pathway generates prostaglandins PGD_2, PGE_2, $PGF_{2\alpha}$, prostacyclin (prostaglandin I_2, PGI_2) and thromboxane A_2 (TXA_2). The prostaglandins induce pain and fever, and prostacyclin is an inhibitor of platelet aggregation. Thromboxane causes vaso- and bronchoconstriction and also enhances inflammatory cell function.

Arachidonic acid can also be metabolized by the enzyme lipooxygenase. This pathway is called the eicosanoid pathway, and it produces the leukotrienes LTB_4 (a chemotactic agent), LTC_4, LTD_4, and LTE_4. The latter group of leukotrienes, called slow-reacting substances of anaphylaxis or SRS-A, stimulate smooth-muscle contraction and increase microvascular permeability.

Corticosteroids inhibit phospholipase A_2 and thus block the formation of all arachidonic acid metabolites. This is one mechanism by which these drugs function as anti-inflammatory agents. Nonsteroidal antiinflammatory drugs such as aspirin, indomethacin, and ibuprofen, on the other hand, inhibit the downstream enzyme, cyclooxygenase, thereby preventing the formation of only prostaglandins and thromboxanes.

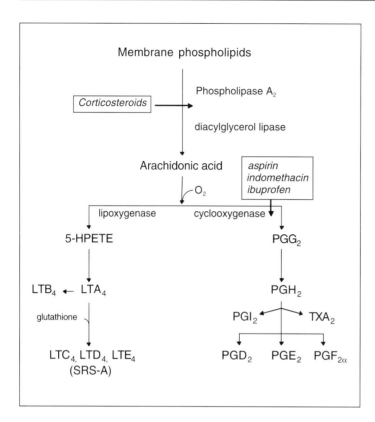

Fig 3-4 Production of prostaglandins and leukotrienes. Arachidonic acid is liberated from membrane phospholipids by enzymes phospholipase A_2 and diacylglycerol lipase. The arachidonic acid is metabolized, through the cyclooxygenase pathway, to prostaglandins, thromboxane, or prostacyclin, or to leukotrienes through the lipooxygenase pathway. Both pathways generate several metabolites, and only those discussed in the text are shown. Corticosteroids inhibit phospholipase A_2 action, therefore, formation of all arachidonic acid metabolites is blocked. On the other hand, nonsteroidal antiinflammatory drugs such as aspirin inhibit the cyclooxygenase pathway and prevent the formation of only prostaglandins and thromboxanes. HPETE: hydroperoxyeicosatetraenoic acid.

Platelet Activating Factor

Platelet activating factor (PAF) is a lipid acylglycerol of variable structure. It is highly potent at promoting platelet aggregation and degranulation, and leukocyte adhesion to endothelium. It also causes vasodilation and increased permeability in the microvasculature.

Cytokines, Chemokines, and Growth Factors

Numerous bioactive polypeptides play a key role in inflammation and wound repair due their ability to influence the activities of many cell types. Among the cytokines, IL-1 and TNF-α are the most significant in inflammation. Although many cell types produce these substances, they are secreted predominantly by the monocytes/macrophages during inflam-

mation. These solubule inflammatory mediators are pyrogens, and they also stimulate the release of PGE_2, PAF, corticotropin, as well as corticosteroids into circulation. These substances also induce other systemic acute-phase reactions. Cytokines affect the synthesis activities and adhesion properties of monocytes, lymphocytes, neutrophils, and fibroblasts.

The chemokines, which are chemotactic agents involved in leukocyte recruitment and trafficking, have been described in the previous section covering chemotaxis.

In addition to the above substances, a battery of polypeptide growth factors that regulate cell proliferation and matrix synthesis during wound healing are also secreted by platelets and macrophages. The activities of growth factors and some cytokines were elaborated in Chapter 2.

Although the various chemical mediators described previously are primarily destined to regulate the course of inflammation, they can be potentially harmful to the host if their activities are not carefully controlled. Therefore, several mechanisms have evolved to restrain and eventually neutralize their activities. For example, prostaglandins and other arachidonic acid metabolites have very short half-lives that range from seconds to minutes; therefore their effects last only for a short period. Peptide mediators are rapidly degraded by proteolytic enzymes, and inhibitors present in the serum and tissues combine with activated serum proteinases and inactivate them. In spite of these control mechanisms, these substances can cause extensive damage to host tissues if the inflammation does not subside and the production of mediators continues, or if any of the control mechanisms is perturbed.

Mediator production and host-tissue destruction are characteristic features associated with chronic inflammatory diseases such as periodontitis and rheumatoid arthritis. More specific details regarding the role of inflammatory mediators in periodontitis are covered in Chapter 9.

Chronic Inflammation

Acute inflammation becomes chronic if the injurious stimulus is not adequately removed, or if repeated bouts of inflammation occur. A variety of factors, including the type and intensity of injury, nutritional status of the host, and underlying metabolic disorders, such as diabetes, also affect the resolution of acute inflammation. Furthermore, in certain instances (eg, during some viral and rickettsial infections), the acute inflammatory response may be bypassed altogether and the histologic features of chronic inflammation are manifested directly. Low-grade immune responses during autoimmune diseases (eg, rheumatoid arthritis and silicosis) also evoke chronic inflammatory responses.

The hallmarks of chronic inflammation are infiltration of mononuclear cells (macrophages, lymphocytes, and plasma cells), proliferation of fibroblasts, and connective tissue formation, which may be mediated by immunologic as well as nonimmunologic mechanisms (see Table 3-1). The macrophages are derived either from the circulation (C5a, fibrin peptides, lymphokines, and growth factors are chemotactic for macrophages), or they replicate locally by proliferation. B and T lymphocytes are the other major cellular participants in chronic inflammation. The B cells interact with antigens, become plasma cells, and produce antibodies locally. The T lymphocytes, which consist of subtypes such as killer, helper, and suppressor cells, participate in activities associated with cell-mediated immunity. The T cells secrete many polypeptide lymphokines that interact with other inflammatory cells and fibroblasts.

Certain fungal infections, including tuberculosis, leprosy, and schistosomiasis, and foreign bodies such as talc and suture materials evoke a specific chronic inflammatory response called chronic granulomatous inflammation. This type of inflammation is characterized by the presence of epithelioid cells, which are actually derived from macrophages but so-named because they resemble epithelial cells in appearance. Predisposing factors for this type of lesion are the presence of indigestible foreign materials and cell-mediated immunity. A characteristic feature of chronic granulomatous inflammation is the presence of granulomas. These are tumorlike bodies caused by inflammation, and consisting of epithelioid cells usually surrounded by a rim of lymphocytes. They may be surrounded by fibroblasts, collagen fibers, plasma cells, and neutrophils. The granulomas may contain multinucleated giant cells formed by fusion of several epithelioid cells. The Langhans' giant cells found in tuberculosis are typical of such cells; up to 50 nuclei are arranged around the periphery of the cytoplasm in a circle or in a horseshoe pattern. Another type of giant cell is foreign body giant cells, which form similarly to Langhans' cells, but the nuclei in the former are scattered in clusters in an irregular pattern throughout the cytoplasm.

Morphologic Variations in Inflammation

The tissue type, site, cause, severity, and type of inflammatory reaction are responsible for morphologic variations in the patterns of inflammation. One of these is the abscess. This is a suppurative or purulent inflammation characterized by formation of pus or purulent exudate, and it is caused by pyogenic bacteria, such as *Staphylococcus aureus, Streptococcus pyogenes,* and *Neisseria gonorrhoeae.* Another type of inflammation is cellulitis, a term that describes the acute inflammation of loose connective tissues caused commonly by β-hemolytic streptococci. An ulcer is a local defect or excavation of the surface (epithelium) of an organ due to sloughing of necrotic tissue. This lesion commonly occurs in the mucosa of the mouth, stomach, intestine, or genitourinary tract, and as a result of subcutaneous infections of lower extremities among older people. Ulcer formation is also a common occurrence in leprosy.

Wound Healing

Wound healing is the process by which an organism attempts to reconstitute a tissue damaged by injury and restore its function. It can be achieved either by regeneration or by repair. In regeneration, lost tissue is replaced by new tissue identical in both architecture and function to the original. However, when this is not possible, the damaged tissue is repaired and the injured tissue is replaced with a fibrous scar. In either case, wound healing requires the coordination of a variety of physiologic processes that follow a specific time sequence. Wound healing involves blood components, soluble mediators, cells, and the extracellular matrix (Clark 1996).

Phases of Wound Healing

Wound healing progresses through three phases that overlap with each other and are interdependent (Clark 1996) (Fig 3-5). The first phase is the inflammatory response that immediately follows injury; the events and processes of this have been described in the previous section. Immediately following injury, a blood clot fills the wound site. The process of blood coagulation is controlled by the inhibition of thrombin and by the degradation of coagulation factors V and VIII by protease C. Subsequently, plasminogen activator activates plasmin and clot lysis begins. The clot, which is rich in fibrin and fibronectin, serves several important functions during this early phase of wound repair. It provides tensile strength and stability to the wound, serves as a provisional matrix for migration and establishment of cells, and it is a source of growth factors.

Demolition. The events involved in healing of most tissues and organs are similar, and they have been delineated using experimental skin wound models. In a typical dermal wound, polymorphonuclear leukocytes migrate into the clot by chemotaxis within 24 hours, and remove dead or damaged tissue and foreign matter by phagocytosis. Monocytes, which are also recruited to the site following the arrival of the polymorphonuclear leukocytes, also participate in the phagocytic process. This phase of wound repair is referred to as demolition. Within 24 to 48 hours, keratinocytes (epithelial cells) migrate from the edges of the wounded epidermis, underneath the fibrin clot, and into the wound site to form a fine covering over the wounded dermis. During this process, the epithelial cells must modify their morphologic

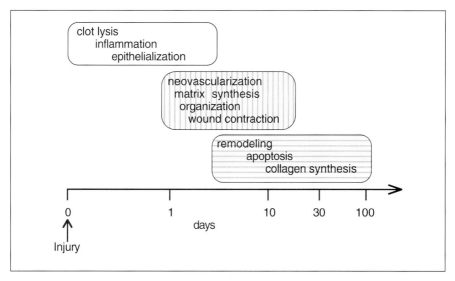

Fig 3-5 A time course of wound repair events. These events are not mutually exclusive, but overlap in time. The time course is arbitrary and the duration of each phase may vary depending upon several factors. The first phase (open box) is inflammation when neutrophils infiltrate, followed later by monocytes and lymphocytes. The PMN and monocytes dispose of dead tissue and bacteria; this phase lasts 2 to 3 days. During this time, epithelial cells originating from wound margins close the epithelial breach. Toward the end of this phase, epithelial cells may also be derived from new division. Peptides derived from lysis of blood-clot and host-tissue matrix and inflammatory cell products serve as mediators, and as chemotactic agents to recruit cells to the wound site. During the next phase (box with vertical bars), endothelial cells actively produce new capillaries. Fibroblasts, which begin to move from the first day, differentiate into myofibroblasts, synthesize collagen, and eventually organize the fibrin clot into granulation tissue. The myofibroblasts also contract the wound. During the final phase (box with horizontal bars), the capillaries and myofibroblasts disappear, and granulation tissue is gradually remodeled into a scar. Collagen synthesis continues for weeks and months until the tensile strength of tissue is restored to near normal levels.

features to become migratory. To this end, they become elongated and flattened, lose the desmosomes in cell junctions, and become phagocytic. The migration of these cells appears to be facilitated by the enzyme collagenase, plasminogen activator, and other bioactive molecules. For example, migrating epithelial cells prominently express receptors for epidermal growth factor (EGF) and transforming growth factor-α (TGF-α), both of which are strongly chemotactic for these cells. One or two days after the injury, epithelial cells at the wound margin proliferate and provide cells for further epithelialization.

A new basement membrane is formed to which epithelial cells attach and differentiate, and eventually continuity of the epithelium is established.

Formation of granulation tissue, organization, and contraction. The next phase in wound healing is the formation of granulation tissue. This is the new stroma that serves as an intermediate tissue, and it involves active angiogenesis and fibroplasia. It begins to form approximately 3 to 5 days after injury, and the framework for its formation is provided by the fibrin clot. Angiogenesis (or neo-

Table 3-4. A Summary of Major Processes and Regulatory Molecules Involved in Wound Repair

Process	Polypeptide*
Chemotaxis	PDGF, TGF-β, FGF, IL-1, matrix products
Adhesion	Fibronectin, collagens, laminin, vitronectin
Proliferation	PDGF, FGF, IGF-I
Differentiation	Matrix (inhibits proliferation, promotes differentiation), growth factors, hormones
Angiogenesis	FGF, TGF-β, angiogenin
Matrix synthesis, remodeling	TGF-β (stimulates synthesis, inhibits degradation) γ-IFN, TNF-α (inhibit synthesis) IL-1 (degradation)

*These are only representative examples that have been shown to play a prominent role; the list is not complete.

vascularization) is the formation of new capillaries by the budding of endothelial cells resident in the surrounding preexisting vessels. These budding cells produce collagenase, which can degrade the basement membranes on which the cells are layered, migrate toward the angiogenic stimulus, proliferate, mature, and finally organize into capillary tubes. Newly formed capillaries are leaky, and thus blood components escape, which accounts for the edema and redness that are characteristic features of granulation tissue. Angiogenesis is promoted by a variety of angiogenic factors, and involves the interaction between the endothelial cell integrin $\alpha_v\beta_3$ and specific extracellular matrix proteins. Prominent angiogenic factors are FGF, TGF-β, VEGF (vascular endothelial cell growth factor), and angiogenin (Table 3-4).

Fibroblasts begin to migrate into the wound after one day and are transformed into myofibroblasts (Desmoulière and Gabbiani 1996; Grinnell 1994). The term myofibroblast refers to certain cells in granulation tissue and fibrotic lesions that manifest morphologic features of both fibroblasts and smooth muscle cells (Darby et al 1990). These cells actively synthesize new matrix components, of which collagen is the major constituent. During the initial stages of healing, type III collagen is the major collagen species produced,

and type I collagen synthesis becomes prominent later. A variety of growth factors, cytokines, and lymphokines, released by inflammatory cells, participate in these processes. Important among these are platelet-derived growth factor (PDGF), which is a major mitogen for mesenchymal cells, and TGF-β, which stimulates matrix synthesis. Conversion of the fibrin clot into a fibrous tissue is commonly referred to as organization.

Another major event occurring during this stage is wound contraction. This is believed to be brought about by the myofibroblasts residing in the granulation tissue (Grinnell 1994). Wound contraction is an especially important and necessary feature in large wounds as it reduces the wound to approximately 5% to 10% of its original size. Besides contracting the wound, the granulation tissue serves as a provisional matrix, and it also prevents excessive epithelial migration.

Remodeling of the newly formed tissues. Remodeling of the granulation tissue represents the final phase of wound repair. During this phase, the newly formed granulation tissue matures and it loses most of its capillaries, and its connective tissue is remodeled and converted into a fibrous scar. Apoptosis of endothelial cells and myofibroblasts accompany the granulation tissue remodeling. At this stage, proteoglycan and collagen synthesis proceed in a coordinated manner. The appearance of hyaluronate, followed by proteoglycans containing chondroitin sulfate and then dermatan sulfate, occur within the first 3 to 5 days. Subsequently, the synthesis of collagen becomes maximal at 7 to 14 days after injury, however, it continues for weeks and months until tensile strength of the wound is restored to near normal levels (see Fig 3-5).

In contrast to injury in adult organisms, fetal wounds appear to heal faster and might not form a scar. This is believed to be due to the preponderance of inflammatory mediators in these tissues. There appears to be no neovascularization, and this may be due to the inhibition of angiogenesis by high levels of hyaluronate. Collagen fibers in the fetal wound are deposited in a reticular pattern similar to normal skin, whereas in adult wounds, the collagens are present as dense fibrils (McCallion and Ferguson 1996).

Cell Types Involved in Wound Healing

Apart from the inflammatory cells that secrete polypeptide mediators, the other major cell types that directly participate in reconstituting the wound include epithelial cells, fibroblasts and other mesenchymal cells that produce the connective tissue matrix, and endothelial cells. The primary role of epithelial cells is to restore the damaged epithelium, whereas endothelial cells are responsible for angiogenesis. Only the microvascular endothelial cells appear to participate in angiogenesis; those from other vessels do not manifest angiogenic responses, and they appear to participate in the denudation of injuries. Among the mesenchymal cells, myofibroblasts are believed to be primarily responsible for wound contraction and matrix synthesis during early wound healing stages. Although these cells are thought to be derived primarily from fibroblasts, they may also form from smooth muscle cells, pericytes, glomerular

mesangial cells, and hepatic sinusoidal cells (Masur et al 1996; Desmoulière and Gabbiani 1996). Based on the presence of cytoskeletal markers, myofibroblasts have been classified as type V, V-D, VA, or VAD (V, vimentin; D, desmin; A, SM-actin). Other mesenchymal cell types involved in wound healing include the fibroblasts in soft tissues, osteoblasts in calcified tissues, and glial cells in the nervous system. These cells are primarily responsible for reconstituting the wound by producing collagens and other matrix components.

Effects of Soluble Mediators on Connective Tissue Cells

Under healthy conditions, connective tissue cells remain quiescent and their synthetic activity is low. Following injury and inflammation, these cells are dislodged from their matrix and are activated to migrate to the wound site, divide, differentiate, and produce a new matrix. The migration, adhesion, proliferation, and differentiation of connective tissue cells and their matrix synthesis are affected by a variety of polypeptide factors present in the local environment (Raines et al 1990; Roberts and Sporn 1990; Slack et al 1993; Sporn and Roberts 1990). Many of these mediators are derived from inflammatory cells during wound healing (Bennett and Schultz 1993a, 1993b). FGF-1 and FGF-2 (these are the currently accepted names for acidic and basic FGF, respectively), TGF-α, and EGF are found in significant amounts at the wound site during early stages, with FGF-1 and FGF-2 concentrations increasing 2- to 10-fold relative to unaffected tissues. The levels of these agents peak by 24 hours and stay high for up to 5 days before returning to basal level in approximately 7 days. The most dramatic change occurs in FGF-7 (the recommended name for keratinocyte growth factor, KGF) concentration, which increases more than 160-fold in 24 hours and stays high even after

7 days (Werner et al 1992). This growth factor is highly specific to keratinocytes, and it is believed to be involved in re-epithelialization. Other growth factors found in the wound include PDGF, especially the PDGF-AA isoform (Soma et al 1992), and TGF-β. Both PDGF and FGF are major mitogenic factors for fibroblasts. The TGF-β, on the other hand, activates the transcription of genes for type I, III, IV, VI, and VII collagens and proteoglycans and, in addition, it coordinately inhibits synthesis of the collagen-degrading enzyme, collagenase (Roberts and Sporn 1990; Slack et al 1993; Sodek and Overall 1992). The appearance of TGF-β in healing wounds and in fibrotic lesions correlates with collagen synthesis (Broekelmann et al 1991). It is secreted by platelets and macrophages, and it is also sequestered in the matrix. Although TGF-β is also angiogenic, it is believed to decrease the diameter of blood vessels owing to its antiproteolytic action. In contrast, the formation of the lumina of blood vessels appears to be due to FGF-2, which generates a proteolytic response. The matrix stimulatory effects of TGF-β are counteracted by PGE_2, IFN-γ, and TNF-α, all of which inhibit collagen synthesis. Another major factor that regulates matrix composition is IL-1; this cytokine appears to be responsible for matrix degradation of both hard (cartilage and bone) and soft connective tissues in rheumatoid arthritis, periodontitis, and other chronic inflammatory diseases. The actions of these and other molecules associated with wound healing are summarized in Table 3-4.

Growth factors and cytokines mediate their influence through specific cell surface receptors. Binding of these agents to receptors activates various signaling events (described in Chapter 2), and the results of these reactions are migration, attachment, DNA synthesis, or other cell functions such as protein synthesis. Frequently, the expression of integrins and other cell surface receptors is also affected by these polypeptides, and cell-matrix and cell-surface interactions are modified accordingly.

The various mediators may affect the growth and synthesis activities of all cells of the resident population, or only particular cell types (Fig 3-6). Even subpopulations of the same cell type may respond differently to specific substances. Such selective interactions are believed to enrich certain cell types and subtypes of cells during the progression of wound healing events, to determine whether healing occurs by repair or by regeneration, and to contribute to connective tissue alterations associated with inflammation and fibrosis (Fries et al 1994; Narayanan and Bartold 1996; Pitaru et al 1994).

The extracellular matrix frequently modifies the manner in which cells respond to growth factors. The role of the matrix in inhibiting proliferation and promoting differentiation of cells was discussed in Chapter 2 (Adams and Watt 1993; Ekblom et al 1986; Hay 1993; Schuppan et al 1994). However, the role of the matrix in regulating cell function can be complex. For example, TGF-β stimulates matrix synthesis, however, once the matrix is formed, this cytokine has no further effect on the cells. Cell responses are also affected by their replicative age and the cell-cycle phase. The presence of more than one mediator can also influence how cells respond, and the combined effects of these mediators may be complementary, contradictory, additive, or synergistic.

Lesions such as hypertrophic scars and fibrosis, and even tumors, can be considered aberrant wound healing responses due to a breakdown in normal regulatory mechanisms (Fig 3-7) (Dvorak 1986). For example, persistence of TGF-β at a wound site can cause excessive connective tissue formation. This possibility is supported by observations that the presence of TGF-β is associated with high collagen synthesis rates and low collagenase levels in cells of evolving fibrotic lesions (Broekelmann et al 1991). Alternatively, other factors such as lack of regulation by collagen synthesis inhibitors, such as IFN-γ, may also

Fig 3-6 Possible interactions between soluble mediators and cells during wound repair. During inflammation, growth factors, cytokines, and other biologically active substances are secreted by inflammatory cells. Degradation products of host matrix proteins are also generated by the actions of PMN and macrophage enzymes. These substances affect the growth and synthesis activities of endothelial cells, epithelial cells (not shown), and fibroblasts. The activities of all resident cells, or only certain cell types or subtypes, may be affected, and the outcome may be proliferation and activation of matrix synthesis. Selective proliferation of certain cell subtypes with disease phenotypes can lead to pathologic conditions (eg, cells with elevated levels of collagen synthesis in scleroderma and phenytoin-induced gingival overgrowth).

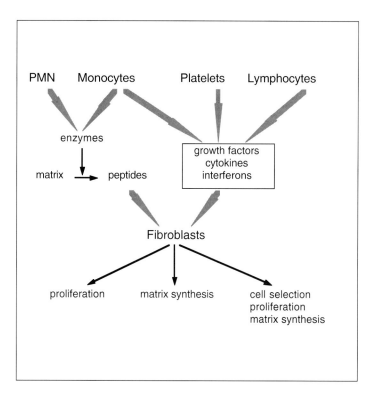

Fig 3-7 Possible outcomes of wound healing response. An injury, if it is minor with little tissue damage, or if it involves labile cells, can be resolved or regenerated. If regeneration is not possible, then the damage is patched with a scar. Aberrations in the wound healing response can lead to pathologic conditions. For example, continuous and unregulated matrix synthesis can lead to a hypertrophic scar or keloid. Fibrosis may be another outcome, and it also is characterized by the accumulation of matrix elements. Both fibrosis and hypertrophic scar are characterized by the accumulation of connective tissue, and may represent a similar response with minor differences.

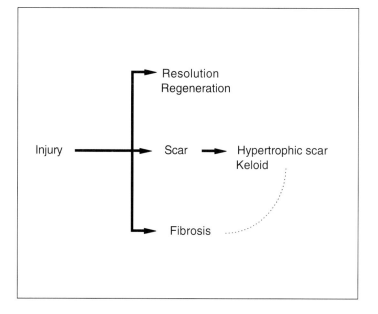

contribute to a fibrotic response (Granstein et al 1990). Aberrations of wound healing may also be caused by other predisposing factors such as diseases (eg, diabetes), nutritional deficiencies (Zn^{++} and vitamin C deficiencies), and infections.

Factors Affecting Wound Healing

Proper wound healing requires the progression of various wound healing events in an ordered and programmed sequence (Clark 1996). One major factor that determines the course of healing is the availability of appropriate cells. As discussed in Chapter 2, cells involved in wound healing may be classified into three types on the basis of their potential to divide. Labile cells (those which continually divide and have considerable division potential throughout postnatal life) are necessary for regeneration, as these cells can populate the wound, divide, differentiate, and restore the original tissue architecture and composition. However, if this is not possible, stable cells that have limited division potential (fibroblasts, endothelial cells, osteoblasts, and chondrocytes) can populate the wound site and produce a scar, which is a repair tissue. Similarly, injuries to tissues containing permanent cells (cells that have exited the cell cycle, differentiated, and do not divide) can only heal by repair, because these cells cannot divide and are replaced by cells that produce only scar tissue. Examples of healing in specialized tissues containing these different types of cells are outlined in the next section.

Besides the type of cells, the matrix scaffolding also may determine whether healing occurs by repair or by regeneration. If the matrix structure is seriously disrupted, the cells repopulating the site have little framework upon which to align themselves, and this significantly affects the type of repair. For example, in hepatitis, complete resolution of the liver occurs because the matrix structure is not affected; however, in alcoholic cirrhosis, the structure of the extracellular matrix is extensively damaged and, in this case, the liver is replaced by fibrotic tissue.

Many other factors also affect the rate of wound healing. For example, old age, lack of blood supply, foreign bodies, persistent inflammation, local pressure, ionizing radiation, glucocorticoids, and antibiotics all retard the healing process. The nutritional status of an individual also has a significant effect on the healing process. Protein deficiencies lead to impairment of granulation tissue and collagen formation. Vitamin C is essential for healing as it is a cofactor for prolyl hydroxylase, the enzyme that converts proline to hydroxyproline in collagen (see Chapter 4). Thus, individuals with vitamin C deficiency (eg, scurvy) demonstrate delayed healing. A variety of pathologic conditions involving various systems, such as hemolytic disorders and diabetes mellitus, also affect the rate of wound healing due to their general effect on the metabolic status of the individual, which influences extracellular matrix production and remodeling.

Healing in Specialized Tissues

The general principles of wound healing described above apply to all tissues. Skin abrasion or erosion, in which only the epithelium is denuded, causes very little damage and healing occurs by regeneration. However, in deeper wounds, healing occurs with very little scarring only if the cut edges are replaced in good apposition. Surgical incisions heal in this manner; this is called healing by primary intention, or primary union. When the wound is large and edges are poorly apposed, a large granulation tissue forms and it heals with a large scar. This is considered healing by secondary intention or secondary union.

In contrast to skin and other soft tissues bone fractures heal by regeneration, as this tissue contains undifferentiated pluripoten stem cells that provide the cells needed for regeneration. Bone regeneration is facilitated by the bone matrix, which sequesters many growth factors. The events of fracture healing follow the general pattern outlined above with minor variations; first a blood clot forms and neovascularization begins, and, in 2 to 4 days, a soft callus fills the fracture site. By the end of the first week, pluripotent mesenchymal cells differentiate into osteoblasts. These cells synthesize spicules of woven bone, and the soft callus is converted into a bony callus. Jagged ends of the cortex are subsequently eroded by osteoclasts and the new bone is realigned with the old bone. Bone regeneration is facilitated by one or more members of a family of at least 20 closely related proteins consisting of 30 or more members called the bone morphogenetic proteins (BMP) or growth and differentiation factors (GDFs) (Reddi and Cunningham 1993). While the regenerative potential of fractured bones is well established, the regeneration of bone lost due to erosive-type disorders in which bone matrix is resorbed and replaced with fibrous tissue (periodontitis and osteoarthritis) is not yet fully understood and is not a predictable process (see Chapter 11).

As mentioned above, the extracellular matrix is essential for liver regeneration. This tissue can regenerate completely, even after removing three fourths of its tissue mass. In contrast, skeletal and smooth muscles have limited regeneration potential, and large defects can heal by scar with significant loss of tissue function. Similarly, myocardial cells in the heart cannot be regenerated, and thus damaged tissue is replaced by fibrous scar tissue. Nerves in the peripheral nervous system have very limited regenerative capacity, and axons can recover if cut ends are apposed and if the nuclei of neurons are not destroyed. However, in the central nervous system, regeneration of axons is limited and nerve cells are replaced by astrocytic and microglial proliferation in a process known as gliosis.

In contrast to most of the body organs, healing of the diseased periodontium poses special problems because it is an integrated system of two soft and two calcified tissues. One major obstacle for periodontal regeneration is the need to form new cementum to replace the old tissue, contaminated by bacterial endotoxins, that is removed. New connective tissue has to be formed and reattached to the cementum, and this is not always possible; therefore, the most common outcome is repair by formation of an epithelial, rather than a connective tissue, attachment. Periodontal healing is affected by many conditions discussed above, among which aging is a major factor. Various aspects of periodontal regeneration are discussed in specific detail in Chapter 11.

Summary

Inflammation and wound healing are two processes that are highly relevant to surgeons and periodontists. Over the last two decades, tremendous advances have been made in understanding the molecular and cellular mechanisms involved in wound healing. In particular, the events involved in the acute phase, granulation tissue formation, and the restoration of tissue function have been elucidated. As a result, many growth factors implicated in wound repair and regeneration, including PDGF, EGF, IGF-I, and TGF-β (either alone or in combination), have been successfully utilized to accelerate wound repair in experimental wound healing and fracture models. These fundamental concepts have significant ramifications for healing and regenerative events occurring in the diseased periodontium. However, for successful regeneration to occur in the periodontium, each of its specific anatomical components must be produced in a coordinated and integrated manner. These requirements pose special problems for the periodontist; these are outlined in more detail in Section III.

References

Adams JC, Watt FM. Regulation of development and differentiation by the extracellular matrix. Development 1993;117:1183.

Albeda SM, Smith CW, Ward PA. Adhesion molecules and inflammatory injury. FASEB J 1994;8:504.

Ben-Baruch A, Michiel DF, Oppenheim JJ. Signals and receptors involved in recruitment of inflammatory cells. J Biol Chem 1995;270:11703.

Bennett NT, Schultz GS. Growth factors and wound healing: Part I. Biochemical properties of growth factors and their receptors. Am J Surg 1993a;165:728.

Bennett NT, Schultz GS. Growth factors and wound healing: Part II. Role in normal and chronic wound healing. Am J Surg 1993b;166:74.

Bevilacqua MP. Endothelial-leukocyte adhesion molecules. Annu Rev Immunol 1993;11:767.

Bevilacqua MP, Butcher E, Furie B, et al. Selectins: A family of adhesion receptors. Cell 1991;67:233.

Bevilacqua MP, Nelson RM. Selectins. J Clin Invest 1993; 91:379.

Broekelmann TJ, Limper AH, Colby TV, McDonald JA. Transforming growth factor β_1 is present at sites of extracellular matrix gene expression in human pulmonary fibrosis. Proc Natl Acad Sci USA 1991;88:6642.

Clark RAF. The Molecular and Cellular Biology of Wound Repair. 2nd ed. New York: Plenum; 1996.

Cotran RS. Pathologic Basis of Disease. 5th ed. Philadelphia: Saunders; 1994.

Cotran RS, Grimbone MP, Bevilacqua MP, Mendrick DL, Pober JS. Induction and detection of a human endothelial antigen in vivo. J Exp Med 1986;164:661.

Darby I, Skalli O, Gabbiani G. α-Smooth muscle actin is transiently expressed by myofibroblasts during experimental wound healing. Lab Invest 1990;63:21.

de Fougerolles AR, Klickstein LB, Springer TA. Cloning and expression of intercellular adhesion molecule 3 reveals strong homology to other immunoglobulin family counter-receptors for lymphocyte function-associated antigen 1. J Exp Med 1993;177:1187.

Desmoulière A, Gabbiani G. The role of the myofibroblast in wound healing and fibrocontractive diseases. In: Clark RAF, ed. The Molecular and Cellular Biology of Wound Repair. 2nd ed. New York: Plenum; 1996:391.

Diamond MS, Staunton DE, deFougerolles AR, et al. ICAM-1 (CD54) as counter receptor for Mac-1 (CD11b/CD18). J Cell Biol 1990;111:3129.

Dvorak HF. Tumors: Wounds that do not heal. New Engl J Med 1986;315:1650.

Ekblom P, Vestweber D, Kemler R. Cell-matrix interactions and cell adhesion during development. Annu Rev Cell Biol 1986;2:27.

Fries KM, Blieden T, Looney RJ, et al. Evidence of fibroblast heterogeneity and the role of fibroblast subpopulations in fibrosis. Clin Immunol Immunopathol 1994;72:283.

Goldberger A, Middleton KA, Oliver JA, et al. Biosynthesis and processing of the cell adhesion molecule PECAM-1 includes production of a soluble form. J Biol Chem 1994;269:17183.

Granstein RD, Flotte TJ, Amento EP. Interferons and collagen production. J Invest Dermatol 1990;95:75S.

Grinnell F. Fibroblasts, myofibroblasts and wound contraction. J Cell Biol 1994;124:401.

Hay ED. Extracellular matrix alters epithelial differentiation. Curr Opin Cell Biol 1993;5:1029.

Ihle JN. Cytokine receptor signalling. Nature 1995; 377:591.

Larsen E, Palabrica T, Sajer S, et al. PADGEM-dependent adhesion of platelets to monocytes and neutrophils is mediated by a lineage-specific carbohydrate, LNF-III (CD-15). Cell 1990;63:467.

Lasky LA. Selectins: Interpreters of cell specific carbohydrate information during inflammation. Science 1990; 258:964.

Masur SK, Dewal HS, Dinh TT, Erenburg I, Petridou S. Myofibroblasts differentiate from fibroblasts when plated at low density. Proc Natl Acad Sci USA 1996;93:4219.

McCallion RI, Ferguson MWJ. Fetal wound healing and the development of antiscarring therapies for adult wound healing. In: Clark RAF, ed. The Molecular and Cellular Biology of Wound Repair. 2nd ed. New York: Plenum; 1996:561.

Narayanan AS, Bartold PM. Biochemistry of periodontal connective tissues and their regeneration: a current perspective. Connect Tissue Res 1996;34:191.

Osborn L, Vassallo C, Benjamin CD. Activated endothelium binds lymphocytes through a novel binding site in the alternatively spliced domain of vascular cell adhesion molecule-1. J Exp Med 1992;176:99.

Pitaru S, McCulloch CA, Narayanan AS. Cellular origins and differentiation control mechanisms during periodontal development and wound healing. J Periodont Res 1994; 29:81.

Pober JS, Bevilacqua MP, Mendrick DL, Lapierre LA, Fiers W, Gimbrone MA. Two distinct monokines, interleukin-1 and tumour necrosis factor, each independently induce biosynthesis and transient expression of the same antigen on the surface of cultured human vascular endothelial cells. J Immunol 1986:136:1680.

Raines EW, Bowen-Pope DF, Ross R. Platelet-derived growth factor. In: Sporn MB, Roberts AB, eds. Peptide Growth Factors and Their Receptors. New York: Springer-Verlag; 1990;173–262.

Reddi AH, Cunningham NS. Initiation and promotion of bone differentiation by bone morphogenetic proteins. J Bone Miner Res 1993;8:S499.

Roberts AB, Sporn MB. The transforming growth factor-βs. In: Sporn MB, Roberts AB, eds. Peptide Growth Factors and Their Receptors. New York:Springer-Verlag; 1990;419–472.

Rosen SD, Bertozzi CR. The selectins and their ligands. Curr Opin Cell Biol 1994;6:663.

Sandhu C, Lipsky B, Erickson HP, et al. LFA-1 binding site in ICAM-3 contains a conserved motif and non-contiguous amino acids. Cell Adhes Commun 1994;2:429.

Schuppan D, Somasundaram R, Dieterich W, Ehnis T, Bauer M. The extracellular matrix in cellular proliferation and differentiation. Ann NY Acad Sci 1994;733:87.

Slack JL, Liska DJ, Bornstein P. Regulation of expression of type I collagen genes. Am J Med Genet 1993;45:140.

Sodek J, Overall CM. Matrix metalloproteinases in periodontal tissue remodeling. Matrix Suppl 1992;1:352.

Soma Y, Dvonch V, Grotendorst GR. Platelet-derived growth factor AA homodimer is the predominant isoform in human platelets and acute human wound fluid. FASEB J 1992;6:2996.

Somersalo K, Carpen O, Saksela E, Gahmberg CG, Nortamo P, Timonen T. Activation of natural killer cell migration by leukocyte integrin-binding peptide from intracellular adhesion molecule-2 (ICAM-2). J Biol Chem 1995;270:8629.

Sozzani S, Locait M, Allavena P, Van-Damme J, Mantovani A. Chemokines: a superfamily of chemotactic cytokines. Int J Clin Lab Res 1996; 26:69.

Sporn MB, Roberts AB, eds. Peptide Growth Factors and Their Receptors, I and II. New York and Berlin: Springer-Verlag; 1990.

Stoolman LM. Adhesion molecules controlling lymphocyte migration. Cell 1989;56:907.

Tedder TF, Penta AC, Levine HB, Freedman AS. Expression of the human leukocyte adhesion molecule, LAM-1. Identity with the TQ1 and leukocyte 8 differentiation antigens. J Immunol 1990;144:532.

Teunissen MB, Koomen CW, Bos JD. Intercellular adhesion molecule-3 (CD50) on human epidermal Langerhans cells participates in T-cell activation. J Invest Dermatol 1995;104:995.

Toothill VJ, Van Mourik JA, Niewenhuis HK, Metzelaar MJ, Pearson JD. Characterization of the enhanced adhesion of neutrophil leukocytes to thrombin-stimulated endothelial cells. J Immunol 1990;145:283.

Vaseaux R, Hoffman PA, Tomita JK, et al. Cloning and characterization of a new intercellular adhesion molecule ICAM-R. Nature 1992;360:485.

Ward P. Role of complement, chemokines and regulatory cytokines in acute lung injury. Ann NY Acad Sci 1996;796:104.

Werner S, Peters KG, Longaker MT, Fuller-Pace F, Banda MJ, Williams LT. Large induction of keratinocyte growth factor expression in the dermis during wound healing. Proc Natl Acad Sci USA 1992;89:6896.

Xie J, Kotovuori P, Vermot-Desroches C, et al. Intercellular adhesion molecule-2 (CD102) binds to the leukocyte integrin CD11b/CD18 through the A domain. J Immunol 1995;155:3619.

Yan HC, Baldwin HS, Sun J, Albelda SM, DeLisser HM. Alternative splicing of a specific cytoplasmic exon alters the binding characteristics of murine platelet/endothelial cell adhesion molecule-1 (PECAM-1). J Biol Chem 1995;270:23672.

Part II

Composition of the Extracellular Matrix

4

Structure, Biosynthesis, and Regulation of Collagens

Introduction

The cells of the periodontium and other connective tissues are embedded in an extracellular matrix that regulates their activities and functions. The connective tissue matrix is composed of several organic constituents including collagens, noncollagenous proteins, and proteoglycans. Among these, the collagens are the principal structural components. The collagen molecule is a rigid, rod-like structure that resists stretching, and fibers made up of collagen have high tensile strength. Therefore, this protein is an important structural component in tissues such as periodontal ligament and tendon in which mechanical forces need to be transmitted without loss. Apart from their structural role, collagens can also influence cell shape, differentiation, and many other cellular activities, thus forming an important group of multifunctional connective tissue proteins that participate in many biologic functions. This chapter reviews the events involved in collagen biosynthesis, how collagen production is regulated, and how the structure and content of collagens are affected under a variety of pathologic conditions. Although the majority of information provided here is derived from non-periodontal model systems, it can apply equally well to the periodontal tissues. Specific information for periodontal connective tissue components is described in Part III.

Structure and Types of Collagens

Structural Features

Collagens are the most abundant proteins in the animal kingdom, and they are found in species ranging from insects to man. The word *collagen* is derived from Greek roots *kolla* (glue) and gene, and in French, the word *collagene* designates glue-producing constituents because collagenous tissues were used as the sources of glue and gelatin. As a group of proteins, the collagens contain a number of characteristic features that distinguish them from other matrix molecules. These features include:

1. The presence of a triple helical structure formed by three polypeptide chains called α chains. The α chains are left-handed helices, which wrap around each other into a right-handed, ropelike triple helical rod. Depending on the type of collagen, the molecule may be made up of either three identical α chains, or two or three different α chains (Ramachandran and Ramakrishnan 1976; Piez 1976). The triple helix may be a continuous stretch, or it may be interrupted by noncollagenous segments.
2. Within the triple helical domain, glycine occupies every third position in the repeating amino acid sequence Gly-X-Y, where X and Y are usually amino acids other than glycine. Glycine is essential for the triple-helical conformation because larger amino acids will not fit in the center of the

triple helix. Proline frequently occupies the X and Y positions.
3. Collagens contain two unique amino acids, hydroxyproline (Hyp) and hydroxylysine (Hyl). In vertebrate collagens, these amino acids are present in the Y position.
4. The collagen molecule is stabilized through the formation of a number of lysine-derived intra- and intermolecular cross-links.

Types of Collagens

The collagens represent a large family of proteins and at least 19 different collagen types have been described so far (Prockop and Kivirikko 1995; van der Rest and Garrone 1991). These are divided roughly into three groups, based on their abilities to form fibrils (Fig 4-1; Table 4-1).

The most easily recognized forms of collagens are those that form banded fibrils, and these are called fibril-forming collagens. Type I, II, III, V, and XI collagens belong to this group. In these molecules, the triple helical domain contains an uninterrupted stretch of 338 to 343 Gly-X-Y triplets in each α chain, and the molecule measures 15 × 3000 Å (Ramachandran and Ramakrishnan 1976; Piez 1976).

The second group of collagens consists of proteins in which collagenous domains are interrupted by noncollagenous sequences; these are found associated with the surface of fibril-forming collagens. This group is called fibril-associated collagens with interrupted triple helices (FACIT), and includes collagen types IX, XII, XIV, and perhaps XVI. The type IX, XII, and XIV collagens are unique in containing glycosaminoglycan components covalently linked to the protein.

All other nonfibrillar collagens form the third group, which includes network-forming collagens (types IV, VIII, and X), those forming beaded (type VI) and anchoring fibrils (type VII) and invertebrate cuticle collagens.

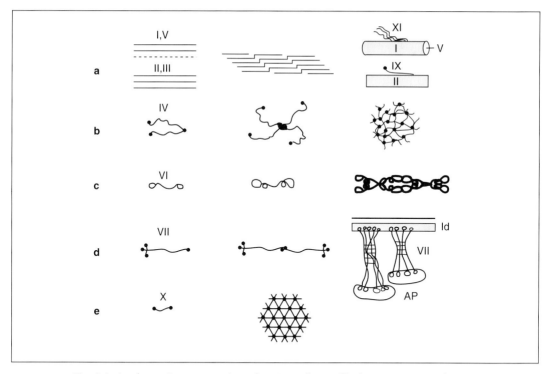

Fig 4-1 A schematic presentation of major collagen fibril structures. **(a)** Three α chains of banded fibril-forming collagens assemble into a triple helix as hetero- (types I and V) and homo-trimers (types II, III, and XI) and aggregate in a quarter-staggered conformation. They are then cross-linked. Fibrils of type I (and III) collagen(s) polymerize around a core of type V, and type XI collagen is on the surface. The type II copolymerizes with type XI (not shown), and the FACIT-type IX and XII collagens. **(b)** Type IV collagen first forms dimers at the C-termini, and four chains form a tetramer at the N-termini. These further form a chicken wire–like network of fibrils. **(c)** Type VI collagen forms beaded fibrils by the assembly of monomers into dimers, dimers into tetramers, and the tetramers into polymers. These fibrils are stabilized by disulfide linkages. **(d)** Type VII collagen has a longer, 4240-Å helix; it first assembles at the C-terminus as antiparallel dimers, and a portion of this end is removed by processing. Fibrils then form and attach to lamina densa (ld) at one end and to anchoring plaques (AP) on the other end. The lamina densa contains type IV collagen, laminin-1, and nidogen. The anchoring plaques contain type IV collagen and laminin-1. **(e)** Type X collagen forms a hexagonal network from monomers (Redrawn with permission from Eckes et al 1996; Prockop and Kiviriko 1995; and Uitto et al 1996).

These collagens form sheets or protein membranes enclosing tissues and organisms.

In addition to the above collagen groups, at least ten noncollagenous proteins incorporating short, triple helical collagen domains have been described. This group of collagen domain–containing nonmatrix proteins includes the C1q component of C1 complement, lung surfactant protein, acetylcholinesterase, conglutinin, and mannose binding protein. These proteins are not considered true collagens because they do not form a part of the extracellular matrix.

Table 4-1. Vertebrate Collagen Types and Their Tissue Distribution

Collagen type	Chain composition*	Gene†	Tissue
Fibrillar collagens			
Type I	$\alpha1(I)_2\alpha2(I)$	COL1A1, COL2A1	Most tissues, including bone
Type II	$\alpha1(II)_3$	COL2A1	Cartilage, vitreous humor
Type III	$\alpha1(III)_3$	COL3A1	Most tissues, fetal tissues
Type V	$\alpha1(V)_3$	COL5A1	Most tissues
Type XI	$\alpha1(XI)\alpha2(XI)\alpha3^{\ddagger}$	COL11A1, COL11A2‡	Cartilage
FACIT collagens			
Type IX	$\alpha1(IX)\alpha2(IX)\alpha3(IX)$	COL9A1, COL9A2, COL9A3	Cartilage, vitreous humor, cornea
Type XII	$\alpha1(XII)_3$	COL12A1	Most tissues
Type XIV	$\alpha1(XIV)_3$	COL14A1	Most tissues
Type XVI	$\alpha1(XVI)_3$	COL16A1	Many tissues
Nonfibrillar collagens			
Type IV	$\alpha1(IV)_2\alpha2;$ $\alpha3,\alpha4,\alpha5,\alpha6^{\S}$	COL4A1–COL4A6§	Basement membranes
Type VI	$\alpha1(VI)\alpha2(VI)\alpha3(VI)$	COL6A1, COL6A2, COL6A3	Most tissues
Type VII	$\alpha1(VII)_3$	COL7A1	Anchoring fibils
Type VIII	$\alpha1(VIII)_3$	COL8A1	Endothelium, Descemet's membrane
Type X	$\alpha1(X)_3$	COL10A1	Hypertrophic cartilage
Type XIII	$\alpha1(XIII)_3$	COL13A1	Many tissues
Type XV	$\alpha1(XV)_3$	COL15A1	Many tissues
Type XVII	$\alpha1(XVII)_3$	COL17A1	Hemidesmosomes in skin
Type XVIII	$\alpha1(XVIII)_3$	COL18A1	Many tissues, liver, kidney
Type XIX	$\alpha1(XIX)_3$	COL19A1	Rhabdomyosarcoma cells

* The arabic numeral identifies the α chain and the roman numeral within parentheses, the collagen type. For example, $\alpha1(I)_2\alpha2$ indicates type I collagen consisting of two $\alpha1$ and one $\alpha2$ chains.

† COL: collagen. The arabic numeral following COL indicates the collagen type. A: α chain of the arabic numeral that follows. Thus, COL4A1 indicates the gene for $\alpha1(IV)$.

‡ $\alpha3(XI)$ is encoded by COL2A1 gene.

§ Major type IV species is $\alpha1(IV)_2\alpha2$; minor species are $\alpha3(IV)_2\alpha4$ and $\alpha5(IV)_2\alpha6$.

Tissue Distribution of Collagens

All tissues contain a mixture of several collagen types, and demonstrate considerable variability in the proportion of the different collagen types as well as their structural organization. The most abundant collagen species in mammalian tissues is type I, which accounts for 65% to 95% of the total collagens. In soft connective tissues, type III is, quantitatively, the second major species, and its proportion ranges from 5% to 30% in adult tissues, and higher in fetal and granulation tissues. These two collagens are codistributed with the minor collagen types V, VI, XII, and XIV. The major function of type I and type III collagens is to provide mechanical strength to the tissues that they comprise.

Among calcified tissues that form dense connective tissues, bone contains predominantly type I collagen, together with very small quantities of types V, III, XII, and XIV. In cartilage, type II collagen is the major fibril-forming collagen present, with other minor species including type XI and the FACIT types IX and XII. Type II collagen is necessary for mechanical strength in these tissues, while type IX collagen appears to permit the cartilage to function at low friction by coating articular surfaces (van der Rest and Garrone 1991). The presence of type X collagen, a shorter molecule with a 1380-Å helix, is limited to the zone of hypertrophic chondrocytes in growing bones.

Type IV collagen is found only in basement membrane structures. It is composed of primarily $\alpha1(IV)$ and $\alpha2(IV)$ chains, although some basement membranes contain small amounts of $\alpha3(IV)$, $\alpha4(IV)$, $\alpha5(IV)$, and $\alpha6(IV)$ chains. This collagen is bound to anchoring fibrils composed of type VII collagen (Sakai et al 1986). In skin, anchoring fibrils are structures that extend to the papillary dermis from the lamina densa, which contains type IV collagen, laminin-1, and nidogen (see Chapter 5). These molecules are attached, by their extremities, to epithelial basement membranes on one end and to anchoring plaques containing type IV collagen and laminin-1 on the other end. The composition and structural features of major collagen types and their tissue distribution are summarized in Figure 4-1 and Table 4-1.

Biosynthesis of Collagens

The collagen molecule is insoluble under physiologic conditions. It contains hydroxyproline and hydroxylysine, two amino acids that are posttranslationally modified from peptidyl prolines and lysines. These modifications can occur only on nascent α chains because the triple helical collagen molecule is not accessible to the modification enzymes. Some collagens contain sugar residues at the triple helical domain, and others have covalently attached glycosaminoglycan chains. For these, as well as other reasons, the collagen

molecule is first synthesized as a larger precursor containing extra amino acids at both N- and C-terminal ends. Synthesis of these pro-α chains, their assembly into procollagen, and their conversion to collagen fibers involve several well-coordinated biosynthetic reactions occurring in the nucleus, cytoplasm, and extracellular space (Byers 1995; Prockop and Kivirikko 1995). Although these reactions have been very well characterized for type I collagen, they are applicable (with some variations) to all collagens.

Gene Expression

Collagen genes are large and range in size from 5 kb for COL1A1, to 130 kb for COL13A1 (see Table 4-1 for terminology; Jacenko et al 1991; Vuorio and de Crombrugghe 1990). They are several times as large as their respective mRNAs. More than 30 genes have been described for collagen types I to XIX. Although differences exist among the various collagen genes, those for fibril-forming collagens have a similar exon arrangement. These genes contain 42 exons for the major triple helical region, separated by introns 80 to 2000 nucleotides long (Fig 4-2a). Most of these exons are composed of 54 bp (or an integral multiple thereof), and start with an intact codon for glycine. This organization is largely conserved and independent of the species or type of fibrillar collagen (Sandell and Boyd 1990). However, the organization of nonfibrillar collagen genes vary. For example, exons for the type IV collagen genes do not conform to the 54-bp rule, and they frequently start with a split codon for glycine. In this collagen, the COL4A1-COL4A2, the COL4A3-COL4A4, and the COL4A5-COL4A6 genes are arranged in a unique head-to-head orientation separated by a nucleotide sequence (see Fig 4-2d). In type IX collagen, the sizes of exons range from 21 to 400 bp, depending upon their location, and in some tissues they contain an alterna-

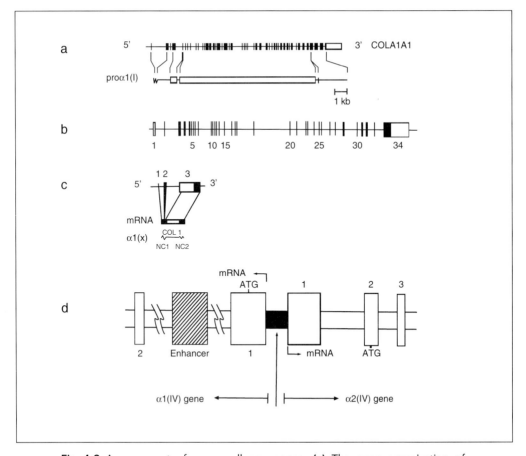

Fig 4-2 Arrangement of some collagen genes. **(a)** The gene organization of COL1A1 is shown at the top, and the protein domains (signal peptide, N- and C-terminal propeptide domains, and triple helical domains) are indicated at the bottom. The exons are designated by solid boxes or vertical lines. **(b)** COL6A1 collagen gene showing the distribution of 34 exons and untranslated mRNA regions (open boxes in exons 1 and 4). **(c)** COL10A1 gene. The gene organization is shown on top and the numbers identify each exon. The boxes represent exons, open areas indicate triple helical domains, and solid areas represent untranslated regions and globular domains. The protein is represented at the bottom. The gene arrangement for type VIII collagen is similar. **(d)** Head-to-head arrangement of COL4A1 and COL4A2 genes separated by a 130-bp bidirectional promoter (black box). The intervening sequence contains a binding site for the transcription factor Sp1. The first two exons (open boxes) are shown; the crosshatched box represents enhancer. a, b, and c are shown roughly on the same scale. Redrawn with permission from Byers 1995 (a); Wälchli et al 1992 (b); Jacenko et al 1991(c); and Burbelo et al 1988 (d).

tive promoter to transcribe a shorter form of type IX. The type VI collagen gene is composed of only 34 exons (see Fig 4-2b), and these exons, as for type IV, are also multiples of 9 bp. The gene arrangement for type X collagen, however, is unlike other collagens. In this gene, the region that encodes its triple helical domain consists of a single 2136-bp exon (see Fig 4-2c).

Translation and Posttranslational Events

Collagen mRNAs are transcribed as precursors and undergo the usual processing reactions described in Chapter 1, including capping, polyadenylation, and splicing. After these nuclear events, the mRNA is translocated to the cytoplasm where it binds to ribosomes and gets translated. The mRNA codes for the pre–pro-α chain, which (in type I, II, and III collagens) contains approximately 1500 amino acids, and includes the signal sequence and extra N- and C-terminal sequences not present in mature α chains. Signal sequences are cleaved during polypeptide chain elongation as the nascent pro-α chains are being transported into the rough endoplasmic reticulum (RER) lumen. As translation of the pro-α (pre–pro-α minus the signal peptide) proceeds, certain prolyl and lysyl residues at the Y position are oxidized to Hyp and Hyl, respectively, by enzymes. Prolyl hydroxylation is performed, predominantly at the C-4 position, by the enzyme prolyl-4-hydroxylase. This enzyme is a tetramer consisting of two α and two β subunits, with molecular masses of 64 and 60 kd, respectively. Some prolyl residues are hydroxylated at C-3 to 3-Hyp by a different enzyme, prolyl-3-hydroxylase. The lysyl hydroxylase is a homodimer of 85-kd subunits. These hydroxylases require O_2, Fe^{++}, α-ketoglutarate, and ascorbic acid (vitamin C) as cofactors. Only nascent pro-α chains act as substrates for these enzymes, not triple helical molecules.

The minimum amino acid sequence requirement for prolyl hydroxylation is X-Pro-Gly. All available prolyl and lysyl residues are not hydroxylated; the extent of hydroxylation depends upon the availability of substrate, type of tissue, and other factors. The relative rate and extent of hydroxylation also vary between collagen types. For example, in type IV collagen, 3-prolyl hydroxylation occurs to a higher degree than in types I, II, and III, with up to 90% of its lysines hydroxylated.

Triple helical type I collagen, with fully hydroxylated 4-hydroxyproline, has a T_m (melting temperature, above which the collagen triple helix is denatured to α chains) of 39°C. However, underhydroxylated molecules melt at lower temperatures, and the T_m of completely unhydroxylated collagen is 25°C (Rosenbloom and Harsch 1973). Therefore, prolyl hydroxylation is essential for collagen thermal stability at physiologic temperature, while underhydroxylated molecules are denatured and degraded. Hydroxylysine residues, on the other hand, serve as specific glycyosylation sites, and form more stable cross-links than lysine. The role of 3-hydroxyproline, however, is unclear.

The pro-α chains undergo glycosylation at certain Hyl and Asn residues during translation, and oligosaccharides rich in galactose, galactose plus glucose (to hydroxylysine), or mannose (to asparagine) are added. Glycosylation occurs at the C-5 oxygen of peptidyl hydroxylysine and it is carried out by the enzymes hydroxylysylgalactosyl transferase and galactosylhydroxylysylglucosyl transferase. These enzymes transfer UDP-galactose and UDP-glucose, respectively. The glycosylation of hydroxylysyl residues takes place in the RER lumen, and oligosaccharides are added to asparagine residues in the ER and Golgi complex.

As soon as the synthesis of pro-α chains is completed, two proα1(I) chains and one proα2(I) in type I, or three proα1 chains in collagen types II and III, associate at the C-terminal ends. This association is stabilized by interchain disulfide bond formation, which is catalyzed by the enzyme protein-disulfide isomerase. Triple helix formation is thus initiated and proceeds from the C-terminal toward the N-terminal end, like a zipper. The rate of collagen folding is limited by the extent of *cis-trans* isomerization of prolyl bonds. Collagen chain assembly and folding of types I and IV collagens involve the heat shock protein Hsp47 as a molecular chaperone. Some procollagens lack large C-terminal domains (eg, type XII), and these procollagens appear to fold by mechanisms not involving the formation of a nucleus at the C-terminus.

The procollagen molecule thus assembled is then translocated to the Golgi complex, where additional glycosylation and phosphorylation may occur. Sulfate (eg, in type V) and phosphate (to type I in bone) groups may also be added to tyrosyl and seryl residues, respectively, located at the N-terminal propeptide domain. The procollagen molecules are then packaged into vesicles, which fuse with cell membrane and release their contents into the extracellular space.

Extracellular Collagen Biosynthetic Events

Conversion of the procollagen into mature collagen fibers occurs in the extracellular space and involves several stages (Fig 4-3). First the propeptide sequences at N- and C-terminal ends are removed by N- and C-procollagen peptidases (also called N- and C-proteinases), respectively. The N-propeptidase cleaves a proline-glutamine bond in proα(I) and proα1(III) chains, and an alanine-glutamine bond in proα2(I). This enzyme requires a triple helical substrate and the pro-N domains are removed en masse. Cleavage at the carboxyl end occurs at alanine-aspartic acid bond in both proα1(I) and proα2(I) chains. Although the propeptides are removed from type I, II, and III procollagens, other collagens may be processed differently or not at

all. For example, N-and C-terminal extensions are not removed in nonfibrillar collagens and they are retained in mature fibrils.

Fibrillar collagens formed in this manner then aggregate spontaneously as ordered fibrils due to the distribution of charged and hydrophobic regions on their surface. Aggregation occurs in a parallel, overlapping lateral array such that adjacent molecules are staggered by approximately one fourth (670 Å) of the length of the molecule (see Fig 4-1a). This quarter-stagger arrangement permits interaction with the side chains of neighboring molecules, and gives tensile strength to the fibrils and fibers formed. Although the aggregation is nonenzymatic, the diameter of the fibrils appears to be regulated by the presence of types V and XI, and type IX procollagens, which copolymerize with type I and type II, respectively. This is illustrated by a deletion mutation in the COL11A1 gene; this results in the formation of extremely thick type II fibrils in the recessive *cho* mice, and these animals develop chondrodysplasia.

Removal of the propeptide extensions is necessary for ordered fibril formation, and their retention, especially at the N-terminus, results in poor apposition of the collagen molecules due to steric hindrance. This prevents normal fibril growth, and the fibrils formed are thinner and disorganized. Such a defect occurs in dermatosparaxis, an inherited disease in cattle, sheep, humans, and cats (see Byers 1995). Retention of the pro-ends is believed to be the reason why type IV collagen does not aggregate into banded fibrils in basement membranes.

The collagen fibrillar array is stabilized by covalent cross-links. Cross-linking requires the enzyme lysyl oxidase. This enzyme oxidatively deaminates the amino groups of lysyl and hydroxylysyl residues to aldehydes, converting these amino acids to allysine and hydroxyallysine, respectively. Lysyl oxidase requires Cu^{++} and pyridoxal phosphate as cofactors (Narayanan et al 1974; Kagan and Trackman 1991). The aldehyde residues in allysines and hydroxyallysines condense spontaneously with each other, or with unmodified lysine or hydroxylysine residues in adjacent α chains forming divalent cross-links with norleucine, hydroxynorleucine, and aldol condensation products. They may be subsequently converted to the more complex cross-links, merodesmosines and hydroxypyridiniums, by forming adducts with additional residues (Fig 4-4) (Eyre et al 1984). In collagen types I, II, and III, four cross-linking loci (lysines) exist, one each at the N- and C-terminal telopeptides (telopeptides are (non-glycine)-X-Y sequences retained at C- and N-terminal ends of mature collagen molecules) and two within the triple helix.

Cross-linked collagen molecules then combine with other extracellular matrix components to form three-dimensional scaffolding. The ultimate organization of collagens into fibers depends upon the specific functional demands of each tissue, and appears to be dictated by the presence of minor collagens and proteoglycans such as decorin. Thus, in tendon and ligament, dense collagen fibers consisting of type I and III collagens are oriented parallel to their long axis, whereas they form branching and anastomosing fibers in the skin. The fibers are arranged into several architecturally distinct forms in the gingiva; in bone they are arranged in layers with the fibers parallel to each other. In the cornea, collagens are present as laminated sheets, with the collagen fibers parallel within each sheet, but perpendicular to those of adjacent layers. Type II collagen forms relatively smaller fibers, oriented randomly in a viscous proteoglycan matrix.

In type IV collagen, the triple helical domain is longer than most collagens, with approximately 1400 amino acids, but is interrupted by short noncollagenous sequences. Both the N- and C-terminal noncollagenous ends are retained in mature type IV collagen. This molecule forms a fine spiderlike network of cords in which two monomers associate into dimers through the C-termini, and at the

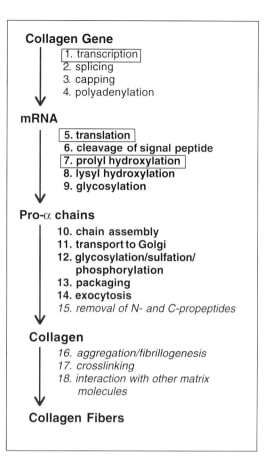

Fig 4-3 Major biochemical events of collagen biosynthesis. Extracellular reactions are shown in italic type; bold type indicates reactions occurring in the cytoplasm. All other reactions occur in the nucleus. Events associated with regulation of synthesis are enclosed in boxes. Although this general scheme is common to all collagens, variations occur for individual collagen species, especially in the removal of propetide. (Reproduced with permission from Bartold and Narayanan 1996.)

N-termini they assemble into tetramers (see Fig 4-1b; Timpl 1989). Type IV collagen is bound to anchoring fibrils, which are formed by the antiparallel assembly of two type VII molecules overlapping at their C-terminal ends (see Fig 4-1d). The C-terminal ends of the type VII molecules are removed by proteolysis, the dimers are then stabilized by disulfide linkage, and these associate laterally to form anchoring fibrils.

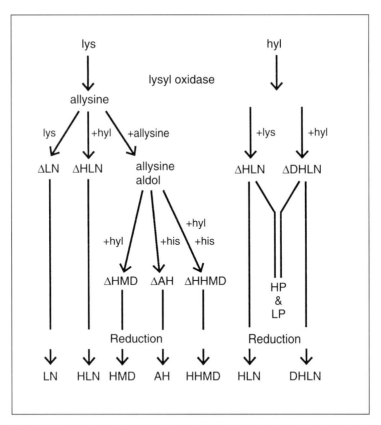

Fig 4-4 Formation of lysine-derived cross-links. Lysyl and hydroxylysyl residues are first oxidatively deaminated to allysine or hydroxyallysine, respectively, by lysyl oxidase. The deaminated products spontaneously condense with other allysines, lysines, or other cross-links already formed to form additional cross-links.

LN, lysinonorleucine; HLN, hydroxylysinonorleucine; DHLN, dihydroxylysinonorleucine; HMD, hydroxymerodesmosine; AH, aldolhistidine; HHMD, histidinohydroxymerodesmosine; HP, hydroxylysyl pyridinoline; LP, lysyl pyridinoline. The prefix ΔH indicates dehydro forms. For chemical formulas and more details, see Eyre et al (1984). Elastin cross-links also form in similar reactions, except that this protein does not have hydroxylysine derived cross-links. (Reproduced with permission from Bartold and Narayanan 1996.)

In Descemet's membrane, which separates corneal endothelial cells from the stroma, type VIII collagen forms a different network structure with the collagen molecules arranged in stacks of hexagonal lattices. Type X collagen also forms a similar structure (see Fig 4-1e).

In contrast to these collagens, type VI collagen forms microfibrils in most soft connective tissues. This collagen molecule is a heterotrimer of α1, α2, and α3 chains, each with a short triple helical domain and larger N- and C-terminal domains. Two type VI monomers form dumbbell-shaped dimers, by antiparallel assembly, which are able to aggregate into tetramers (see Fig 4-1c). One distinguishing feature of these fibers is their stabilization by disulfide bonds such that the structure has a high degree of stability.

Regulation of Collagen Biosynthesis

Because collagens are the major structural components of connective tissues, and each tissue contains a typical mixture of collagen types, the quantity and proportion of collagens within each tissue need to be precisely regulated to maintain tissue integrity. Regulation is necessary, not only to control the amount of collagens produced, but also to control the fiber architecture. This is illustrated by the differences noted in the properties of connective tissue during the course of wound healing (see Chapter 3). After injury, the wound bed is first replaced by a granulation tissue and then with either normal tissue or a scar. The connective tissue in all three cases may contain the same matrix constituents, yet they have different tensile strengths. Thus, although they can supplement tissue properties to some extent, scar and granulation tissue cannot function as well as the normal tissue.

The most important step at which regulation of collagen production occurs is at the level of gene transcription. Collagen gene expression is regulated in a cell- and tissue-specific manner during both normal development and homeostasis. Regulation of transcription rates is mediated primarily through promoters and enhancer elements. In the type I collagen gene, short promoter and enhancer sequences are present in the first intron of the COL1A2 gene. In the mouse COL1A2 gene, these sequences are the CCAAT motif localized between −84 and −80, a CAGA sequence at −250 to −247, and a GCCAAG sequence between −315 and −295, all relative to the transcription initiation site (Karsenty et al 1988; Ramirez and Di Liberto 1990). The last sequence represents a binding site for the nuclear factor NF1, which is an intracellular mediator for DNA replication and a transcription factor. TGF-β has been noted to up-regulate collagen gene transcription through this sequence (Rossi et al 1988). The first intron of the human COL1A1 gene contains a negative regulatory sequence domain located at +820 to +1093 that contains the transactivator protein-1 (AP-1) binding motif GCCC-CGCCCC and a viral core enhancer sequence (GTGGTTAGC) (Bornstein and McKay 1988; Bornstein and Sage 1989).

In type IV collagen, the pair of genes for COL4A1 and COL4A2 (COL4A3 and COL4A4, and COL4A5 and COL4A6) are each arranged in a unique head-to-head arrangement separated by a short 130-bp segment (see Fig 4-2d), with a binding site for SP1 at its center. The intervening sequence interacts with enhancer and negative regulatory elements located in COL4A1 and COL4A2 genes, respectively, and regulates the expression of both genes (Burbelo et al 1988).

Developmental expression of collagens is regulated in a temporal-, tissue-, and cell type–specific manner. For example, interruption of the first intron of the COL1A1 gene in mouse germ line, by integration of the MoMLV viral gene, causes transcriptional inactivation of the COL1A1 gene. Through this mechanism, type I collagen cannot be made and homozygous embryos die at 12 to 14 days. However, in these animals, tooth rudiments synthesize normal amounts of type I collagen, indicating that in odontoblasts, unlike fibroblasts, type I collagen is regulated by a domain different from intron 1 (Kratochwil et al 1989). Tissue-specific expression of type IX collagen appears to be achieved by utilizing different transcription initiation sites located 20 kb apart. In cartilage, transcription starts at exon 1, however, in cornea it starts downstream at the 3′ end of the intron 6. After splicing, the product in the cornea has skipped exons up to 7, therefore, the α1(IX) chain produced in cornea is shorter than the chain in cartilage α1(IX) (Nishimura et al 1989).

The magnitude of collagen synthesis is dependent upon the levels of the mRNA for its α chains. Although these levels are largely determined by the rate of transcription, some

Table 4-2. Some Mediators That Affect Collagen Synthesis

Mediator	Major Source	Collagen Synthesis
Growth factors		
PDGF	Platelets, macrophages, smooth muscle cells, epithelium	↑
TGF-β*	Platelets, macrophages	↑
FGF	Platelets, macrophages, matrix	↑
IGF	Serum, matrix	↑
Cytokines/lymphokines		
IL-1$_{\alpha,\beta}$[†]	Macrophages, most cells	↓
IFN-γ	Lymphocytes	↓
TNF-α	Monocytes/macrophages	↓
Hormones		
Glucocorticoids[‡]	...	↓
Others		
PGE$_2$	Monocytes/macrophages	↓

* Stimulates synthesis of other matrix components as well, and TIMP; decreases MMP synthesis.
† Enhances matrix degradation through MMP synthesis.
‡ Increases elastin and fibronectin synthesis.

substances, such as TGF-β, elevate mRNA levels by increasing their stability.

Collagen synthesis can, in theory, be regulated posttranslationally by the extent of prolyl hydroxylation because an underhydroxylated collagen molecule is unstable at physiologic temperature and is degraded rapidly. Prolyl underhydroxylation appears to contribute to connective tissue changes in scurvy, a disease in which prolyl hydroxylase activity is impaired due to vitamin C deficiency. The synthesis of collagen may also be inhibited by the N-propeptide released from proα1(I), as this peptide is an inhibitor of protein translation in vitro (Hörlein et al 1981). However, whether this mode of feedback inhibition is physiologically significant is unclear.

During development, inflammation, and wound repair, the synthesis of collagens is influenced by a variety of growth factors, hormones, cytokines, and lymphokines. Prominent among these is TGF-β, which stimulates the production of collagens and other matrix components. This growth factor has also been implicated in the evolution of fibrotic lesions. Among the different TGF-β isoforms, TGF-β$_1$ appears to be the species that plays a major role in wound repair and fibrosis (Roberts and Sporn 1990). In contrast to TGF-β, collagen genes are down-regulated by the inflammatory cytokine TNF-α and by the lymphokine interferon gamma (IFN-γ) (Armendariz-Borunda et al 1992; Bornstein and Sage 1989; Czaja et al 1987). Many growth factors and cytokines affecting collagen synthesis are secreted by platelets, macrophages, keratinocytes, and fibroblasts during inflammation, and their presence at the foci of inflammation and wound sites generally correlates with changes in collagen synthesis (Table 4-2) (Clark 1996). How collagen synthesis is regulated in periodontal tissues has been studied using cells derived from periodontal components. These studies have revealed that the regulation of type I and III collagens, as well as proteoglycans and hyaluronate, by various growth factors and cytokines follows the general mechanisms described for other cells (Narayanan and Bartold 1996).

Degradation and Remodeling of Collagens

Degradation of collagen and other matrix elements is a key component of normal tissue remodeling, including ovulation, embryo implantation, and involution of the uterus and mammary glands. Nevertheless, degradation of the extracellular matrix also contributes greatly to pathologic alterations. For example, matrix degradation is the major cause of connective tissue destruction in periodontitis, rheumatoid arthritis, and other chronic inflammatory diseases, whereas hyperplasias and fibroses are associated with low levels of degradation. Enzymes capable of degrading the matrix aid in tumor invasion by metastasizing cancer cells.

Although several enzymes are involved in the destruction of matrix components, collagen degradation is mediated primarily by the collagenases. These are specialized enzymes that have evolved specifically to hydrolyze collagens because their triple helical collagen structure is resistant to most common proteinases. The collagenases belong to a family of enzymes, called matrix metalloproteinases (MMP), that consists of at least 13 members with closely related domain structures and discrete functions. All have a 21-kd catalytic domain that contains a Zn^{++} binding site. Based on their substrate specificity, they have been classified as collagenases, gelatinases, stromelysins, and matrilysins (Mignatti et al 1996; Woessner 1991). Three interstitial collagenases capable of degrading native matrix collagen fibrils have been described so far, all of which cleave $\alpha 1(I)$ and $\alpha 2(I)$ chains at the glycine$_{775}$-isoleucine$_{776}$ and glycine$_{775}$-leucine$_{776}$ bonds, respectively. The cleavage of these susceptible peptide bonds, located approximately one quarter of the length from the C-terminus, therefore results in the release of cleavage fragments three quarters and one quarter of the chain's original size. The released fragments have a lower T_m than the intact collagen molecule at physiologic temperature, and therefore they become denatured and subsequently are degraded by other proteinases.

Collagenase-1 (also called MMP-1 or fibroblast type collagenase) is produced by a variety of human epithelial and mesenchymal cell types including keratinocytes, fibroblasts, and macrophages. This enzyme can hydrolyze type I, II, III, VI, VIII, and X collagens and gelatin (Birkedal-Hansen et al 1993). It hydrolyzes type III molecules faster than it does type I. Another enzyme, collagenase-2 (also called polymorphonuclear leukocyte [PMN]-type collagenase or MMP-8), also hydrolyzes type I and III collagens, but this enzyme degrades type I faster than it does type III. Collagenase-2 is found only in the granules of polymorphonuclear leukocytes. Collagenase-3 is a recently described enzyme found in breast cancer.

The gelatinase group of MMPs has two prominent members, the 72-kd (gelatinase-A, MMP-2) and 92-kd (gelatinase-B, MMP-9) gelatinases. Both of these enzymes have a high affinity for gelatin, but they also degrade type IV, VII, X, and XI collagens and elastin. These enzymes cleave the Gly-X peptide bond, where X = Val, Leu, Glu, Asn, or Ser. The 92-kd gelatinase is produced by eosinophils, macrophages, and keratinocytes, and it is stored in PMN granules. Its gene (and those of MMP-1 and stromelysin-1 as well) contains AP-1 binding motifs, and therefore its synthesis is regulated by several inflammatory mediators. In contrast, the gene for the 72-kd gelatinase lacks the AP-1 binding motif; therefore, it is not regulated by most mediators other than TGF-β. This enzyme is constitutively produced by most cell types.

Stromelysins have broad specificity with the ability to degrade proteoglycans, basement membrane, laminin, and fibronectin, in addition to collagens. Three stromelysins, stromelysin-1 (MMP-3), stromelysin-2 (MMP-10), and stromelysin-3 have been described so far. Matrilysin (MMP-7) and metalloelastase

Table 4-3. Specificities and Source of Collagenases and Other Matrix Metalloproteinases

Enzyme	MMP Type	Source	Specificity
Collagenases			
Collagenase-1	MMP-1	Connective tissue cells, macrophages	Type I, II, III, VII, VI collagens
Collagenase-2	MMP-8	PMN	Same as collagenase-1
Gelatinases			
72-kd, gelatinase-A	MMP-2	Connective tissue cells	Gelatin, types IV–VII, X, XI, elastin
92-kd, gelatinase-B	MMP-9	Connective tissue cells	Same as gelatinase-A
Stromelysins			
SL-1	MMP-3	Many cells, tumor cells	Proteoglycans, laminin, collagen types III–V, IX, X
SL-2	MMP-10	Many cells, tumor cells	Same as SL-1
SL-3	MMP-11	Tumor cells, stromal cells	?
Others			
PUMP-1 (matrilysin)	MMP-7 Macrophages	Connective tissue cells	Fibronectin, laminin, type IV collagen, gelatin, proteoglycans
Metalloelastase	MMP-12	Macrophages	Elastin, fibronectin
Membrane type MMP	MT-MMP	Cell membrane	Progelatinase-A

(MMP-12) are other MMPs. In addition, another group of MMPs, called membrane-type metalloproteinases (MT-MMPs), has recently been identified. These enzymes incorporate a transmembrane domain in their primary structure, and they are located on the cell surface. The MT-MMPs are believed to activate progelatinase-A for tumor cell invasion. They also play a role in early embryogenesis, tissue remodeling, and wound healing (Sato et al 1994; Takino et al 1995; Yang et al 1996). The properties of MMPs are summarized in Table 4-3.

The destructive propensity of the MMPs in vivo is kept under control by at least three different mechanisms (Birkedal-Hansen et al 1993). These enzymes are normally present in tissues as inactive precursors, and conversion to an active form requires activation by plasmin, trypsin, or other proteinases. The activating proteinases are themselves activated when conditions demand (eg, during inflammation), and they are also regulated by other proteins such as tissue plasminogen activator. The second mechanism by which MMP activity is regulated is through modulation of its synthesis. MMP synthesis is induced by numerous mediators such as growth factors, cytokines, or other similar mediators by activation of MMP gene expression. Two key regulators of MMP expression are IL-1 and TGF-β, and these substances are present in abundance in inflamed tissues (Sodek and Overall 1992). In these and other tissues, IL-1, TNF-α, and PGE$_2$ increase MMP production by fibroblasts and keratinocytes. TGF-β also increases MMP synthesis in fibroblasts, but decreases it in keratinocytes. In macrophages, MMP production is stimulated by lipopolysaccharides (LPS), and production is inhibited by IFN-γ, IL-4, and IL-10. Glucocorticoids and retinoid hormones also suppress MMP production (Birkedal-Hansen et al 1993). In all these cases there is a time lag between the exposure of a cell to these molecules and enzyme release. However, collagenase-2 is an exception to this rule because it is readily released on demand as it is stored in the PMN granules. Finally, the activities of MMPs are neutralized by inhibitors present in serum and tissues. A major serum inhibitor is α_2-macroglobulin, which covalently cross-links with collagenases and other susceptible proteolytic enzymes and inactivates them. In particular, α_2-macroglobulin acts as a potent inhibitor of the collagenase MMP-1 by binding to this MMP with a greater avidity than does collagen, which is the natural substrate for MMP-1 (Enghild et al 1989). Tissues contain another group of inhibitors, each called a tissue inhibitor of metalloproteinases (TIMP), which are distributed widely in many tissues and body fluids. To date, three such members of the TIMP family have been described. Among these, TIMP-1 and TIMP-2 have been well studied and found to be more effective towards interstitial collagenases and gelatinases, respectively (Howard et al 1991).

In contrast to the vertebrate enzymes, bacterial collagenases degrade native collagen molecules to small peptides. These enzymes are highly potent and have broad specificities, and they can degrade all native collagen fibrils regardless of the collagen type.

Diseases Associated with Collagen Alterations

Because most tissues contain a mixture of collagen types, any change in the structure, content, or proportion of collagen types can be expected to lead to functional abnormalities of the tissues containing these collagens. Three types of alterations can affect collagens and lead to connective tissue changes: a defect in the structure of collagen genes, a molecular defect in the processing enzymes, and mecha-

nisms affecting the expression of collagen genes due to pathologies of acquired diseases. Diseases due to molecular defects are inherited, and those associated with acquired diseases, although they may involve one or more genetic components, are induced by a variety of physiologic and environmental factors.

Inherited Diseases of Collagen Structure and Biosynthesis

These diseases arise due to point mutations, deletions, or insertions in the structural genes for collagens or their posttranslational processing enzymes. The severity of these diseases depends on several factors. For type I collagen, mutations that affect the assembly of proα1(I) chains can be lethal, whereas those affecting proα2(I) assembly are not. This difference arises because homotrimers of α1(I) formed in the absence of proα2(I) are stable at physiologic temperature, whereas the $\alpha2(I)_3$ formed in the absence of α1(I) is not stable and gets degraded. Thus, large deletions, insertions, or mutations near the C-terminus of pro-α1(I), which affect its assembly into collagen, are often lethal. Replacement of glycine with other amino acids decreases the rate of collagen folding, its thermal stability, and secretion; therefore, such mutant molecules are retained intracellularly for a longer period and are degraded. Mutations associated with the genes of collagen-processing enzymes, however, are usually not lethal, even though they lead to functional abnormalities of constituent tissues (Byers 1995).

Almost 200 mutations have been characterized in COL1A1 and COL1A2 genes so far, and many of these mutations have been associated with various forms of osteogenesis imperfecta (OI) and Ehlers-Danlos syndrome (EDS) (Table 4-4). Osteogenesis imperfecta is a heterogeneous group of disorders associated with bone fragility, dentinogenesis imperfecta, hearing loss, blue sclera, and soft tissue dys-

Table 4-4. Some Inherited Diseases and the Collagen Genes That Are Affected

Disease	Affected Gene	Biochemical Defect
Osteogenesis imperfecta		
Type I	COL1A1	Decreased type I procollagen production; glycine substitution in helical domain
Type II	COL1A1, COL1A2	Substitution of glycine near C-terminus, deletion, rearrangement of genes
Type III	COL1A1, CO1A2	Point- and frameshift mutations
Type IV	COL1A2, COL1A1	Point mutation mostly in α2(I), deletion
Ehlers-Danlos syndrome		
Type IV (vascular)	COL3A1	Glycine substitution, exon skipping, small deletions affecting type III structure, synthesis, and secretion
Type VI (ocular)	Lysyl hydroxylase	Lysine underhydroxylation in type I and III
Type VIIA, B	COL1A1, COL1A2	Defective procollagen-collagen conversion; mutation at cleavage site (exon 6)
Type VIIC, dermatosparaxis	N-proteinase	Defective procollagen to collagen conversion (N-proteinase)
Type VIII periodontal	Unknown	Unknown
Type IX, X-linked cutis laxa	ATP7A*	Defective copper distribution, low lysyl oxidase activity
Chondrodysplasias	COL2A1	Glycine substitution, deletion, partial duplication
Alport's syndrome	COL4A5	Point mutations, exon deletion
Epidermolysis bullosa, dystrophic form	COL7A1	Glycine substitution, premature termination

* Also known as MNK.

plasia. It is subdivided into four major subclasses. Osteogenesis imperfecta type I is a dominantly inherited form with blue sclera, but normal teeth and near-normal stature. It is caused most commonly by mutations that decrease type I procollagen production because of mutations that lead to null COL1A1 alleles. Other molecular defects identified in this disease include substitution of glycine by cysteine, especially near the N-terminal end. Osteogenesis imperfecta type II is lethal in the perinatal period, and this disease is associated with new dominant mutations. This form arises due to mutations that affect procollagen assembly by substitution of glycine near the C-terminal end, rearrangement of multiple exons (resulting in loss of a large segment of amino acids), or mutations at the C-terminal propeptide of

proα(I). Osteogenesis imperfecta type III is a genetically heterogeneous disease most commonly inherited in autosomal dominant, and rarely as recessive, forms, and it is a progressively deforming variety. Point mutations in proα1(I) genes, and mutations in proα2(I) that prevent its inclusion in collagen molecules, have been identified as some of the causes for this disease. Osteogenesis imperfecta type IV is a dominantly inherited disease caused by point mutations and small deletions in the α2(I) gene; a common feature of this type of osteogenesis imperfecta is dentinogenesis imperfecta.

The Ehlers-Danlos syndrome represents another heterogeneous group of connective tissue diseases characterized by skin fragility and hyperextensibility, and hypermobility of the joints. Among these, the Ehlers-Danlos syndrome type IV (the vascular, or ecchymotic, type) is characterized by arterial rupture and spontaneous rupture of the colon, and the defects identified in this disease are mutations or multiple exon deletions within the COL3A1 gene. In Ehlers-Danlos syndrome type VI (ocular form in which blindness and kyphoscoliosis are major features), lysyl hydroxylase activity is severely depressed, and lysines in type I and III collagens, but not in type II and IV, are underhydroxylated. In Ehlers-Danlos syndrome type VII, the defect is impairment of the procollagen-to-collagen conversion. In this disease, the assembly of collagens into functional fibrils is affected due to steric hindrance by the retained pro-peptide domain. The conversion may be impaired due to mutations at the N-propeptidase cleavage site (exon 6 of COL1A1 or COL1A2); this is the defect in Ehlers-Danlos syndrome forms VIIA and B. Alternatively, the enzyme itself may be affected; this is the defect in Ehlers-Danlos syndrome form VIIC (dermatosparaxis). Ehlers-Danlos syndrome type VIII is an autosomal dominant form characterized by periodontal involvement and loss of teeth; the molecular defect responsible for this disease has not yet been identified. Marked reduction in the activity of lysyl oxidase due to defective intracellular distribution of copper, a cofactor for lysyl oxidase, gives rise to Ehlers-Danlos syndrome type IX (cutis laxa or occipital horn syndrome). This is an X-linked recessive disease.

In the type II collagen gene (COL2A1), approximately 50 mutations that lead to chondrodysplasias have been reported. The chondrodysplasias are a heterogeneous group of diseases characterized by abnormal growth or development of cartilage, and their severity ranges from mild symptoms to perinatal death. Three major forms of this group of disorders are achondrogenesis/hypochondrogenesis, spondyloepiphyseal dysplasia, and Stickler syndrome (Byers 1995). Individuals affected by these diseases exhibit abnormalities in type II collagen–containing tissues such as growth plates, nucleus pulposus, and vitreous humor. The type of mutations identified in these diseases are similar to those for type I collagen, and include a glycine-to-aspartate substitution in a Kniest dysplasia, an arginine-to-cysteine conversion, and an interesting G-to-T transversion that interferes with splicing and results in the deletion of 18 amino acids (Byers 1995; Eyre et al 1991; Tiller et al 1995a, 1995b). Mutations in type X collagen, a product of hypertrophic chondrocytes, cause a form of dwarfism known as Schmid metaphyseal chondrodysplasia in humans.

Molecular defects have also been described in the basement membrane collagens. Alport syndrome is a progressive hereditary nephritis associated with sensoneuronal deafness and ocular abnormalities. It has an X-linked inheritance pattern, and it is characterized by splitting and thinning of the glomerular basement membrane. This condition has been linked to defects on the COL4A5 gene. Point mutations in triple helical and C-propeptide domains and multiple exon deletions have been identified as the causes.

Mutations have also been identified in COL7A1 gene in individuals affected by the dominantly or recessively inherited forms of dystrophic epidermolysis bullosa. In this disease dermal-epidermal integrity is affected due to abnormal or absent anchoring fibrils, and the molecular defects are in the type VII collagen gene (Christiano et al 1996; Uitto and Christiano 1994).

The extent of involvement of periodontal structures in collagen molecular diseases ranges from slight to significant and, with the exception of dentinogenesis imperfecta, molecular defects in other diseases have not been investigated in detail.

Acquired Diseases

While inherited diseases arising due to defects in collagen structural genes are relatively rare, acquired connective tissue disorders are much more common. Indeed, most diseases in higher animals, including humans, affect the connective tissues directly and indirectly. Chronic inflammatory diseases and fibroses are two of the most common acquired diseases. These diseases, especially systemic diseases affecting connective tissues, involve the periodontium. Two examples are Crohn's disease and progressive systemic sclerosis. The acquired diseases differ from inherited diseases in several respects. In these disorders, the gene expression is affected, not the gene structure. The underlying cause in these diseases is often unknown; the diseases are caused by a variety of factors, and all matrix components, including collagens and proteoglycans, are affected (Narayanan and Page 1983). The proportions, as well as quantities, of the different collagen types undergo alterations in these diseases. For example, type V collagen is enriched in atherosclerosis and periodontal disease, and type I and III collagen content decreases in inflammation (see Chapter 9). These changes may be caused either by increased production of a particular collagen type, or by the different susceptibilities of various collagen types to degradation by collagenases. For example, type V collagen is more resistant to collagenase than is type I, while type III is less resistant (Birkedal-Hansen et al 1993; Narayanan and Page 1983).

The connective tissue alterations in acquired diseases are brought about by interactions of connective tissue cells, chiefly fibroblasts, with numerous inflammatory mediators and cytokines released by inflammatory cells or derived from blood plasma and damaged tissues. As discussed earlier in this chapter, these substances act on multiple levels of protein synthesis by affecting the rate of expression of collagen and collagenase genes, mRNA stability, and production of collagenase inhibitors. The sum total of the effects of these soluble mediators depends upon their types and concentrations present at any one instance (Narayanan and Page 1983; Slack et al 1993). These factors may affect the activities of all resident cells, or only those of a subpopulation. In acquired diseases, selective enrichment of certain subpopulations of resident cells with a particular property (eg, abnormally high levels of collagen synthesis) may be a mechanism that leads to a disease phenotype. Presence of such cells is believed to be one reason for the alterations of matrix constituents during wound repair in periodontal diseases and in scleroderma (LeRoy 1972; Narayanan and Page 1983).

Summary

Collagens are fascinating proteins not only because they are unique in structure and function, but also because of their ubiquitous distribution throughout the animal kingdom. Most diseases in higher animals involve collagen-containing connective tissues either directly or indirectly. The collagens represent a family of at least 20 closely related types that have various distribution patterns and functions in different connective tissues. They are synthesized in a complex series of biochemical events and their syntheses are highly regulated. Synthesis and turnover of collagens are prominent activities associated with wound healing when the matrix undergoes cycles of degradation and remodeling. Mechanisms that regulate collagen synthesis have a direct bearing on periodontal structures in which the connective tissues, especially collagens, undergo dramatic changes during periodontitis and drug-induced gingival hyperplasias. Periodontal regeneration is also intertwined with events associated with collagen production and degradation.

References

Armendariz-Borunda J, Katayama K, Seyer JM. Transcriptional mechanisms of type I collagen gene expression are differentially regulated by interleukin-1, tumor necrosis factor α, and transforming growth factor β in Ito cells. J Biol Chem 1992;267:14316.

Bartold PM, Narayanan AS. The biochemistry and physiology of the periodontium. In: Wilson TG, Kornman KS eds. Fundamentals of Periodontics. Chicago: Quintessence; 1996:61-107.

Birkedal-Hansen H, Moore WGI, Bodden MK, et al. Matrix metalloproteinases: A Review. Crit Rev Oral Biol Med 1993;4:197.

Bornstein P, McKay J. The first intron of the α1(I) collagen gene contains several transcriptional regulatory elements. J Biol Chem 1988;263:1603.

Bornstein P, Sage H. Regulation of collagen gene expression. Prog Nucl Acid Res Mol Biol 1989;37:67.

Burbelo PD, Martin GR, Yamada Y. α1(IV) and α2(IV) collagen genes are regulated by a bidirectional promoter and a shared enhancer. Proc Natl Acad Sci USA 1988;85:9679.

Byers PH. Disorders of Collagen Biosynthesis and Structure. In: Scriver CR, Beaudet AL, Sly WS, Valle D, eds. The Metabolic Basis of Inherited Disease. 7th ed. New York: McGraw-Hill; 1995:Chapter 134.

Christiano AM, McGrath JA, Tan KC, Uitto J. Glycine substitutions in the triple-helical region of type VII collagen result in a spectrum of dystrophic epidermolysis bullosa phenotypes and patterns of inheritance. Am J Hum Genet 1996;58:671.

Clark RAF, ed. The Molecular and Cellular Biology of Wound Healing. 2nd ed. New York: Plenum; 1996:1.

Czaja MJ, Weiner FR, Eghbali M, Giambrone M-A, Eghbali M, Zern MA. Differential effects of γ interferon on collagen and fibronectin gene expression. J Biol Chem 1987; 262:13348.

Eckes B, Aumailey M, Krieg T. Collagens and the re-establishment of dermal integrity. In: Clark RAF, ed. The Molecular and Cellular Biology of Wound Healing. New York: Plenum; 1996:493.

Enghild JJ, Salvesen G, Brew K, Nagase H. Interaction of human rheumatoid synovial collagenase (matrix metalloproteinase 1) and stromelysin 1 (matrix metalloproteinase 3) with human α2-macroglobulin and chicken ovostatin. J Biol Chem 1989;264:8779.

Eyre DR, Paz MA, Gallop PM. Cross-linking in collagen and elastin. Annu Rev Biochem 1984;53:717.

Eyre DR, Weis MA, Moskowitz RW. Cartilage expression of type II collagen mutation in an inherited form of osteoarthritis associated with a mild chondrodysplasia. J Clin Invest 1991;87:357.

Hörlein D, McPherson J, Goh SH, Bornstein P. Regulation of protein synthesis: Translational control by procollagen-derived fragments. Proc Natl Acad Sci USA 1981; 78:6163.

Howard EW, Bullen EC, Banda MJ. Preferential inhibition of 72- and 92 kDa gelatinases by tissue inhibitor of metalloproteinases-2. J Biol Chem 1991;266:13070.

Jacenko O, Olsen BR, LuValle P. Organization and regulation of collagen genes. Crit Rev Eukaryot Gene Exp 1991; 1:327.

Kagan HM, Trackman PC. Properties and function of lysyl oxidase. Am J Respir Cell Mol Biol 1991;5:205.

Karsenty G, Golumbek P, de Crombrugghe B. Point mutations and small substitution mutations in three different upstream elements inhibit the activity of the mouse alpha2(I) collagen promoter. J Biol Chem 1988;263:13909.

Kratochwil K, von der Mark K, Kollar EJ, et al. Retrovirus-induced insertional mutation in Mov13 mice affects collagen I expression in a tissue-specific manner. Cell 1989;57:807.

LeRoy EC. Connective tissue synthesis by scleroderma skin fibroblasts in cell culture. J Exp Med 1972;135:1351.

Mignatti P, Rifkin DB, Welgus HG, Parks WC. Proteinases and tissue remodeling. In: Clark RAF, ed. The Molecular and Cellular Biology of Wound Repair. 2nd ed. New York: Plenum; 1996:427.

Narayanan AS, Bartold PM. Biochemistry of periodontal connective tissues and their regeneration: A current perspective. Connect Tissue Res 1996;34:191.

Narayanan AS, Page RC. Connective tissues of the periodontium: A summary of current work. Collagen Relat Res 1983;3:33.

Narayanan AS, Siegel RC, Martin GR. Stability and purification of lysyl oxidase. Arch Biochem Biophys 1974; 162:231.

Nishimura I, Muragaki Y, Olsen BR. Tissue specific forms of type IX collagen-proteoglycan arise from the use of two widely separated promoters. J Biol Chem 1989;264:20033.

Piez KA. Primary structure. In: Ramachandran GN, Reddi AH, eds. Biochemistry of Collagen. New York: Plenum; 1976;1.

Prockop DJ, Kivirikko KI. Collagens: Molecular biology, diseases and potential for therapy. Annu Rev Biochem 1995;64:403-434.

Ramachandran GN, Ramakrishnan C. Molecular structure. In: Ramachandran GN, Reddi AH, eds. Biochemistry of Collagen. New York: Plenum; 1976:45.

Ramirez F, Di Liberto M. Complex and diversified regulatory programs control the expression of vertebrate collagen genes. FASEB J 1990;4:1616.

Roberts AB, Sporn MB. The transforming growth factor-βs. In: Sporn MB, Roberts AB, eds. Peptide Growth Factors and Their Receptors. Berlin: Springer; 1990;1:419.

Rosenbloom J, Harsch M, Jimenez S. Hydroxyproline content determines the denaturation temperature of chick tendon collagen. Arch Biochem Biophys 1973;158:478.

Rossi P, Karsenty G, Roberts AB, Roche NS, Sporn MB, de Crombrugghe, B. A nuclear factor 1 binding site mediates the transcriptional activation of type I collagen promoter by transforming growth factor-β. Cell 1988;52:405.

Sakai LY, Keene DR, Morris NP, Burgeson RE. Type VII collagen is a major structural component of anchoring fibrils. J Cell Biol 1986;103:1577.

Sandell LJ, Boyd CD. Conserved and divergent sequence and functional elements within collagen gene. In: Sandell LJ, Boyd CD. Extracellular Matrix Genes. New York: Academic Press; 1990:1.

Sato H, Takino T, Okada Y, et al. A matrix metalloproteinase expressed on the surface of invasive tumor cells. Nature 1994;370:61.

Slack JL, Liska DJ, Bornstein P. Regulation of expression of the type I collagen genes. Am J Med Genet 1993;45:140.

Sodek J, Overall CM. Matrix metalloproteinases in periodontal tissue remodeling. Matrix Suppl 1992;1:352.

Takino T, Sato H, Shinagawa A, Seiki M. Identification of the second membrane-type matrix metalloproteinase (MT-MMP-2) gene from a human placenta cDNA library. J Biol Chem 1995;270:23013.

Tiller GE, Polumbo PA, Weis MA, et al. Dominant mutations in the type II collagen gene, COL2A1, produce spondyloepimetaphyseal dysplasia, Strudwik type. Nat Genet 1995a;11:87.

Tiller GE, Weis MA, Polumbo PA, et al. An RNA-splicing mutation (G+5IVS20) in the type II collagen gene (COL2A1) in a family with spondyloepiphyseal dysplasia congenita. Am J Hum Genet 1995b;56:388.

Timpl R. Structure and biological activity of basement membrane proteins. Eur J Biochem 1989; 180:487-502.

Uitto J, Christiano AM. Molecular basis of the dystrophic forms of epidermolysis bullosa: mutations in the type VII collagen gene. Arch Dermatol Res 1994;287:16.

Uitto J, Mauviel A, McGrath J. The dermal-epidermal basement membrane zone in cutaneous wound healing. In: Clark RAF, ed. The Molecular and Cellular Biology of Wound Healing. 2nd ed. New York: Plenum: 1996:513.

van der Rest M, Garrone R. Collagen family of proteins. FASEB J 1991;5:2814.

Vuorio E, de Crombrugghe B. The family of collagen genes. Annu Rev Biochem 1990;59:837.

Wälchli C, Koller E, Trueb J, Trueb B. Structural comparison of the chicken genes for α1(VI) and α2(VI) collagen. Eur J Biochem 1992;205:583.

Woessner JF Jr. Matrix metalloproteinases and their inhibitors in connective tissue remodeling. FASEB J 1991; 5:2145.

Yang M, Hayashi K, Hayashi M, Fujii JT, Kurkinen M. Cloning and developmental expression of a membrane-type matrix metalloproteinase from chicken. J Biol Chem 1996;271:25548.

5

Noncollagenous Proteins and Receptors for Matrix Proteins

Introduction

Apart from collagens and proteoglycans, several other protein components are also present in connective tissues. These molecules not only contribute to the structural architecture of tissues, they also play important roles in regulating cellular activities and tissue function. Therefore, as their roles in the functions of the extracellular matrix are elucidated, they will undoubtedly be found to be just as important as the collagens and proteoglycans. The noncollagenous matrix proteins possess several common features. They share similar interactive components as part of their modular compositions. These modular domains are associated with cell surface binding, growth factor binding, matrix binding, and other biologic activities. In addition, these molecules often form multimeric aggregates through the formation of disulfide bonds or noncovalent interchain aggregation. Finally, within a given group of matrix macromolecules, considerable structural and functional heterogeneity may exist due to alternative splicing of their precursor mRNA.

The proportions of different noncollagenous proteins vary from tissue to tissue depending upon their functional demands. For instance, laminin and nidogen are found only in basement membrane structures, whereas osteocalcin and bone sialoprotein are restricted to the bone matrix. Most of these proteins are produced locally by connective tissue cells; however, vitronectin, which is found in the extracellular matrix, is actually a serum protein. In this chapter, the biology of several noncollagenous proteins of the extracellular matrix and their cell surface receptors found in periodontal structures is reviewed. Some of these proteins are quantitatively very minor components; nevertheless, we discuss these molecules because they are important to periodontal development, wound repair, and pathology.

Noncollagenous Proteins

Elastin

The physiologic function of many tissues in higher organisms demands elasticity. For example, elasticity is required during expansion of the heart and arteries and for their recoil during diastole, during inspiration and expiration of the lungs, and for weight bearing in the nuchal ligament of grazing animals. In vertebrates, this function is provided by the fibrous protein, elastin. This protein may constitute minimal amounts in tissues such as the periodontal ligament, moderate amounts (2%–4%) in skin, or may account for more than half of tissue protein, even exceeding collagens, in tissues such as the aorta and nuchal ligament. Changes in the content and structure of elastic tissue are seen in many diseases including atherosclerosis, emphysema, hypertension, solar dermatosis, and aging (Sandberg et al 1981).

Normal elastic tissue is composed of two distinct morphologic components, an amorphous component lacking any regular structure and constituting 90% of the protein elastin, and a variable amount of fine microfibrillar structures, 10 to 12 nm in diameter, located mostly around the periphery of the amorphous component (Fig 5-1). The microfibrils appear to encase the amorphous elastin, and they are believed to participate in elastogenesis by determining the structure of the mature elastic fiber. The precise biochemical composition of microfibrils is still unclear, but they contain many glycoproteins, including fibrillin (Cleary 1987; Rosenbloom et al 1993; Sakai et al 1986).

In its tissue form, elastin is one of the most insoluble proteins known. This feature made early characterization of elastic tissues very difficult. The amino acid composition of elastin is unique in that approximately 33% of the residues are glycine, similar to collagens. It also contains hydroxyproline, but no hydroxylysine. The nonpolar amino acids glycine, proline, alanine, valine, phenylalanine, isoleucine, and leucine make up the majority of its amino acids. The elastin molecule consists of alternating hydrophobic and lysine-rich domains. The lysines usually occur in pairs, and these represent cross-link sites. There are multiple repeats of VPGVG (in bovine elastin, GVGVAP in human elastin) and PGVGVA sequences. These repeating peptide sequences are believed to form β-turn conformation that allows the elastin chain to fold back on itself. Regions near cross-link sites are rich in alanine and the common sequence motifs are AAK and AAAK (Sandberg et al 1981).

Like collagens, elastin is synthesized as a soluble precursor, however the precursor does not have long propeptide extensions. The precursor, called tropoelastin, is a 72-kd molecule that is insoluble at physiologic temperature. Therefore, it precipitates and is cross-linked in the extracellular space by lysyl oxidase, the same enzyme that cross-links collagen. The lysyl oxidase enzyme oxidizes lysines to allysines, and then allysine-lysine

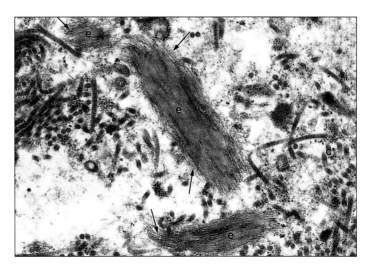

Fig 5-1 Section of nuchal ligament demonstrating the relationship between the central core of elastin, surrounded by the microfibrils. e, amorphous elastin; c, collagen. Arrows indicate microfibrils. (Courtesy of Dr JS Kumaratilake, University of Adelaide.)

pairs from two adjacent polypeptide chains condense nonenzymatically to form the cross-links shown in Fig 4-4. In addition to these cross-links, two unique cross-links, desmosine and isodesmosine, are formed, each of which is derived from four lysines (Kagan and Trackman 1991).

The elastin gene occurs as a single copy localized in chromosome 7q11,1-21.1. It consists of 36 exons; hydrophobic and cross-link domains are encoded by separate exons. As noted in collagen genes, glycine is usually found at exon-intron junctions. Exon-intron borders have split codons; thus, the first nucleotide is at the 3′ end of first exon, and the second and third nucleotides are at the 5′ end of the following exon. This structure permits alternative splicing and maintains the reading frame. Splicing of the elastin gene involves exclusion or exclusion of complete exons, while exon division occurs only occasionally. The elastin gene does not have canonical TATA boxes, but it contains CAAT and GC-rich sequences. The absence of TATA boxes indicates the presence of multiple transcription initiation sites for the elastin gene. However, many other regulatory elements are present, and these include multiple Sp1 and AP-2 binding sites, and response elements for glu-

cocorticoids (GREs), cyclic AMP (CRE), and 12-O-tetradecanoylphorbol-13-acetate (TRE). The transcription of the elastin gene is regulated by many substances. Glucocorticoids and insulinlike growth factor-I enhance the transcription, while TNF-α decreases it (Rosenbloom et al 1993, 1995). The induction and maintenance of elastogenesis is largely regulated by transcriptional mechanisms, while the cessation of tropoelastin expression is controlled by a posttranslational mechanism (Swee et al 1995).

Numerous cells, including vascular smooth muscle cells, endothelial cells, and fibroblasts are capable of synthesizing elastin. The deposition of microfibrils within the extracellular matrix adjacent to the cell surface is one of the earliest events in elastogenesis. Subsequent to the appearance of the microfibrils, amorphous elastin material is deposited within the collections of microfibrils. Further growth of the elastic fibers occurs by accrual of additional amorphous material in such a manner that the growing amorphous mass is continually surrounded by a rim of microfibrils. Thus, the microfibrils are an integral component of the elastic fiber, probably serving to help align tropoelastin molecules in a specified manner to permit cross-linking regions to be aligned prior to oxidation by lysyl oxidase (Mecham and Heuser 1992). The microfibrils contain a 31-kd glycoprotein called microfibrillar associated glycoprotein, and a 350-kd glycoprotein called fibrillin (Gibson et al 1991; Rosenbloom et al 1993; Sakai et al 1986). In addition to these glycoproteins, lysyl oxidase, amine oxidase, and several other less-characterized glycoproteins contribute to the structure of the elastin fiber (Gibson et al 1989).

Although the principal function of the elastic fiber is to impart elasticity to tissues that have a requirement for distensibility, elastin and its peptides have chemotactic activity toward monocytes and fibroblasts, and these cells may have cell surface receptors for these molecules (Senior et al 1980). In addition, several pathogenic bacteria can bind to a portion of the amino terminus of the elastin molecule (Park et al 1991), and this might be of significance in the establishment of infections in elastin-rich tissues such as lung, skin, and blood vessels.

Fibronectin

Fibronectin is one of the most studied extracellular matrix glycoproteins to date. In general, two major forms of fibronectin exist: a soluble dimeric form found in plasma (pFN), and a dimeric or multimeric cross-linked form deposited as fibrils in the extracellular matrix of most tissues (cellular fibronectin, cFN). While pFN is considered to be synthesized principally by hepatocytes, cFN is produced by many different cell types including epithelial cells, fibroblasts, and most other cells of mesenchymal tissues. Wounds contain fibronectin of which the major source is macrophages.

The fibronectin gene is highly conserved among species; it is transcribed from a single promoter into a single primary transcript. There appears to be only one copy of the gene in humans, and it is approximately 50-kb

long. It contains about 50 exons coding for the type I, II, and III repeat sequences and produces an 8-kb mRNA (Schwarzbauer 1990). Many different forms of fibronectin have been identified; these vary in their biologic properties. Much of this variability is due to alternative mRNA splicing, which can occur at three sites along the fibronectin transcript. In humans, the alternative splicing of the fibronectin exons leads to the formation of at least 20 different variants of the molecule (Kornblihtt et al 1996). It has been suggested that variations in splicing may correlate both spatially and temporally with periods of morphogenesis, cell migration, cell attachment, and wound repair, and possibly with fibronectin fibril formation (Kornblihtt et al 1996).

Both the plasma and cellular forms of fibronectin exist as disulfide-bonded dimers composed of similar polypeptide chains of approximately 250 kd. The molecule is made up of multiple repeats of three types of structural modules, called types I, II, and III repeats (Fig 5-2). These have been identified by selective proteolytic fragmentation and recombinant DNA analyses. These repeats are arranged in globular domains and are associated with diverse biologic functions (Mosher 1989; Schwarzbauer 1990). The type I repeats are located at the C- and N- termini of the molecule, and these contain domains that bind to fibrin, fibrin and heparin, and collagens. The type II repeats are located adjacent to the type I repeats at the N-terminus of the molecule, and contain the collagen/gelatin binding domain. The bulk of the fibronectin molecule is made up of between 15 to 17 type III repeats that contain the binding sites for cells, heparin, and DNA, but not for collagens. The plasma form of fibronectin appears to be lacking two repeat sequences, called ED-A and ED-B, within the type III repeat domain. These extra domains may also be differentially expressed by a variety of cell types. An additional domain, called IIICS, can be included within the type III repeat domain. The IIICS sequence is expressed in fibronectins from dif-

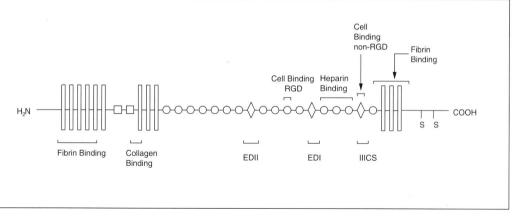

Fig 5-2 Schematic representation of fibronectin showing various domains. IIICS, connecting segment; EDI and EDII, extra domains I and II found in cellular fibronectin but not plasma fibronectin.

erent sources, and alternative splicing of this domain can produce five different sequence patterns.

The fibronectin molecule can be glycosylated, phosphorylated, and sulfated. The unglycosylated molecule has cell adhesion activity; it is, however, more sensitive to proteolysis. Glycosylation also reduces fibronectin's binding avidity to collagen.

Within the extracellular matrix, fibronectin acts as a bridge between cells and the collagen matrix by its ability to act as a substratum for cell adhesion. The interaction between cells and fibronectin appears to facilitate not only cell adhesion, but also cellular spreading and migration. The protein also provides migratory pathways for embryonic cells, it promotes monocyte chemotaxis, and it regulates cell growth and gene expression. Thus, fibronectin plays a significant role in growth and development, wound repair, and oncogenic transformation (Hynes and Yamada 1982). Fibronectin has at least six sites capable of mediating cell adhesion; these are located at the central cell binding domain, the alternatively spliced IIICS region, and the heparin binding domain (Pierschbacher and Ruoslahti 1984; McCarthy et al 1990). Interest-

ingly, these are not generic binding sites and they can be rather cell-specific. For example, the alternatively spliced adhesion sites of the IIICS region mediate binding of cells such as lymphocytes and neural crest cells, but not fibroblasts (Mould et al 1991). The cell binding sequence, RGDS, is localized at the cell binding type III repeat domain in which RGD are the most essential residues. A second synergy sequence, PHSRN, located at the previous type III repeat also participates in cell binding, and this sequence appears to be necessary for affinity to the $\alpha_5\beta_1$ integrin receptor. The RGD sequence is important for several biologic functions, and synthetic RGD peptide inhibits gastrulation and migration of neural crest cells.

Proteolytic fragments of fibronectin are present in wounds; these are chemotactic to monocytes, while intact fibronectin has very little activity. Wounded tissues also have molecules with alternatively spliced IIICS sequences; these promote the adhesion of lymphocytes and embryonic cells better than do fibroblasts. Fibronectin may also play other roles in the wound. It can interact with fibrin in clots and thicken fibrin fibers, probably by cross-linking through transglutaminase. It also serves as an opsonin, and mediates clearance of fibrin from inflamed sites. It also contains heparin binding domains and collagen binding sequences; however, it binds strongly to gelatin, but not efficiently to collagen (Yamada and Clark 1996). It can also serve as a reservoir for cytokines and growth factors such as TGF-β and TNF-α.

Interaction of fibronectin with specific integrin receptors induces transmembrane signaling events that initiate the clustering of receptors, cytoskeletal rearrangement, and other signaling events (Juliano and Haskill 1993). Fibronectin also has specific domains to bind to a number of matrix components, including heparin and fibrin (Yamada 1992). As a consequence, fibronectin is considered to play a significant role in matrix assembly and stabilization.

Laminins

Many cells are attached to, or are surrounded by, a basement membrane structure that forms stable sheets that interact with cell surface receptors. Through this interaction, the basement membrane regulates the cytoskeletal organization of cells. Therefore cell shape, gene expression, migration, differentiation, and apoptosis can all be affected by basement membranes. In addition, the basement membrane may bind growth factors and modulate their availability to cells (Timpl 1996; Dziadek 1995). Basement membranes are composed of type IV collagen, laminin, nidogen, and other proteins including fibulin, and perlecan (a heparan sulfate proteoglycan, see Chapter 6). Of these components, laminins are the major noncollagenous protein component of the basement membrane.

The laminins are a group of structurally related glycoprotein heterotrimers. These large multidomain glycoproteins are composed of three genetically distinct polypeptide chains. The first laminin to be characterized (laminin-1) was isolated from the Engelbreth-

Holm-Swarm (EHS) tumor (Timpl et al 1979). Subsequently, laminin-1 has been found to be distributed in most mammalian basement membranes. This molecule is composed of an α1 (400 kd), a β1 (215 kd), and a γ1 (215 kd) chain. These chains aggregate at the C-terminal globular end with a coiled coil α helix to form a cruciform structure stabilized by disulfide linkages (Fig 5-3). All three chains are composed of at least 6 common domain structures. Domains I and II are comprised of α helices containing haptad repeats, III and V have characteristic cysteine-rich repeat segments, and IV and VI have globular domains. In addition to these domains, the β1 chain has a short cysteine-rich domain located between domains I and II, while the α1 chain has an additional globular domain at its carboxy terminus (Engel et al 1981; Beck et al 1993). Since the first isolation of laminin-1, more than ten different isoforms have been identified on the basis of their three constituent chains (Table 5-1) (Dziadek 1995). Unlike fibronectin variants, which result from alternative splicing, laminin variants appear to be the result of the assembly of a number of closely related gene products to form a single heterogeneous family of molecules. These isoforms appear to have selective distributions throughout various tissues, and may have a number of varied functions.

Laminin is a highly interactive molecule that contributes to the network structure of basement membrane through its interactions with type IV collagen, nidogen (entactin), perlecan, and other matrix molecules (Yurchenco and Schittny 1990; Tryggvason 1993). Most of these interactions are mediated through specific sequence domains within the laminin structure. The interaction between nidogen and laminin is very strong, and is mediated through epidermal growth factor–like (EGF-like) repeats in domain III of the γ1 chain. Since laminin does not bind directly with type IV collagen, or to the protein core of perlecan but nidogen does, the nidogen-laminin complex provides an important link for complex

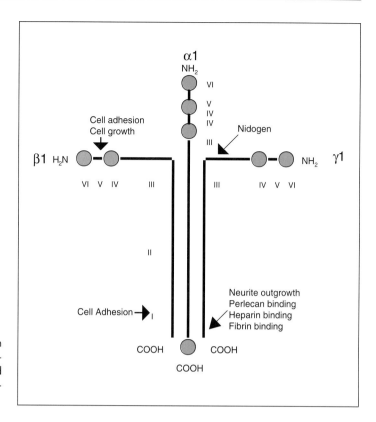

Fig 5-3 Schematic representation of laminin. Various domains are indicated by roman numerals and functional sites are marked according to their recognized function.

Table 5-1. Composition and Distribution of Various Laminins*

Laminin Isoform	Chain Composition	Tissue Distribution
Laminin-1 (EHS laminin)	$\alpha1\beta1\gamma1$	Most, but not all tissues
Laminin-2 (merosin)	$\alpha2\beta1\gamma1$	Heart, placenta, Schwann cells, muscle
Laminin-3 (s-laminin)	$\alpha1\beta2\gamma1$	Neuromuscular synapses, kidney
Laminin-4 (s-merosin)	$\alpha2\beta2\gamma1$	Myotendinous junction, trophoblast
Laminin-5 (kalinen/nicein)	$\alpha3\beta3\gamma2$	Epidermal anchoring filaments
Laminin-6 (K-laminin)	$\alpha3\beta1\gamma1$	Epidermal anchoring filaments
Laminin-7 (K-laminin)	$\alpha3\beta2\gamma1$	Epidermal-dermal junction

* Adapted from Dziadek, 1995.

formation between laminin and type IV collagen, and between laminin and perlecan (Aumailley et al 1989; Battaglia et al 1992). Interactions between laminin and heparin, heparan sulfate, and fibulin-1 have been located at the globular domain near the carboxy terminus of the long arm ($\alpha1$ chain) of laminin-1 (Kluge et al 1990; Battaglia et al 1992).

In addition to interactions with components of the extracellular matrix, laminin is an important regulatory molecule for the attachment, proliferation, and migration of numerous cell types including epithelial cells, endothelial cells, and neurites (Beck et al 1990). Adhesive interactions between laminins and cell surfaces are mediated through several integrins. At least six different integrins bind to the laminins, among which $\alpha_6\beta_1$ is specific to laminins; it recognizes laminin-1, -2, -4, and -5 (Dziadek 1995). Two cell adhesion sites have been identified within the laminin complex. One cell adhesion site has been located near the junction of the globular domain and the rigid coiled coil of the carboxy terminus globular domain of the long arm ($\alpha 1$ chain) of laminin. Another binding domain, containing RGD and other active peptide sites, which has been located near the center of the laminin cross, may include portions of all three chains (Aumailley et al 1990; Graf et al 1987; Skubitz et al 1990). In addition to proteins, various carbohydrate components of the laminins can also interact with cell surface receptors (Tanzer et al 1993). It has been proposed that matrix-cell signaling may operate via various signal transduction pathways according to the type of laminin isoform present and the type of integrin being expressed (Dziadek 1995).

Another important feature of the laminins is the presence of a number of EGF-like repeats (Panayotou et al 1989). The biologic significance of these repeats is still unclear. However, since proteolytic fragments of laminin containing the EGF-like repeat can stimulate cells containing EGF receptors, it is possible that laminin may act as a reservoir of EGF activity that could be released in vivo during tissue damage (for example, during inflammation) and promote cell growth (Yamada 1992).

The most extensively studied laminin is laminin-1. One of the most recently described species is laminin-5, which appears to be involved in the attachment of keratinocytes to basement membranes through anchoring filaments (see Chapter 4). It binds to $\alpha_3\beta_1$ and $\alpha_6\beta_4$ integrins, and it interacts with hemidesmosomes (Uitto et al 1996).

Nidogen

Nidogen (entactin) is a 150-kd sulfated glycoprotein originally isolated from parietal endoderm cells in vitro (Carlin et al 1981); it was subsequently found to be identical to a protein found in most basement membranes (Paulsson et al 1986). To date, no isoforms or alternatively spliced variants of nidogen have been reported. Nidogen, which is O-sulfated on at least one tyrosine residue, also contains two N-linked and seven O-linked oligosaccharides (Fujiwara et al 1993).

Nidogen forms a stable noncovalent complex with laminin (Paulsson et al 1987). Indeed, following extraction of laminin from basement membranes, it is usual to find nidogen present in highly stable 1:1 aggregates with laminin. This high-affinity complex hindered early attempts to determine the structure of nidogen, since any attempts to separate it from laminin resulted in irreversible structural changes (Paulsson et al 1986). However, with the development of molecular cloning techniques, recombinant forms of nidogen were produced and found to consist of three globular domains of variable mass (31–35 kd) interconnected by a stiff-rod and a flexible-link segment (Fig 5-4) (Fox et al 1991). Disulfide bonds within globules 2 and 3 help stabilize their structure and contribute to their binding properties. The rod portion of the molecule contains five EGF-like repeat sequences of which two have high-affinity calcium binding sequences. The N-terminal G1 domain also contains some calcium binding sites, while zinc binding sites have been noted in the G2 and G3 domains. There appears to be a complex modulation of nidogen binding to other basement membrane proteins by some, but not all, transition metals (Reinhardt et al 1993).

Nidogen interacts with both cell surface proteins and extracellular matrix proteins. Limited cell binding properties have been noted for this protein. Whether this is mediated through an RGD sequence in one of th

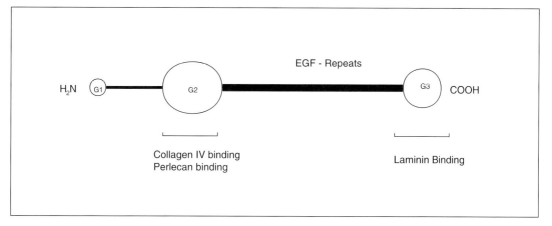

Fig 5-4 Schematic representation of nidogen.

EGF-like domains or elsewhere in the molecule is unclear (Dziadek 1995). Through multiple interactions with other basement membrane components, nidogen appears to play a crucial role in basement membrane organization and stabilization (Aumailley et al 1993). In particular, the G3 domain contains the principal laminin binding site (Fox et al 1991). The G2 domain has two distinct sites that can bind both the protein core of perlecan and type IV collagen (Reinhardt et al 1993). In addition, the laminin binding G3 domain contains lower affinity binding sites for perlecan and type IV collagen which may compete for laminin binding (Reinhardt et al 1993). Through these multiple interactions, nidogen is thought to not only contribute to the supramolecular organization of the basement membrane matrix, but also to participate in the presentation of the binding domains of other matrix glycoproteins to cell surface receptors, and thereby mediate matrix-cell communication.

Tenascin

Tenascin was simultaneously identified from a variety of tissues, and thus has had numerous names ascribed to it, including glioma mesenchymal extracellular matrix (GMEM) protein, myotendinous antigen, hexabrachion, cytotactin, and J1. In general, however, tenascin is considered to be a large oligomeric glycoprotein located principally in developing embryonic tissues (Erickson and Bourdon 1989).

Early nomenclature referred to tenascin as a hexabrachion due to the presence (rotary shadowing electron microscopy) of six spindly arms. These six arms correspond to the six-subunit oligomers of tenascin that are joined through disulfide bonds to form the characteristic star-shaped complex of approximately 1900 kd (Fig 5-5). Each arm of this molecule is 86-nm long and able to span a distance of 150 nm. The hexabrachion is characterized by a number of striking features (see Fig 5-5): (1) a terminal knob on each arm, (2) a thick distal segment, (3) a thin proximal segment, (4) a T-junction where three arms join to form a trimer, and (5) a central knob where two trimers join to form the hexamer (Erickson and Bourdon 1989). Each subunit has a molecular mass of between 190 and 230 kd and is characterized by several domains (Jones et al 1988; Pearson et al 1988; Spring et al 1989). At the amino terminus, there is a cysteine-rich domain that permits disulfide bonding between aggregating chains. Adjacent to the amino terminus is a domain containing 13

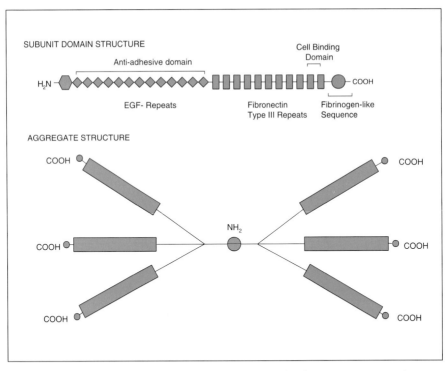

Fig 5-5 Schematic representation of tenascin, showing the domain structure and aggregate form of the molecule.

EGF-like repeats, followed by 8 to 16 fibronectin type III repeats. A globular domain is located at the carboxy terminus, similar to fibrinogen, containing a calcium binding region. The different number of fibronectin type III repeats, located between repeats 6 to 12 inclusive, are the result of alternative splicing of the mRNA and the expression of alternatively spliced variants may be under the control of TGF-β (Zhao and Young 1995). Each of the tenascin subunits appears to be moderately glycosylated.

At least two sites are available for interactions between tenascin and cells, however, these interactions are rather weak and may not represent a major function of tenascin. Cell binding sites have been located in the third fibronectin type III repeat, which acts as the binding site for the $\alpha_9\beta_1$ integrin (Yokasaki et al 1994), and in the 10th and 11th fi-

bronectin type III repeats near the carboxyl terminus (Spring et al 1989). An RGD sequence has also been located in the third fibronectin type III repeat (Schnapp et al 1995). In addition to promoting cell attachment, tenascin can also inhibit cell attachment to both fibronectin and laminin (Chiquet-Ehrismann et al 1988; Spring et al 1989). This antiadhesive property has been mapped to the EGF-like repeat domain next to the amino terminus. It has been proposed that the existence of two contrary functions within the one molecule might be responsible for the versatile features of tenascin (Spring et al 1989).

Because of the large number of fibronectin type III repeats in tenascin, there would appear to be considerable potential for this molecule to interact with other extracellular matrix components. However, to date, the only molecule found to have a definite interactive capacity with tenascin is a chondroitin sulfate proteoglycan. Tentative identification of this proteoglycan suggests that it may be versican (Perides et al 1993) or the large chondroitin sulfate proteoglycans (possibly neurocan or brevican) found in brain tissue. Although an association between tenascin and fibronectin that inhibits cell attachment and migration on fibronectin has been demonstrated, the association is very weak and readily reversible (Lightner and Erickson 1990). No significant binding between tenascin and various collagens, fibronectin, or laminin has been noted using solid-phase ELISA assays (Lightner and Erickson 1990).

The distribution of tenascin is widespread in embryonic development. In particular, tenascin is found within mesenchymal condensations at sites of epithelial-mesenchymal interaction and is intimately associated with morphogenesis (Erickson and Bourdon 1989). The expression of this molecule is very restricted in adult tissues, but it may be expressed during wound healing and tumorigenesis (Yamada et al 1996). It appears maximally in the wound during the formation of granulation tissue (Haapasalmi et al 1995). A very strong relationship between tenascin expression and epithelial-mesenchymal interactions has been noted during tooth morphogenesis (Chapter 7). The production of tenascin has been shown to be induced by serum, TGF-β, interleukins, and TNF-α (Sakai et al 1994). This may be important in tumorigenesis as well as in the appearance of tenascin during wound healing, where it may possibly facilitate the migration of epithelial cells. Tenascin does not appear to be present in scar tissue.

Thrombospondins

The thrombospondins are a family of glycoproteins produced by platelets and many other cells; they are distributed throughout the extracellular matrix. These proteins participate in platelet aggregation and affect the attachment, spreading, migration, and proliferation of many other cells, especially polymorphonuclear leukocytes and macrophages (Mosher 1990; Lawler et al 1993a).

To date, four genes have been identified that encode for members of the thrombospondin family, called thrombospondins 1, 2, 3, and 4. While the thrombospondins show significant structural homology, there are sufficient subtle differences to indicate that they have different structures and functions. All the thrombospondins share a similar domain structure (Fig 5-6). At the amino terminus, there is a globular domain that binds avidly to heparin and also acts as a cell attachment region. A central linear portion of the molecule contains several type II (EGF-like) repeats. At the carboxy terminus, there is another domain that contains up to seven type III (Ca^{++} binding) repeats that contain the RGD cell attachment sequence. In addition to these domains, other portions of the molecule share homology with procollagen, fibronectin, and von Willebrand's factor. These molecules aggregate to form a trimeric glycoprotein complex linked together by interchain disulfide bonding (see Fig 5-6).

Thrombospondin 1 and thrombospondin 2 have very similar structures, and analysis of their gene structures indicates their close evolutionary relationship and that they perform overlapping but distinct functions (Shingu and Bornstein 1994). Thrombospondin 3 has similar structural features to thrombospondins 1 and 2, but has several important differences. For example, it has four, rather than three, type II repeats, it lacks both the type I repeat sequence and the sequence containing homology with procollagen, and it has a different structure in the amino terminal domain. Thrombospondin 4 also differs significantly from thrombospondins 1 and 2 and appears to be more homologous with thrombospondin 3 (Bornstein et al 1993; Lawler et al 1993b). Thrombospondin 1, but not

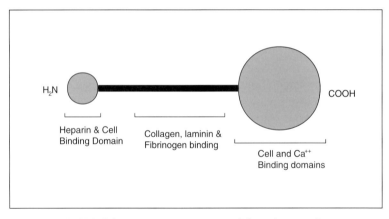

Fig 5-6 Schematic representation of thrombospondin.

thrombospondins 2 or 3, is expressed in the neural tube, head mesenchyme, and mega-karyocytes, while thrombospondin 2 is found mostly in connective tissues and myoblasts. Thrombospondin 3 is restricted to the brain, cartilage, and lung, while thrombospondin 4 is found in heart and skeletal muscle.

The synthesis of thrombospondin is stimulated by platelet-derived growth factor (PDGF), TGF-β, heparin, and heat shock. It appears at the wound edges in 12 hours and its concentration peaks in 2 to 3 days. At the site of inflammation it can bind to fibronectin, proteases, plasmin, neutrophil elastase, urokinase-type plasminogen activator (uPa), and bacteria. It also modulates platelet aggregation and inhibits angiogenesis. As mentioned previously, it can mediate and modulate spreading of certain cell types such as the keratinocytes, but it has an opposite effect on endothelial cells and fibroblasts. In addition to its cell binding properties, thrombospondin interacts with several components of the extracellular matrix. Thrombospondin molecules may aggregate with heparan sulfate proteoglycans to form large (100–300 nm) spherical granules that may interact with fibronectin. In addition, various portions of the thrombospondin molecule have been found to interact with collagen types I and V, fibrinogen, and laminin (Bacon-Baguley et al 1990; Takagi et al 1993; Cockburn and Barnes 1991).

Vitronectin

Vitronectin, also known as complement S protein, serum spreading factor, and epibolin, is an acidic glycoprotein found in plasma and in extracellular matrices; it was initially discovered as a cell attachment factor that bound strongly to glass (*vitro:* glass). This is a multifunctional glycoprotein produced by the liver and present in serum. It has a molecular mass of around 75 kd and may be purified from tissues either as the intact molecule or as a smaller, proteolytically converted 65 kd molecule, linked by a disulfide bond to a 10-kd peptide fragment (Kubota et al 1988). Approximately 15% of the vitronectin molecule is glycosylated with N-linked oligosaccharides. The vitronectin gene spans approximately 3 kb of genomic DNA, and consists of 8 exons and 7 introns of variable length (Jenne and Stanley 1987). It has been located at the centromic region of the long arm of chromosome 17, at 17q11 (Seiffert et al 1993).

As with many other interactive matrix glycoproteins, vitronectin has several domains

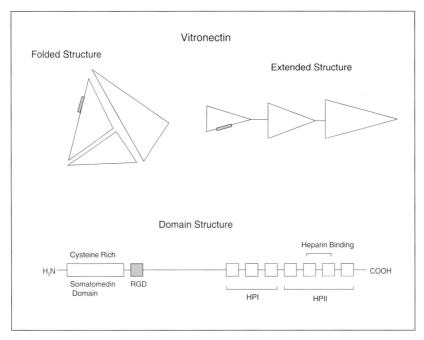

Fig 5-7 Schematic representation of vitronectin, demonstrating the folded and extended structures together with the domain structure of the molecule.

that contain a variety of peptide sequences responsible for its interactive features (Fig 5-7). At the amino terminus there is a somatomedin B sequence that is highly disulfide-linked, resistant to proteolysis, and that may act as a trypsin inhibitor. Following this domain is an RGD cell attachment sequence that is recognized by several integrins, including $\alpha_V\beta_3$, $\alpha_{IIb}\beta_3$, and $\alpha_V\beta_5$. The interaction between vitronectin and its receptors is commonly located at focal adhesion sites, where it can be localized with vinculin, talin, paxillin, and other cytoskeletal proteins. It is believed to provide an important means of cell-matrix communication (Dejana et al 1988).

The structure of vitronectin is complex; it has a hingelike conformation that enables it to unravel to expose various domains (see Fig 5-7). A connector domain links the RGD sequence to two hemopexinlike sequences. In the second hemopexinlike sequence, a heparin binding sequence is located in the second and third repeats. The heparin binding site is cryptic and is only exposed following denaturation of the protein with chaotropic agents or adsorption onto a surface (Tomasini and Mosher 1991). Adjacent to the second hemopexinlike sequence is the 10-kd peptide (containing the carboxy terminus) that can be released following proteolysis and form a disulfide-bonded aggregate with the parent 65-kd molecule.

Apart from associating with cytoskeletal proteins, vitronectin has several additional functions (Felding-Habermann and Cheresh 1993). It promotes cell adhesion and mediates cell spreading and migration. Vitronectin is found in the stroma of the wound and may participate in wound-related functions. For example, it can affect host immune function by binding to the soluble C5b-9 complex (membrane attack complex) of the complement cascade and inhibit the cytolytic action. It also binds to several serine protease inhibitors of the serpin family, including

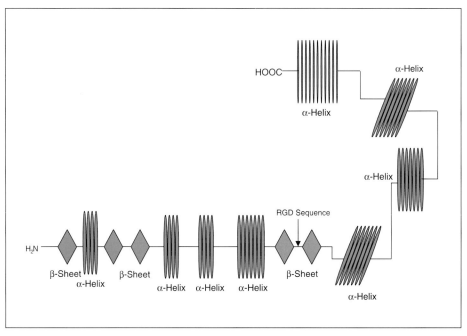

Fig 5-8 Schematic representation of the structure of osteopontin.

antithrombin III, plasminogen activator-inhibitor I (PAI-I), heparin cofactor II, and the protease nexin (Preissner 1991; Tomasini and Mosher 1991). Certain cells, especially the polymorphonuclear leukocytes, migrate on vitronectin substrates. Vitronectin may also play a role in platelet activation through its ability to control the final stages of complement activation, and as an adhesion molecule for platelets via interaction with the $\alpha_{IIb}\beta_3$.

Osteopontin

Osteopontin is a glycosylated phosphoprotein with a molecular mass of 41.5 kd and is unusual because of its high content of serine, asparagine, and glutamate (Denhardt and Guo 1993). It is present in significant amounts in bone at mineralization fronts and at cement lines where bone formation follows resorption. It is also found in the kidney in the loop of Henle and in distal convoluted tubules,

and in virtually all other tissues. It was originally called secreted phosphoprotein 1 (SPP-1), and bone sialoprotein I to distinguish it from another glycosylated bone phosphoprotein called bone sialoprotein II (now called bone sialoprotein; see p. 109).

Osteopontin has a 32-kd polypeptide backbone, and it has several characteristic structural features (Oldberg et al 1986; Prince 1989). The amino and carboxy terminal ends contain eight α helices that constitute approximately 41% of its 301 amino acids. The middle of the molecule contains a very acidic region with a typical RGD cell attachment domain flanked on both sides by two segments of β-sheet structures (Fig 5-8). Toward the amino terminus, there is a highly acidic region that contains nine consecutive aspartic acid residues. Other features of the molecule may include a calcium binding loop and two heparin binding sites. The human osteopontin gene consists of seven exons, six of which contain the coding sequence, and spans approximately 4.8 kb (Crosby et al 1995; Yamamoto et al 1995). Initial studies on the osteopontin gene structure indicated that multiple forms existed. These were presumed to arise from alternative splicing of the primary transcript, and accounted for the distinct forms of protein that had been noted (Young et al 1990). Further analysis of the osteopontin gene has indicated that there are two classes of osteopontin transcripts with different 5′ ends but identical coding regions from exon II to exon VII (Saavedra et al 1995). These transcripts do not appear to result from alternative splicing of the coding exons; therefore, it has been suggested that the differences in osteopontin protein structure are most likely a result of differences in posttranslational modification. Osteopontin binds to calcium and hydroxyapatite through aspartic acid–rich sequences located at the N-terminus (Chen et al 1992; Ritter et al 1992). It covalently binds to fibronectin catalyzed by the enzyme transglutaminase. It contains the RGDS cell attachment sequence, therefore it is recognized by several integrins that bind to this sequence. Integrin $\alpha_V\beta_3$ is the major receptor for this molecule, and this integrin is abundant in osteoclasts (Ross et al 1993; Reinholt et al 1990). However, not all of the binding capacity of osteopontin can be ascribed to the presence of the RGD sequence. Indeed, only half of the binding activity of osteopontin can be inhibited by the addition of synthetic RGD sequences in attachment assays.

Although it was once considered to be a principal component of bone, osteopontin is found in several nonmineralized tissues including kidney, arterial smooth muscle cells, and at the luminal surface of epithelial cells of ductal tissues (Denhardt and Guo 1993). It is synthesized by many cell types including osteocytes, osteoblasts, osteoclasts, smooth muscle cells, and epithelial cells. Highest levels of osteopontin expression are observed in preosteoblastic cells early in bone formation, and by mature osteoblasts at sites of bone re-

modeling. It is expressed earlier than the bone-specific glycoprotein, bone sialoprotein. In particular, osteopontin is considered to play a significant role in both mineralization and resorption of bone (Boskey 1992). Secreted osteopontin is present in concentrated amounts in areas of bone formation (Mark et al 1988), and it has been implicated in the recruitment and stimulation of macrophages and lymphocytes in response to nonspecific infections (McKee and Nanci 1996). The synthesis of osteopontin is up-regulated by osteotropic hormones such as vitamin D_3. While these observations are indicative of its role in bone formation, it is a major ligand for osteoclasts to which it is chemotactic; thus it appears to be involved in bone remodeling (Boskey 1992). In the bone it is synthesized in two molecular forms, as a 55-kd low-phosphorylated species produced by preosteoblasts that form a cement matrix, or as a 44-kd highly phosphorylated species that binds to hydroxyapatite (Sodek et al 1995). The latter form is produced by osteoblasts.

Osteopontin also appears to play a role in wound healing. It is produced and secreted in response to injury by macrophages, activated T lymphocytes, and smooth muscle cells. Substances present in the wound site, PDGF, TGF-β, and interleukin-2, as well as EGF and bone morphogenetic protein-7, up-regulate its synthesis. Osteopontin is also found in atherosclerotic plaques and it is also produced by transformed cells. It is expressed during cementogenesis.

SPARC (Osteonectin)

SPARC (secreted protein acidic and rich in cysteine) is a Ca^{++} binding glycoprotein associated with the extracellular matrix of many tissues, especially bone. It is secreted by a variety of proliferating cells in vitro and expressed

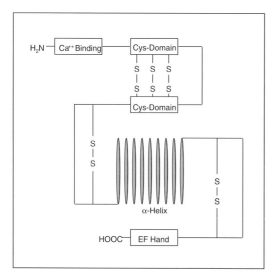

Fig 5-9 Schematic representation of the structure of SPARC (osteonectin).

bone (Bianco et al 1988), it is widely expressed in many tissues and synthesized and secreted by many cell types. It is expressed at high levels in tissues undergoing morphogenesis and during early development in nonossifying tissues. Fibroblasts, including periodontal fibroblasts, synthesize osteonectin (Wasi et al 1984). It may play an important role in wound healing; for example, this protein is synthesized by macrophages at sites of wound repair, and it is also released by platelet degranulation.

SPARC does not support cell attachment, and, like thrombospondin and tenascin, it is antiadhesive and an inhibitor of cell spreading. It disrupts focal adhesion in fibroblasts. It also regulates the proliferation of some cells, especially the endothelial cells, and it may mediate this effect through its ability to bind to cytokines and growth factors (Young et al 1992). Osteonectin has also been found to decrease DNA synthesis in cultured bone cells (Lane and Sage 1994). The biosynthesis of extracellular matrix components, especially the matrix metalloproteinases and PAI-I, appear to be influenced by the SPARC. The expression of osteonectin can be regulated by many growth factors, cytokines, and environmental stimuli including TGF-β, calcitriol, retinoic acid, cyclic AMP, and culture shock conditions (Young et al 1992).

in high levels in tissues undergoing morphogenesis, remodeling, and repair. SPARC is a 32-kd protein also known as osteonectin, endothelial "culture shock" glycoprotein, and a basement membrane protein known as BM-40 (Bolander et al 1988; Swaroop et al 1988). The human SPARC gene is 26.5-kb long and contains 10 exons and 9 introns, of which 9 exons, separated by 8 introns, code for the mature protein. The primary transcript of this gene codes for 284 to 287 amino acids of mature protein together with a 17-residue amino terminal hydrophobic signal peptide. Several domains within the molecule have been identified (Fig 5-9), including Ca^{++} binding domains near the glutamic acid–rich amino terminus (domain I), a cysteine-rich domain II, an α helical domain III and an EF-hand domain in the C-terminal region (domain IV) (Villarreal et al 1989).

SPARC is a highly conserved, 40- to 44-kd molecule that can bind to several cations, collagens, hydroxyapatite, albumin, and thrombospondin (Lane and Sage 1994; Young et al 1990), and it may be phosphorylated. Although it is found as an abundant protein in

Osteocalcin

Osteocalcin (also known as bone Gla protein) is a member of a family of extracellular mineral binding proteins present in the bone (Hauschka et al 1989; Neugebauer et al 1995). It is generally found in the bone matrix and specifically localizes to developing bone (Bronkers et al 1987). It is a small protein, with a molecular mass of approximately 6 kd, containing 49 amino acids. The amino acid sequence is remarkably well conserved throughout most species, and minor differences in amino acid composition most likely result from point mutations in the genomic DNA (Shimomura et al 1984). A notable feature of osteocalcin is the presence of three γ-carboxyglutamic acid residues, which are associated with potent calcium binding properties (Shimomura et al 1984; Hauschka et al 1989). The γ-carboxyglutamic acid residues interact with the mineral phase of bone and lead to its incorporation into the bone matrix (Atkinson et al 1995). Structural studies indicate that osteocalcin has two antiparallel α helices that are connected by a β turn and stabilized by a disulfide bond (Fig 5-10). In solution, the molecule does not seem to adopt a single conformation, but rather has a flexible structure that is believed to be essential for the function of the protein (Atkinson et al 1995). The osteocalcin gene is a 953-nucleotide sequence consisting of four exons and three introns and may be localized on chromosome 3 (Lian et al 1989; Desbois et al 1994). Originally identified as a single copy gene, recent data indicate that, in mice and rats, multiple copies of the osteocalcin gene exist clustered together (Rahman et al 1993). The gene is regulated by a promoter with multiple basal and enhancer elements that are responsive to a number of physiologic mediators such as TGF-β, glucocorticoids, and vitamin D (Heinrichs et al 1993; Banerjee et al 1996). Osteocalcin is produced by osteoblasts and odontoblasts, and it is one of the most abundant proteins synthesized by these cells. Only fully differentiated cells express this protein. The protein is synthesized and secreted into the bone matrix at the time of mineralization. One of the three isoforms of osteocalcin is expressed in kidneys, where it is believed to be involved in Ca^{++} removal. The synthesis of osteocalcin is up-regulated by vitamin D through a vitamin D responsive element, VDRE. The γ-carboxylation by the carboxylase requires vitamin K, and the carboxylation is inhibited by warfarin.

The precise biologic function of the osteocalcin is unclear. Its properties, developmental expression, and the serum level reflecting new

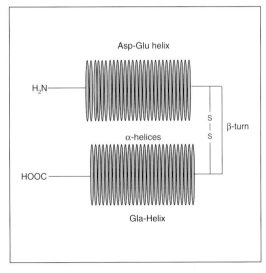

Fig 5-10 Schematic representation of the structure of osteocalcin.

bone synthesis indicate a role in bone formation (Boskey 1992). The serum osteocalcin level correlates with histomorphometric analysis of new bone. However, osteocalcin binds to osteopontin that interacts with osteoclasts; therefore, it may be involved in recruiting osteoclasts to sites of newly formed bone and thus may function as a negative regulator (Desbois and Karsenty 1995).

Bone Sialoprotein

Bone sialoprotein (originally called bone sialoprotein II to distinguish it from bone sialoprotein I, now known as osteopontin) is a highly glycosylated and acidic phosphoprotein with a high sialic acid content (Fisher et al 1983). It is a major structural protein of the bone matrix, and it is, like the osteocalcin, specifically expressed by fully differentiated osteoblasts (Shapiro et al 1993; Young et al 1992). This glycoprotein is one of the predominant matrix proteins of hard tissues, where it accounts for some 15% of the noncollagenous proteins.

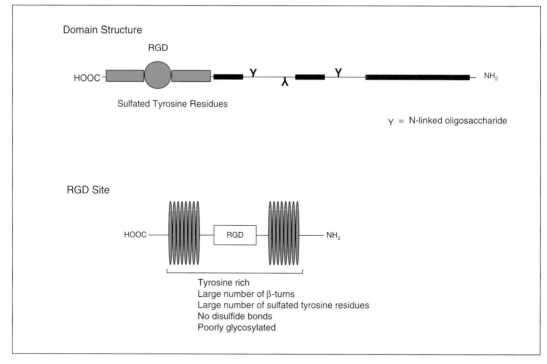

Fig 5-11 Schematic representation of bone sialoprotein, showing the domain structure, as well as the detailed structure of the RGD cell binding site.

Human bone sialoprotein is coded by a single copy 15-kb gene located on chromosome 4q28-q31 (Fisher et al 1990; Kerr et al 1993; Kim et al 1994). There appears to be considerable homology (~80%) for bone sialoprotein among various species (Chenu et al 1994; Fisher et al 1990; Shapiro et al 1993). Isolates of cDNA for human bone sialoprotein indicate it to be synthesized as a precursor protein of 317 amino acids with a molecular mass of 33 kd containing a 16–amino acid leader signal. It undergoes extensive posttranslational modification prior to secretion and up to 50% of the secreted 75-kDa product may contain carbohydrates (Fisher et al 1990; Shapiro et al 1993).

Several well-conserved domains have been noted in the bone sialoprotein (Fig 5-11). Up to three regions rich in acidic amino acids have been located toward the middle of the molecule; two of these contain poly(glutamic acid) domains that are potential sites for hydroxyapatite binding (Shapiro et al 1993). In addition, three regions rich in tyrosine residues, and a domain toward the carboxy terminus containing an RGD cell attachment sequence have been noted (Fisher et al 1990; Shapiro et al 1993). Other conserved sequences include a number of serine, threonine, and tyrosine residues that are potential sites for glycosylation and phosphorylation, as well as for tyrosine sulfation (Shapiro et al 1993).

Interestingly, bone sialoprotein appears to contain no cysteine (Fisher et al 1990). Whether multiple forms of bone sialoprotein exist is unclear, however, one report has demonstrated a close, if not identical, relationship in protein between bone sialoprotein and keratan sulfate proteoglycan in rabbit bone (Kinne and Fisher 1987). On the basis of its primary structure, predictions for the secondary structure for bone sialoprotein have been made, and these appear to include an open flexible structure with the potential to form significant numbers of α helices and some β sheets (Shapiro et al 1993).

Based on its structural features, bone sialoprotein has been implicated in several functions. Due to the presence of an RGD sequence, bone sialoprotein is thought to play an important role in osteoblast attachment to mineralized tissues. Cell attachment to bone sialoprotein appears to be mediated through the vitronectin receptor (Oldberg et al 1988). Numerous sites within the molecule have the potential to bind to hydroxyapatite, thus providing an anchoring mechanism for bone cells to attach to mineralized tissues (Boskey 1992). Immunolocalization and in situ hybridization studies have shown that the distribution of bone sialoprotein is restricted to bone, while osteopontin and SPARC are present in the cartilage matrix and in soft tissues (Bianco et al 1991; Chen et al 1993). Bone sialoprotein is found in reversal lines of rapidly remodeling bone, and it is produced by osteoblasts and odontoblasts actively forming bone (Chen et al 1992, 1993). It is expressed during the early formation of dentin and alveolar bone when it accumulates in peritubular dentin and bone matrix. It is also expressed by cementoblasts during cementogenesis (Chen et al 1992). Bone sialoprotein has been found to be closely associated with differentiated osteoblasts found on the surfaces of new forming bone trabeculae. It has been implicated in nucleation of hydroxyapatite during bone formation de novo and in the initial mineralization of newly formed bone.

Recent studies on the promoter region for bone sialoprotein gene have demonstrated the presence of *cis*-acting elements that may be involved in hormonal regulation and the developmentally regulated, tissue-specific expression of this protein (Ogata et al 1995; Kim et al 1994). These include inverted a TATA box, GRE half sites, VDRE, and a putative AP-1

site (Kim et al 1996). Bone sialoprotein expression is up-regulated by dexamethasone and suppressed by vitamin D (Kim et al 1996; Ogata et al 1995; Yamauchi et al 1996).

Receptors for Matrix Proteins

The attachment of cells to their surroundings is important in determining cell shape and in maintaining proper cell function and tissue integrity. Thus, cell surface receptors that mediate cell-cell and cell-substratum interactions have been the subject of intense investigation during the past decade. The list of matrix components capable of interacting with cell surfaces is expanding rapidly. However, many of these molecules are related and, as a result of recombinant DNA technology, several groups have been identified on the basis of their structural and biochemical profiles (see Table 5-2). To date, three families of adhesion molecules are recognized: (1) the integrins, (2) the selectins, and (3) the immunoglobulin gene superfamily. All of these molecules are composed of a variety of structural domains that dictate their different functions. Through their interactions with molecules on other cells, or in the surrounding extracellular matrix, intracellular signaling mechanisms are activated that lead to functional responses by the cells. This chapter focuses only on the interaction between cell surface receptors and components of the extracellular matrix as mediated through the integrins. The selectins and CAMs have been described previously (see Chapter 3).

Integrins

The term integrin was first used to describe a variety of molecules located on cell surfaces that were thought to link the extracellular matrix with the cytoskeleton (Hynes 1987). Over time, many different types of integrins

Table 5-2. Interactions Between the α and β Subunits of Integrins

	β1	β2	β3	β4	β5	β6	β7	β8
α1	X							
α2	X							
α3	X							
α4	X						X	
α5	X							
α6	X			X				
α7	X							
α8	X							
αL		X						
αM		X						
αX		X						
αV	X		X		X	X		X
αIIb			X					
αIEL							X	

have been identified and studied. Today, the integrins constitute a large group of related heterodimeric glycoproteins composed of structurally unrelated α and β subunits that span mammalian cell membranes (Garratt and Humphries 1995).

To date, eight β chains and 16 α chains have been identified. It is likely that, in the future, the number of members of this family will increase. Since the α chains can associate with several different β chains, the number of permutations for different types of intergins is large (Table 5-2). Nonetheless, several sub-groupings of integrins have been noted on the basis of their ligand affinity and β-chain composition (Table 5-3). For example, integrins containing the β1 chain are largely involved in interactions between cell surfaces and extracellular matrix molecules such as collagens, laminin, and fibronectin. The integrins containing the β2 chain are largely involved in inflammatory cell interactions with the matrix and other cells and are often referred to as the leukocyte integrins. The integrins containing the β3 chain are mainly involved in cell surface interactions with components of the vas-

cular system such as thrombospondin, vitronectin, and fibrinogen (Hynes 1992).

Structure of Integrins

As is common with many cells surface glycoproteins, both subunits of the integrins are composed of three domains, which include a large extracellular domain, a membrane-spanning domain, and a short cytoplasmic domain (Fig 5-12).

The α subunits range in size from 1200 to 1800 amino acids and, among the 14 α subunits identified to date, share between 20% and 70% homology with each other (Hynes 1992). At the N-terminus, the α subunits contain seven repeating domains that have homology with the cation binding EF-hand motif (Tuckwell and Humphries 1993). This region accounts for the earlier observations that the α chains have several calmodulinlike Ca^{++} and Mg^{++} binding sites within their extracellular domains. This repeat domain is interrupted in some α chains (α1, α2, αL, and αX) by the insertion of an additional domain

Table 5-3. Integrin Family of Adhesion Receptors

Name	Ligand
Beta-1 integrins	
α1β1	Collagen, laminin
α2β1	Collagen, laminin
α3β1	Collagen, entactin, fibronectin, laminin
α4β1	Fibronectin
α5β1	Fibronectin
α6β1	Laminin
α7β1	Laminin
αvβ1	Fibronectin, vitronectin
Beta-2 integrins	
(leukocyte adhesion receptors)	
α2β2	
αMβ2	iC3b, fibrinogen, factor X, ICAM-1
αXβ2	iC3b, fibrinogen
αLβ2	ICAM-1, ICAM-2
Beta-3 integrins	
(Cytoadhesins)	
αvβ3	Bone sialoprotein, fibrinogen, fibronectin, thrombospondin, vitronectin, von Willebrand's factor
αIIbβ3	Fibrinogen, fibronectin, thrombospondin, vitronectin, von Willebrand's factor
Beta-4 integrins	
α6β4	Laminin
Beta-5 integrins	
αvβ5	Fibronectin
Beta-6 integrins	
αVβ6	Fibronectin
Beta-7 integrins	
α4β7	Fibronectin

(I-domain) between the second and third EF-hand–containing repeats. Although the structure of the I-domain is unclear, it shares homology with complement factor B, type VI collagen, and the A-domain of von Willebrand's factor (Larson et al 1989). In the region between the EF-hand repeat domains and the short transmembrane domain, most α chains show little conservation. However the α3, α5, α6, α7, α8, αIIb, αV, and aIEL chains may undergo posttranslational proteolytic cleavage at a conserved site. The resultant two chains remain covalently bound through a disulfide bond (Hynes 1992). The intracellular domain of the α subunits is relatively small, spanning some 30 amino acids.

In general, the β subunits, composed of approximately 800 amino acids, are smaller than the α subunits (Tuckwell and Humphries 1993). An exception to this is the β4 chain, which has an extended cytoplasmic domain at its carboxy terminus (Hogervorst et al 1990).

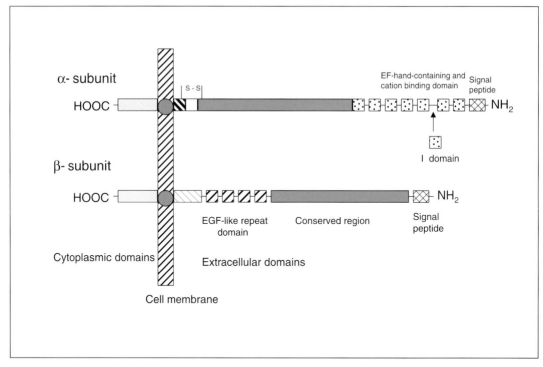

Fig 5-12 Schematic representation of the integrin α- and β-subunits, demonstrating the cytoplasmic and extracellular domains.

The amino terminus for most β subunits appears to be a well-conserved region of approximately 200 residues. A single cation binding site with features similar to the EF-hand domain may be present in this region (Loftus et al 1990). Closer to the transmembrane domain, the extracellular domain contains a cysteine-rich region that is composed of four EGF-like domains. The intracellular domain is relatively short (except for β4) and can be quite variable due to alternative splicing and posttranslational proteolytic cleavage (Giancotti et al 1992).

In order for effective ligand-binding to occur, the α and β chains must associate with each other through noncovalent interactions mediated via divalent cations and the extracellular domains. The intracellular domains appear to have little role in the heterodimer formation (Tuckwell and Humphries 1993).

Integrin-Ligand Binding

In recent years the relationship between integrin structure, ligand binding, and cytoplasmic signaling has become well established (Garratt and Humphries 1995). Ligand binding appears to be dependent upon the presence of bound cations, usually calcium or magnesium (Gailet and Ruoslahti 1988; Kishimoto et al 1989). Interestingly, some binding processes appear to be specific for particular cations. For example, only magnesium can support an integrin-ligand binding reaction between β1αV and fibronectin, and also between β1α2 and collagen, yet both magnesium and calcium may be involved in the interaction between β3αV and vitronectin (Kirchhofer et al 1991). Apart from the need for the presence of divalent cations, integrin-ligand binding requires other specific portions of both the α and β subunits. Given the highly conserved nature of the amino terminus of the extracellular domains of the α and β subunits, it seems likely that sequences within these regions are involved in the binding process (Tuckwell and Humphries 1993). In particular, the EF-hand domains and the I-domain have been implicated in ligand binding. The role of the intracellular portion of integrins in ligand binding is unclear. However, it has been reported that the cytoplasmic portion of the β1 integrins is necessary for functional ligand binding (Hayashi et al 1990).

Of particular interest to the interaction of integrins with their ligands has been the identification of a common amino acid sequence among the ligands. Within the sequence of many of these proteins is a tripeptide sequence of Arg-Gly-Asp (RGD) that appears to be responsible for many cell attachment interactions (Humphries 1990). This RGD sequence appears unique in that other peptides do not permit attachment. Indeed, if the RGD sequence is changed by even one amino acid, the promotion of attachment is eliminated (Pierschbacher and Ruoslahti 1987). Despite this uniformity in amino acid sequence within the attachment region of the various adhesive proteins, cells can recognize the proteins individually through a variety of integrins, each of which is capable of recognizing only a single RGD-containing protein ligand (Pierschbacher and Ruoslahti 1987). Nonetheless, the relationship between ligand and integrin is often nonspecific in that one integrin has the ability to bind several different molecules. For example, the β1α1 integrin can bind several collagens in addition to laminin. Similarly, a single ligand may bind to numerous integrins, as seen for laminin, which can bind to the β1α1, β1α2, β1α3, and β1α6 integrins.

While the presence of RGD sequences is necessary for many cell-matrix interactions, not all molecules that contain RGD sequences act as adhesion molecules. Indeed, data banks indicate that many hundreds of molecules contain such sequences, yet do not play a role in cell adhesion. Of those molecules that do contain RGD sequences and are involved in cell adhesion, those involved in platelet aggregation (fibrinogen, von Willebrand's factor, fibronectin, vitronectin, and thrombospondin) and fibroblast attachment (collagen, fibronectin, and laminin) have been well studied (Pierschbacher and Ruoslahti 1987). Other RGD-containing molecules have been identified in extracts of bone, including osteopontin and bone sialoprotein, which may function in regulating osteoblast adhesion.

Integrin-mediated cell adhesion may occur through three different modes, including direct interaction with components of the extracellular matrix to mediate cell-matrix interactions, binding to components of cell membrane proteins to effect cell-cell interactions, or with soluble adhesion proteins as required for platelet aggregation. These different mechanisms reflect the different needs and functions of cells. For example, adherent cells (eg, fibroblasts) that rely on cell matrix interactions for their normal function express integrins that are constitutively activated. However, cells that require a variable ability to interact with matrix components or other cells (eg, leukocytes and platelets) express a range of integrins that require some form of activation prior to their ability to undergo adhesive interactions.

Functions of Integrins

These integral cell surface components are implicated in white blood cell diapedesis, leukocyte migration, T cell–macrophage interactions, clot formation, epithelial cell migration, fibroblast migration, and fibroblast adhesion. Many of the integrins are expressed in high proportions during wound healing and tumorigenesis (Abelda 1993; Larjava et al 1996). Indeed, the role of integrins in matrix deposition and maturation is recognized as crucial. An initial step in matrix repair is the binding of fibroblasts to fibronectin through the $\beta 1\alpha 5$ integrin. Whether the binding to fibronectin leads to the deposition of insoluble fibronectin followed by further assembly of extracellular matrix components is not yet clear.

The integrins also provide a valuable link between the extracellular matrix and the cytoskeleton (Schwartz 1992; Giancotti and Mainiero 1994). The mechanisms by which receptors transmit external messages to intracellular effector pathways are complex. Given their strategic location and near-ubiquitous distribution, it is not surprising that the integrins have been strongly implicated in signal transduction. One common response to ligand binding is phosphorylation of intracellular proteins. This is a process in which integrins have been significantly implicated. Another mechanism of signal transduction through integrins may include small changes in intracellular pH following ligand binding.

Thus, the integrins provide an important link between the matrix and the cytoskeleton and intracellular messenger systems, and are clearly implicated in the intricate feedback loops of matrix and gene expression.

Summary

The noncollagenous proteins of extracellular matrices form a diverse and important group of molecules. Advances in molecular biologic techniques have lead to detailed studies concerning their structure, function, and genetic regulation. With future developments, more detailed understanding of the roles that these components play in pathology will be forthcoming. In addition, through specific genetic "knockout" experiments and recombinations, it will be possible to control expression of these components in whole animals. These exciting developments will have considerable ramifications with respect to management of specific diseases, as well as directing regeneration of tissues damaged as a result of pathology or injury.

The adhesive interactions between cells and the surrounding matrix mediate the attachment and migration of cells, as well as induce a range of intracellular signaling mechanisms that enable the cells to communicate with their environment and respond to any changes. With recent advances in molecular biologic techniques, there have been significant advances in our understanding of the structure and function of the molecules involved in these interactions. Cell-matrix interactions are central to normal development, inflammation, wound healing, and tissue repair. As such, a more detailed understanding of the molecules involved in cell-matrix interactions is needed to enable an effective means of manipulating tissue responses, to manage tissue destruction, and to promote tissue regeneration.

References

Abelda SM. Role of integrins and other cell adhesion molecules in tumor progression and metastasis. Lab Invest 1993;68:4.

Atkinson RA, Evans JS, Hauschka PV, et al. Conformations studies of osteocalcin in solution. Eur J Biochem 1995;232:515.

Aumailley M, Battaglia C, Mayer U, et al. Nidogen mediates the formation of ternary complexes of basement membrane components. Kidney Int 1993;43:7.

Aumailley M, Gerl M, Sonnenberg A, Deutzmann R, Timpl R. Identification of the Arg-Gly-Asp sequence in laminin A chain as a latent cell-binding site being exposed in fragment P1. FEBS Lett 1990;262:82.

Aumailley MM, Wiedemann H, Mann K, Timpl R. Binding of nidogen and the laminin-nidogen complex to basement membrane collagen type IV. Eur J Biochem 1989;184:241.

Bacon-Baguley T, Ogilvie ML, Gartner TK, Walz DA. Thrombospondin binding to specific sequences within the A alpha- and B beta-chains of fibrinogen. J Biol Chem 1990;265:2317.

Banerjee C, Stein JL, Van Wijnen AJ, Frenkel B, Lian JB, Stein GS. Transforming growth factor-beta 1 responsiveness of the rat osteocalcin gene is mediated by an activator protein-1 binding site. Endocrinology 1996;137:1991.

Battaglia C, Mayer U, Aumailley M, Timpl R. Basement membrane heparan sulfate proteoglycan binds to laminin by its heparan sulfate chains and to nidogen by sites in the protein core. Eur J Biochem 1992;208:359.

Beck K, Dixon TW, Engel J, Parry DA. Ionic interaction on the coiled coil domain of laminin determine the specificity of chain assembly. J Mol Biol 1993;231:311.

Beck K, Hunter I, Engel J. Structure and function of laminin: anatomy of a multidomain glycoprotein. FASEB J 1990;4:148.

Bianco P, Fisher LW, Young MF, Termine JD, Gehron-Robey P. Expression of bone sialoprotein (BSP) in developing human tissues. Calcif Tissue Res 1991;49:421.

Bianco P, Silvestrini G, Termine JD, Bonucci E. Immunohistochemical localization of osteonectin in developing human and calf bone using monoclonal antibodies. Calcif Tissue Int 1988;43:155.

Bolander ME, Young MF, Fisher LW, Yamada Y, Termine JD. Osteonectin cDNA sequence reveals potential binding regions for calcium and hydroxyapatite and shows homologies with both a basement protein (SPARC) and a serine proteinase inhibitor (ovomucoid). Proc Natl Acad Sci USA 1988;85:2919.

Bornstein P, Devarayalu S, Edelhoff S, Disteche CM. Isolation and characterization of the mouse thrombospondin 3 (Thbs3) gene. Genomics 1993;15:607.

Boskey AL. Mineral–matrix interactions in bone and cartilage. Clin Orthop 1992;281:244.

Bronkers ALJJ, Gay S, Finkelman RD, Butler WT. Developmental appearance of Gla proteins (osteocalcin) and alkaline phosphatase in tooth germs and bones of the rat. J Bone Miner Res 1987;2:361.

Carlin B, Jeffe R, Bender B, Chung AE. Entactin, a novel basal lamina-associated sulfated glycoprotein. J Biol Chem 1981;256:5209.

Chen Y, Bal BS, Gorski JP. Calcium and collagen binding properties of osteopontin, bone sialoprotein and bone acidic glycoprotein-75 from bone. J Biol Chem 1992;267:24871.

Chen J, McCulloch CA, Sodek J. Bone sialoprotein in developing porcine dental tissues: cellular expression and comparison of tissue localization with osteopontin and osteonectin. Arch Oral Biol 1993;38:241.

Chenu C, Ibaraki K, Gehron-Robey P, Delmas PD, Young MF. Cloning and sequence analysis of bovine bone sialoprotein cDNA: conservation of acidic domains, tyrosine sulfation consensus repeats, and RGD cell attachment domain. J Bone Miner Res 1994;9:417.

Chiquet-Ehrismann R, Kalla P, Pearson CA, Beck K, Chiquet M. Tenascin interferes with fibronectin action. Cell 1988;53:383.

Cleary EG. The microfibrillar component of the elastic fibers. Morphology and biochemistry. In: Uitto J, Pereja A Jr, eds. Connective Tissue Disease. Molecular Pathology of the Extracellular Matrix. New York: Marcel Dekker; 1987:55.

Cockburn CG, Barnes MJ. Characterization of thrombospondin binding to collagen (type I) fibres: role of collagen telopeptides. Matrix 1991;11:168.

Crosby AH, Edwards SJ, Murray JC, Dixon MJ. Genomic organization of the human osteopontin gene: exclusion of the locus from a causative role in the pathogenesis of dentinogenesis imperfecta type II. Genomics 1995;27:155.

Dejana E, Colella S, Conforti G, Abbadini M, Gaboli M, Marchisio PC. Fibronectin and vitronectin regulate the organization of their respective Arg-Gly-Asp adhesion receptors in cultured human endothelial cells. J Cell Biol 1988;107:1215.

Denhardt DT, Guo X. Osteopontin: a protein with diverse functions. FASEB J 1993;7:1475.

Desbois C, Karsenty G. Osteocalcin cluster: implications for functional studies. J Cell Biochem 1995;57:379.

Desbois C, Seldin MF, Karsenty G. Localization of osteocalcin gene cluster on mouse chromosome 3. Mamm Genome 1994;5:321.

Dziadek M. Role of laminin-nidogen complexes in basement membrane formation during embryonic development. Experientia 1995;51:901.

Engel J, Odermatt E, Engel A, et al. Shapes, domain organizations and flexibility of laminin and fibronectin, two multifunctional proteins of the extracellular matrix. J Mol Biol 1981;150:97.

Erickson HP, Bourdon MA. Tenascin: An extracellular matrix protein prominent in specialized embryonic tissues and tumors. Annu Rev Cell Biol 1989;5:71.

Felding-Habermann B, Cheresh DA. Vitronectin and its receptors. Curr Opin Cell Biol 1993;5:864.

Fisher LW, McBride OW, Termine JD, Young MF. Human bone sialoprotein. Deduced protein sequence and chromosomal localization. J Biol Chem 1990;265:237.

Fisher LW, Whitson SW, Avioli LV, Termine JD. Matrix sialoprotein of developing bone. J Biol Chem 1983;258:12723.

Fox JW, Mayer U, Nischt R, et al. Recombinant nidogen consists of three globular domains and mediates binding of laminin to collagen type IV. EMBO J 1991;10:3137.

Fujiwara S, Shinkai H, Mann K, Timpl R. Structure and localisation of O- and N-linked oligosaccharide chains on basement membrane protein nidogen. Matrix 1993;13:215.

Gailet J, Ruoslahti E. Regulation of the fibronectin receptor affinity by divalent cations. J Biol Chem 1988;263:12927.

Garratt AN, Humphries MJ. Recent insights into ligand binding, activation and signalling by integrin adhesion receptors. Acta Anat (Basel) 1995;154:34.

Giancotti FG, Mainiero F. Integrin-mediated adhesion and signalling in tumorigenesis. Biochim Biophys Acta 1994;1198:47.

Giancotti FG, Stepp MA, Suzuki S, Engvall E, Ruoslahti E. Proteolytic processing of endogenous and recombinant β4 integrin subunit. J Cell Biol 1992;118:951.

Gibson MA, Kumaratilake JS, Cleary EG. The protein components of the 12-nanometer microfibrils of elastic and non-elastic tissues. J Biol Chem 1989;264:4590.

Gibson MA, Sandberg LB, Grosso LE, Cleary EG. Complimentary cDNA cloning establishes microfibril-associated glycoprotein (MAGP) to be a discrete component of the elastin-associated microfibrils. J Biol Chem 1991;266:7596.

Graf J, Iwamoto Y, Sasaki M, et al. Identification of an amino acid sequence in laminin mediating cell attachment, chemotaxis, and receptor binding. Cell 1987;48:989.

Haapasalmi K, Makela M, Oksala O, et al. Expression of epithelial adhesion proteins and integrins in chronic inflammation. Am J Pathol 1995;147:193.

Hauschka PV, Lian JB, Cole DE, Gundberg CM. Osteocalcin and matrix gla protein: Vitamin K-dependent proteins in bone. Physiol Rev 1989;69:990.

Hayashi Y, Haimovich B, Reszka A, Boettiger D, Horwitz A. Expression and function of chicken integrin β1 subunit and its cytoplasmic domain mutants in mouse NIH 3T3 cells. J Cell Biol 1990;110:175.

Heinrichs AA, Banerjee C, Bortell R, Owen TA, Stein JL, Lian JB. Identification and characterization of two proximal elements in the rat osteocalcin gene promoter that may confer species-specific regulation. J Cell Biochem 1993; 53:240.

Hogervorst F, Kuikman I, von dem Borne AEG, Sonnenberg A. Cloning and sequence analysis of β4 cDNA: an integrin subunit that contains a unique 118 kd cytoplasmic domain. EMBO J 1990;9:765.

Humphries MJ. The molecular basis and specificity of integrin-ligand interactions. J Cell Sci 1990;97:585.

Hynes RO. Integrins: a family of cell surface receptors. Cell 1987;48:549.

Hynes RO. Integrins: versatility, modulation and signalling in cell adhesion. Cell 1992;69:11.

Hynes R, Yamada K. Fibronectins: multifunctional modular glycoproteins. J Cell Biol 1982;95:369.

Jenne D, Stanley KK. Nucleotide sequence and organization of the human S-protein gene: Repeating peptide motifs in the "pexin" family and a model for their evolution. Biochemistry 1987;26:6735.

Jones FS, Burgoon MP, Crossin KL, Cunningham BA, Edelman GM. A cDNA clone for cytotactin contains sequences similar to epidermal growth factor-like repeats and segments of fibronectin and fibrinogen. Proc Natl Acad Sci USA 1988;85:2186.

Juliano RL, Haskill S. Signal transduction from the extracellular matrix. J Cell Biol 1993;120:577.

Kagan H, Trackman P. Properties and function of lysyl oxidase. Am J Respir Cell Mol Biol 1991;5:206.

Kerr JM, Fisher LW, Termine JD, Wang MG, McBride OW, Young MF. The human bone sialoprotein gene (IBSP): genomic localization and characterization. Genomics 1993;17:408.

Kim RH, Li JJ, Ogata Y, Yamauchi M, Freedman LP, Sodek J. Identification of a vitamin D3-response element that overlaps a unique inverted TATA box in the rat bone sialoprotein gene. Biochem J 1996;318:219.

Kim RH, Shapiro HS, Li JJ, Wrana JL, Sodek J. Characterization of the human bone sialoprotein (BSP) gene and its promoter sequence. Matrix Biol 1994;14:31.

Kinne RW, Fisher LW. Keratan sulfate proteoglycan in rabbit compact bone is bone sialoprotein II. J Biol Chem 1987;262:10206.

Kirchhofer D, Grzesiak J, Pierschbacher MD. Calcium as a potential physiological regulator of integrin-mediated cell adhesion. J Biol Chem 1991;266:4471.

Kishimoto TK, Larson RS, Corbi AL, Dustin ML, Staunton DE, Springer TA. The leukocyte integrins. Adv Immunol 1989;46:149.

Kluge M, Mann K, Dziadek M, Timpl R. Characterization of a novel calcium-binding 90 kDa glycoprotein (BM-90) shared by basement membranes and serum. Eur J Biochem 1990;193:651.

Kornblihtt AR, Pesce CG, Alonso CR, et al. The fibronectin gene as a model for splicing and transcription studies. FASEB J 1996;10:248.

Kubota K, Katayama S, Matsuda M, Hayashi M. Three types of vitronectin in human blood. Cell Struct Funct 1988;13:123.

Lane TF, Sage H. The biology of SPARC, a protein that modulates cell-matrix interations. FASEB J 1994;8:163.

Larjava H, Haapasalmi K, Salo T, Wiebe C, Uitto VJ. Keratinocyte integrins in wound healing and chronic inflammation of the human periodontium. Oral Dis 1996;2:17.

Larson RS, Corbi AL, Berman L, Springer T. Primary structure of the leukocyte function-associated molecule-1 α subunit: an integrin with an embedded domain defining a protein superfamily. J Cell Biol 1989;108:703.

Lawler J, Douquette M, Urry L, McHenry K, Smith TF. The evolution of the thrombospondin gene family. J Mol Evol 1993a;36:509.

Lawler J, Duquette M, Whittaker CA, Adams JC, McHenry K, DeSimone DW. Identification and characterization of thrombospondin-4, a new member of the thrombospondin gene family. J Cell Biol 1993b;120:1059.

Lian J, Stewart C, Puchacz E, et al. Structure of the rat osteocalcin gene and regulation of vitamin D-dependent expression. Proc Natl Acad Sci USA 1989;86:1143-1147.

Lightner VA, Erickson HP. Binding of hexabrachion (tenascin) to the extracellular matrix and substratum and its effect on cell adhesion. J Cell Sci 1990;95:263.

Loftus JC, O'Toole TE, Plow EF, Glass A, Frelinger AC, Ginsberg MH. A β3 integrin mutation abolishes ligand binding and alters divalent cation-dependent comformation. Science 1990;249:915.

Mark MP, Butler WT, Prince CW, Finkelman RD, Ruch V. Developmental expression of 44 kDa bone phosphoprotein (osteopontin) and bone carboxyglutamic acid (Gla)-containing protein (osteocalcin) in calcifying tissues of rat. Differentiation 1988;37:123.

McCarthy JB, Skubitz AP, Qi Z, et al. RGD-independent cell adhesion to the carboxy-terminal heparin-binding fragment of fibronectin involves heparin-dependent and -independent activities. J Cell Biol 1990;110:777.

Mecham RP, Heuser JE. The elastic fiber. In: Hay ED, ed. Cell Biology of the Extracellular Matrix. New York: Plenum; 1992:79.

Mosher D. Physiology of thrombospondin. Annu Rev Med 1990;21:85.

Mosher DF, ed. Fibronectin. New York: Academic Press; 1989.

Mould AP, Komoriya A, Yamada KM, Humphries MJ. Affinity chromatographic isolation of the melanoma adhesion receptor for the IIICS region of fibronectin and its identification as the integrin $\alpha4\beta1$. J Biol Chem 1991; 265:4020.

Neugebauer BM, Moore MA, Broess M, Gerstenfeld LC, Hauschka PV. Characterization of structural sequences in the chicken osteocalcin gene: expression of osteocalcin by maturing osteoblasts and by heterotrophic chondrocytes in vitro. J Bone Miner Res 1995;10:157.

Ogata Y, Yamauchi M, Kim RH, Li JJ, Freedman LP, Sodek J. Glucocorticoid regulation of bone sialoprotein (BSP) gene expression. Identification of a gluocorticoid response element in the bone sialoprotein gene promoter. Eur J Biochem 1995;230:183.

Oldberg A, Franzen A, Heinegard D. Cloning and sequence analysis of rat bone sialoprotein (osteopontin) cDNA reveals an Arg-Gly-Asp cell-binding sequence. Proc Natl Acad Sci USA 1986;83:8819.

Oldberg A, Franzen A, Heinegard D, Pierschbacher M, Ruoslahti E. Identification of a bone sialoprotein receptor in osteosarcoma cells. J Biol Chem 1988;263:19433.

Panayotou G, End P, Aumailley M, Timpl R, Engel J. Domains of laminin with growth factor activity. Cell 1989; 66:93.

Park PW, Roberts DD, Grosso LE, et al. Binding of tropoelastin to *Staphylococcus aureus*. J Biol Chem 1991; 266:2399.

Paulsson M, Aumailley M, Deutzmann R, Timpl R, Beck K, Engel J. Laminin-nidogen complex. Extraction with chelating agents and structural characterization. Eur J Biochem 1987;166:11.

Paulsson M, Deutzmann R, Dziadek M, et al. Purification and structural characterization of intact and fragmented nidogen obtained from a tumor basement membrane. Eur J Biochem 1986;231:467.

Pearson CA, Pearson D, Shibahara S, Hofsteenge J, Chiquet-Ehrismann R. Tenascin cDNA cloning and induction by TGF-beta. EMBO J 1988;7:2677.

Perides G, Erickson HP, Rahemtulla F, Bignami A. Colocalization of tenascin with versican, a hyaluronate-binding chondroitin sulfate proteoglycan. Anat Embryol (Berl) 1993;188:467.

Pierschbacher MD, Ruoslahti E. Cell attachment activity of fibronectin can be duplicated by small synthetic fragments of the molecule. Nature 1984;309:30.

Pierschbacher MD, Ruoslahti E. New perspectives in cell adhesion: RGD and integrins. Nature 1987;238:491.

Preissner K. Structure and biological role of vitronectin. Annu Rev Cell Biol 1991;7:275.

Prince CW. Secondary structure predictions for rat osteopontin. Connect Tissue Res 1989;21:15.

Rahman S, Oberdorf A, Montecino M, et al. Multiple copies of the bone-specific osteocalcin gene in mouse and rat. Endocrinology 1993;133:3050.

Reinhardt D, Mann K, Nischt R, et al. Mapping of nidogen binding sites for collagen type IV, heparan sulfate proteoglycan and zinc. J Biol Chem 1993;268:10881.

Reinholt FP, Hultenby K, Oldberg A, Heinegard D. Osteopontin—A possible anchor of osteoclasts to bone. Proc Natl Acad Sci USA 1990;87:4473.

Ritter NM, Farach-Carson MC, Butler WT. Evidence for the formation of a complex between osteopontin and osteocalcin. J Bone Miner Res 1992;7:877.

Rosenbloom J, Abrams WA, Indik A, Yeh H, Ornsten-Goldstein N, Bashir MM. Structure of the elastin gene. Ciba Foundation Symposium 1995;192:59.

Rosenbloom J, Abrams WA, Mecham R. Extracellular matrix 4: The elastin fiber. FASEB J 1993;7:1208.

Ross FP, Chappel J, Alverez JI, et al. Interactions between the bone matrix proteins osteopontin and bone sialoprotein and the osteoclast integrin $\alpha v\beta 3$ potentiate bone resorption. J Biol Chem 1993;268:9901.

Saavedra RA, Kimbro SK, Stern DN, et al. Gene expression and phosphorylation of mouse osteopontin. Ann N Y Acad Sci 1995;760:35.

Sakai LW, Keene DR, Engvall E. Fibrillin, a new 350 kDa glycoprotein, is a component of extracellular microfibrils. J Cell Biol 1986;103:2499.

Sakai T, Kawakatsu H, Ohta M, Saito M. Tenascin induction in tenascin nonproducing carcinoma cell lines in vivo and by TGF-beta 1 in vitro. J Cell Physiol 1994;159:561.

Sandberg LB, Soskel NT, Wolt TB. Elastin structure, biosynthesis and relation to disease states. New Engl J Med 1981;304:566.

Schnapp LM, Hatch N, Ramos DM, Klimanskaya IV, Sheppard D, Pytela R. The human integrin alpha 8 beta 1 functions as a receptor for tenascin, fibronectin and vitronectin. J Biol Chem 1995;270:23196.

Schwartz MA. Transmembrane signalling by integrins. Trend Cell Biol 1992;2:304.

Schwarzbauer J. The fibronectin gene. In: Sandell LJ, Boyd CD, eds. Extracellular Matrix Genes. New York: Academic Press; 1990:195.

Seiffert D, Poenninger J, Binder BR. Organization of the gene encoding mouse vitronectin. Gene 1993;134:303.

Senior RM, Griffen GL, Mecham RP. Chemotactic activity of elastin-derived peptides. J Clin Invest 1980;304:859.

Shapiro HS, Chen J, Wrana JL, Zhang Q, Blum M, Sodek J. Characterization of porcine bone sialoprotein: primary structure and cellular expression. Matrix 1993;13:431.

Shimomura H, Kanai Y, Sanada K. Primary structure of cat osteocalcin. J Biochem (Tokyo) 1984;96:405.

Shingu T, Bornstein P. Overlapping Egr-1 and Sp1 sites function in the regulation of transcription of the mouse thrombospondin 1 gene. J Biol Chem 1994;269:32551.

Skubitz APN, McCarthy JB, Zhao Q, Yi X, Furcht LT. Definition of a sequence, RYVVLPR within laminin peptide F-9 that mediates metastatic fibrosarcoma cell adhesion and spreading. Cancer Res 1990;50:7612.

Sodek J, Chen J, Nagata T, et al. Regulation of osteopontin expression in osteoblasts. Ann NY Acad Sci 1995; 760:223.

Spring J, Beck K, Chiquet-Ehrismann R. Two contrary functions of tenascin: dissection of the active sites by recombinant tenascin fragments. Cell 1989;59:325.

Swaroop A, Hogan BLM, Francke U. Molecular analysis of the cDNA for human SPARC/osteonectin/BM-40: sequence, expression and localization of the gene to chromosome 5q31-q33. Genomics 1988;1:37.

Swee MH, Parks WC, Pierce RA. Developmental regulation of elastin production. Expression of tropoelastin pre-mRNA persists after down regulation of steady-state mRNA levels. J Biol Chem 1995;270:14899.

Takagi J, Fujisawa T, Usui T, Aoyama T, Saito Y. A single chain 19 kDA fragment from bone thrombospondin binds to type V collagen and heparin. J Biol Chem 1993; 268:15544.

Tanzer ML, Chandrasekaran S, Dean JW, Giniger MS. Role of laminin carbohydrates on cellular interactions. Kidney Int 1993;3:66.

Timpl R. Macromolecular organization of basement membranes. Curr Opin Cell Biol 1996;8:618.

Timpl R, Rohde H, Gehron-Robey P, Rennard SL, Foidart JM, Martin GR. Laminin—a glycoprotein from basement membrane. J Biol Chem 1979;254:9933.

Tomasini B, Mosher D. Vitronectin. Prog Hemost Thromb 1991;10:269.

Tryggvason K. The laminins family. Curr Opin Cell Biol 1993;5:877.

Tuckwell DS, Humphries MJ. Molecular and cellular biology of integrins. Crit Rev Oncol Hematol 1993;15:149.

Uitto J, Mauviel A, McGrath J. The dermal-epidermal basement membrane zone in cutaneous wound healing. In: Clark RAF, ed. The Molecular Biology of Wound Repair. New York: Plenum; 1996:512.

Villarreal XC, Mann KG, Long GL. Structure of human osteonectin based upon analysis of cDNA and genomic sequences. Biochemistry 1989;28:6483.

Wasi S, Otsuka K, Yao KL, et al. An osteonectin-like protein in porcine periodontal ligament and its synthesis by periodontal ligament fibroblasts. Can J Biochem Cell Biol 1984;62:470.

Yamada KA. Fibronectin. In: Hay ED, ed. Cell Biology of the Extracellular Matrix. New York: Plenum; 1992:111.

Yamada KM, Clark RAF. Provisional matrix. In: Clark RAF, ed. The Molecular Biology of Wound Repair. New York: Plenum; 1996:51.

Yamamoto S, Hijiya N, Setoguchi M, et al. Structure of osteopontin gene and its promoter. Ann NY Acad Sci 1995;6760:44.

Yamauchi M, Ogata Y, Kim RH, Li JJ, Freedman LP, Sodek J. AP-1 regulation of the rat bone sialoprotein gene transcription is mediated through a TPQ response element within a glucocorticoid response unit in the gene promoter. Matrix Biol 1996;15:119.

Yokasaki Y, Palmer EL, Prieto AL, et al. The integrin alpha 9 beta 1 mediates cell attachment to a non-RGD site in the third fibronectin type II repeat of tenascin. J Biol Chem 1994;269:26691.

Young MF, Kerr JM, Ibraki K, Heegard A-M, Gehron-Robey P. Structure, expression and regulation of the major noncollagenous matrix proteins of bone. Clin Orthop 1992;281:275.

Young MF, Kerr JM, Termine JD, et al. cDNA cloning mRNA distribution and heterogeneity, chromosomal location, and RFLP analysis of human osteopontin (OPN) Genomics 1990;7:491.

Yurchenco P, Schittny JC. Molecular architecture of basement membranes. FASEB J 1990;4:1577.

Zhao Y, Young SL. TGF-beta regulates expression of tenascin alternative-splicing isoforms in fetal rat lung. Am J Physiol 1995;268:L173.

Proteoglycans

Introduction

The term mucopolysaccharide was first used to describe molecules that were "hexosamine containing polysaccharides of animal origin either in a pure state or as protein salts." (Meyer 1958). Later classifications of the mucopolysaccharides were based on their component sugars as well as the presence or absence of sulfate residues. While the term mucopolysaccharide may occasionally be found in the literature, it is largely an outdated term based on histochemical rather than biochemical data. In 1960, a universally accepted terminology was developed in which the term glycosaminoglycan (GAG) was to replace the use of mucopolysaccharide (Jeanloz 1960).

Although many different types of GAG have been isolated from tissues, it is important to note that these molecules (with the exception of hyaluronan) are always found in vivo attached to a protein core. Accordingly, the molecule en masse is called a proteoglycan. The term proteoglycan was first introduced in 1967 to describe a family of macromolecules composed of one or more glycosaminoglycans covalently bound to a protein core (Balazs 1967). Prior to this, these molecules had been called protein-polysaccharide complexes or chondromucoproteins.

Protein-polysaccharide complexes were first described in the late 1950s as long proteins with up to 60 attached chondroitin sulfate chains (Mathews and Lozaityte 1958; Partridge et al 1961). Interestingly, this simple model still holds true for many of the different proteoglycans that have been subsequently identified. However, other proteoglycans do differ significantly in their structure from this early model. For example, numerous glycosaminoglycans (apart from hyaluronan) may make up the chemical composition of proteoglycans. Furthermore, the proportion of carbohydrate to protein may vary from one glycosaminoglycan chain to over 150 chains per core protein molecule (Hardingham and Fosang 1992).

General Structure and Composition

Glycosaminoglycans

Glycosaminoglycans are the principal carbohydrate component of proteoglycans (Fransson 1985; Jackson et al 1991). Glycosaminoglycans are composed of repeating disaccharide units of uronic acid (either D-glucuronic acid or L-iduronic acid) and hexosamine (either D-glucosamine or D-galactosamine). Keratan sulfate is an exception to this generalization in that it contains D-galactose in the place of uronic acid. As a consequence of the negatively charged ester sulfates, sulfamino groups, and carboxyl groups, all glycosaminoglycans are polyanionic. Apart from hyaluronan, all glycosaminoglycans are sulfated to varying degrees (Table 6-1).

Chondroitin sulfate is composed of repeating disaccharide units of O-sulfated N-acetyl-galactosamine and D-glucuronic acid, and may be sulfated on either the C-4 or the C-6 of the N-acetylgalactosamine moiety. In some cases, the degree of sulfation may vary from an undersulfated form containing less than one sulfate per disaccharide to an oversulfated form with multiple sulfate groups per disaccharide unit. The 4- and 6-sulfated isomers are widely distributed throughout mammalian tissues, and are particularly predominant in cartilage.

Dermatan sulfate is very similar to chondroitin sulfate except that the uronic acid residue is epimerized forming L-iduronic acid. Thus, the repeating disaccharide unit of dermatan sulfate consists of 4- or 6-sulfated N-acetylgalactosamine and L-iduronic acid. Within the polysaccharide chain of dermatan sulfate, not all uronic acid residues are epimerized, resulting in blocks of glucuronic acid– and iduronic acid–containing disaccharide sequences. The sulfate ratio per disaccharide unit may be greater than one with sulfate residues located at either the C-4 or the C-6 position, as well as at C-2 of the L-iduronic acid residue. Dermatan sulfate is also widely distributed throughout mammalian tissues, but occurs predominantly in fibrous connective tissues such as skin and tendon.

Heparin and heparan sulfate are two extreme forms of a broad range of molecules called heparinlike polysaccharides. Heparin may be found intracellularly (mast cells and basophils) and extracellularly within blood and connective tissues. The heparin molecule is strongly acidic and highly charged; its most significant biologic property is the ability to react electrostatically with proteins. For example, the ability of heparin to bind various growth factors has given it a prime role in regulation of tissue and cellular functions such as growth, development, and repair. Heparan sulfate is found extracellularly in most mammalian connective tissues. It is primarily located in basement membranes, the microenvi-

Table 6-1. Composition of Glycosaminoglycans

Glycosaminoglycan	Previous Name	Sugars in Disaccharide Unit	Other Sugars	Acidic Group	Sulfate	Sulfates per Disaccharide	Sulfate Position
Hyaluronan	Hyaluronic acid Hyaluronate	N-acetylglucosamine D-glucuronic acid	None	Carboxyl	None	0	None
Chondroitin-4-sulfate	Chondroitin sulfate A	N-acetylgalactosamine D-glucuronic acid	D-galactose D-xylose	Carboxyl Sulfate	O-sulfate	0.2–1.0	4
Chondroitin-6-sulfate	Chondroitin sulfate C	N-acetylgalactosamine D-glucuronic acid	D-galactose D-xylose	Carboxyl Sulfate	O-sulfate	0.2–2.3	6
Dermatan sulfate	Chondroitin sulfate B	N-acetylgalactosamine D-glucuronic acid L-iduronic acid	D-galactose D-xylose	Carboxyl Sulfate	O-sulfate	1.0–2.0	4 and 6
Heparan sulfate	Heparitin sulfate	N-acetylglucosamine N-sulfylglucosamine D-glucuronic acid L-iduronic acid	D-galactose D-xylose	Carboxyl Sulfate	N-sulfate O-sulfate	2.0–3.0	2, 3, and 6
Heparin	None	N-acetylglucosamine N-sulfylglucosamine D-glucuronic acid L-iduronic acid	D-galactose D-xylose	Carboxyl Sulfate	N-sulfate O-sulfate	0.2–2.0	2, 3, and 6
Keratan sulfate	Keratosulfate	N-acetylglucosamine D-galactose	D-galactosamine D-mannose L-fucose Sialic acid	Sulfate	O-sulfate	0.9–1.8	6

ronment of cells, and within cell membranes. Structurally, these molecules are characterized by the presence of N-sulfate groups on the glucosamine residues, in addition to O-sulfate modification of C-2 and C-6, as well as possibly at C-3. Heparin consists of alternating uronic acid (L-iduronic acid or D-glucuronic acid) and D-glucosamine residues. The glucosamine residues may have either sulfated or acetylated amino groups. Most of the glucosamine units are O-sulfated at C-6 and most, but not all, of the iduronic acid residues are sulfated at C-2. Heparan sulfate contains less sulfate and iduronic acid than does heparin, but more N-acetyl groups and glucuronic acid.

Keratan sulfate is distinct from other glycosaminoglycans, in that it does not contain any uronic acid. The disaccharide units of keratan sulfate are composed of *N*-acetylglucosamine and D-galactose, both of which may be variably sulfated at C-6 (Fransson 1985). Keratan sulfate also appears to contain small amounts of D-galactosamine, D-mannose, L-fucose, and sialic acid. In addition to these features, keratan sulfate exists in two principal forms, one is KS I, which is found mainly in cornea, and the other is KS II, which is found mainly in skeletal tissues. These two forms of keratan sulfate may be distinguished by their mode of linkage to their respective proteoglycan core proteins (see later). KS I and KS II also show minor differences in their composition; keratan sulfate II contains small amounts of *N*-acetylgalactosamine and sialic acid replacing the mannose in keratan sulfate I.

Hyaluronan has several unique features that distinguish it from the other glycosaminoglycans (Laurent and Fraser 1992). This is the only nonsulfated glycosaminoglycan composed of repeating disaccharide units of D-glucuronic acid and *N*-acetyl-D-glucosamine. While its molecular mass is quite polydisperse, hyaluronan has by far the largest molecular size, with an average M_r (relative molecular mass) of sev-

eral million. It is also the only glycosaminoglycan that does not bind covalently to a protein core to form a proteoglycan molecule. The biosynthesis of hyaluronan is also unique among the glycosaminoglycans. Rather than being made in the Golgi apparatus, hyaluronan is synthesized via hyaluronan synthase (located at the plasma membrane) through the addition of sugars to the reducing end of the molecule, with the reducing end projecting into the pericellular environment (Prehm 1989).

The distribution of hyaluronan is virtually ubiquitous and hyaluronan is synthesized by most cells. Its functions are many and varied; it is important in tissue hydration, aggregation with other matrix components (aggrecan, CD44), cell surface–matrix interactions, cell migration, tissue development, inflammation, and wound healing (Laurent and Fraser 1992).

Oligosaccharides

In addition to the glycosaminoglycan chains, smaller oligosaccharides have been identified in most proteoglycans. These components may be bound by either O-glycosidic or N-glycosidic linkages to the proteoglycan core protein. The O-linked oligosaccharides are found primarily in the chondroitin/dermatan sulfate–rich portion of proteoglycans, while the N-linked types are usually found within the portion of those core proteins capable of binding to hyaluronan (Thonar and Sweet 1977; DeLuca et al 1980; Lohmander et al 1980). The precise role of these oligosaccharides is unclear, although it is possible that the O-linked oligosaccharides may act as primers for the addition of keratan sulfate chains on proteoglycans in mature tissues (Kuettner and Kimura 1985).

Glycopeptide Linkage

The nature of the linkage of glycosaminoglycans to the proteoglycan core protein has

A. Linkage region sequence for chondroitin sulfates 4 & 6, dermatan sulfate, and heparan sulfate:

Serine - xyl - gal - gal - [GlcUA - GlcNAc(GalNAc)] -

B. Linkage region sequence for keratan sulfate I:

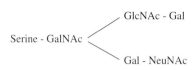

Man - GlcNAc - Gal - GalNAc

Asparagine - GlcNAc - GlcNAc - Man

Man - GlcNAc - Gal - GlcNAc

C. Linkage region sequence for keratan sulfate II:

GlcNAc - Gal

Serine - GalNAc

Gal - NeuNAc

Fig 6-1 Composition of glycosaminoglycan linkage region to proteoglycan core protein. xyl, xylosyl; gal, galactosyl; GlcUA, glucuronic acid; GalNAc, N-acetyl galactosamine; Man, mannose; NeuNAc, neuraminic acid.

been extensively reviewed for proteoglycans of animal, plant, and bacterial origin (Lindahl and Roden 1972). In all cases, the reducing end of the terminal glycosaminoglycan monosaccharide is covalently bound, via a specific carbohydrate sequence, to an amino acid in the core protein (Fig 6-1). The notable exception to this is hyaluronan, which appears to be synthesized without covalent attachment to a core protein.

The sulfated glycosaminoglycans chondroitin sulfate (4- and 6-sulfated isomers), dermatan sulfate, and heparan sulfate share a common carbohydrate linkage sequence to the core protein (see Fig 6-1a). This sequence includes two galactose residues bound in tandem to a terminal uronic acid moiety in the glycosaminoglycan chain. Xylose is bound to the second galactose residue, which provides the O-glycosidic link between the carbohydrate chain and a hydroxyl group of serine in the protein core.

The linkage of keratan sulfate to its core protein is different (see Figs 6-1b, c). Keratan sulfate I (corneal keratan sulfate) has a branched conformation composed of three mannose residues and two *N*-acetylglucosamine residues, resulting in its linkage via an N-glycosidic bond between *N*-acetylglucosamine and asparagine (Nilsson et al 1983; Baker et al 1975). This structure is similar to the linkage of N-linked oligosaccharides described above. The linkage region of keratan sulfate II (skeletal keratan sulfate) to its core protein is also branched, with the *N*-acetylgalactosamine capped with sialic acid at C-3, and linking the keratan sulfate chain through C-6 of this residue. Linkage of this region to the core protein occurs via an O-glycosidic bond between the *N*-acetylgalactosamine residue, and either serine or threonine in the core protein (Bray et al 1967; Hopwood and Robinson 1974).

Core Proteins

Proteoglycans have very heterogeneous protein contents. For example, aggrecan contains between 2% and 18% protein, while the protein content of decorin may be as high as 50% (Hassel et al 1986). This variability is largely associated with differences in core protein size and available sites for glycosaminoglycan attachment. Thus, proteoglycan core proteins have been reported to range in size from 10 to 300 kd with one to several hundred attached glycosaminoglycan chains. Early attempts to determine the amino acid sequences of most proteoglycan core proteins were hampered by their high level of glycosylation. However, with subsequent developments in molecular biology, the sequences for many proteoglycans have now been determined and these confirm the expected diversity in content, structure, and conformation.

Within the amino acid sequences of the proteoglycan core proteins, several specific regions have been identified that relate to hydrophilic, hydrophobic, and globular domains. Each of these sequences appear to correlate with a particular proteoglycan's location and supposed function.

Current evidence indicates that there is considerable diversity in the proteoglycan core proteins; each belongs to its own gene family, and they do not appear to be genetically related. Thus, unlike many other matrix molecules, the proteoglycans do not belong to a single supergene family.

Proteoglycan Synthesis

The biosynthesis of proteoglycans follows a relatively normal pathway consistent with the synthesis of most glycoproteins (Hascall et al 1992). Initially the protein core is synthesized in the rough endoplasmic reticulum (RER) with a hydrophobic N-terminal leader sequence that is removed during ongoing translation of the RNA. Addition of the glycosaminoglycan chain only occurs after the specific glycopeptide linkage has been formed (see above), and later modifications to the glycosaminoglycan chains eventually lead to completion of the synthetic process.

The addition of glycosaminoglycan chains is a complex process involving many enzymes and a variety of sugars (Fig 6-2). Initiation of glycosaminoglycan chain elongation occurs through the sequential addition of sugars that are transported to the Golgi as uridine diphosphate (UDP) complexes and are formed in the cytosol of the cell. With the exception of keratan sulfate, the addition of all other sulfated glycosaminoglycan chains is initiated by the addition of xylose to serine via the enzyme xylosyl transferase in the early Golgi or late RER compartments. For the addition of glycosaminoglycan chains to occur, some specificity in the acceptor site amino acid sequence appears to be necessary. The xylosyl transferase preferentially adds xylose onto serine residues within the sequences:

1. glutamic acid (aspartic acid) – X-serine-glycine
2. $[-serine-glycine-serine-glycine-]_n$

The xylosyl transferase does not operate at 100% efficiency since only 10% to 15% of the available serines in the aggrecan core protein, and a similar small percentage in biglycan, are eventually glycosylated (Hascall 1988).

After the addition of the xylose, two galactose residues are added by two different galactosyl transferases to complete the glycopeptide linkage sequence. The addition of the disaccharide repeating units of uronic acid and hexosamine is carried out by a battery of galactosamine transferase and glucuronic acid transferase enzymes (Roden 1980). In this sequence, glucuronic acid is added to the second galactose residue in the linkage sequence. Chain elongation then proceeds via sequential addition of N-acetylgalactosamine and glucuronic acid to the nonreducing end of the growing chain.

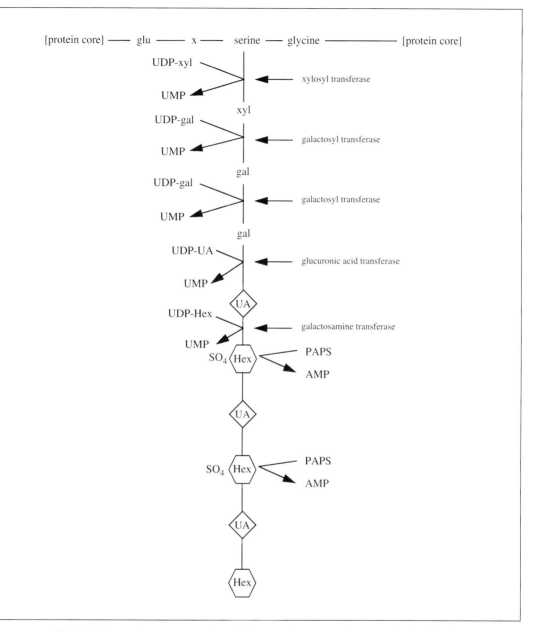

Fig 6-2 Schematic representation of the steps in proteoglycan synthesis. Uronic acid and hexosamine components of glycosaminoglycan chains are added to the trisaccharide sequence, xyl-gal-gal. The xylose is added to specific serine residues within the proteoglycan core protein. Numerous enzymes including xylosyl-galactosyl–, glucuronic acid–, and galactosamine-transferase aid in the assembly of the glycosaminoglycans. During chain elongation, sulfate groups are added along with several other posttranslational modifications. Glu, glutamic acid; xyl, xylosyl; gal, galactosyl; UA, uronic acid; Hex, hexosamine; UDP-xyl, uridine 5′-pyrophosphate-xylose; UMP, uridine 5′-phosphate; UDP-gal, uridine 5′-pyrophosphate-galactose; UDP-UA, uridine 5′-pyrophosphate-uronic acid; UDP-Hex, uridine 5′-pyrophosphate-hexosamine; PAPS, phosphoadenosinephosphosulfate; AMP, adenosine 5′-phosphate.

Table 6-2. Proteoglycans as Matrix Organizers or Space Fillers

Name	Monomer Molecular Mass/kd	Protein Molecular Mass/kd	GAG*	Location and Interaction
Aggrecan	$1–4 \times 10^6$	2.5×10^5	CS/KS	Cartilage, interacts with hyaluronate
Versican	1×10^6	4×10^5	CS	Fibroblasts, interacts with hyaluronate
Perlecan	7×10^5	4×10^5	HS	Basement membrane
Decorin	2×10^5	4×10^4	DS/CS	Soft connective tissues, bone, cartilage. Interacts with collagen I and II, fibronectin and TGF-β
Biglycan	3.5×10^5	4×10^4	DS/CS	Soft connective tissues, bone, cartilage. Interacts with some matrix components and cell surfaces, but not with collagen
Fibromodulin	1×10^5	6×10^4	KS	Interacts with collagen I
Lumican	$7–8 \times 10^4$	4×10^4	KS	Cornea, aorta (?). Interacts with collagen
Collagen type IX	. . .		CS	Cartilage and vitreous. Cross-links with other collagens
Testican	. . .	5.0×10^4	HS/CS	Sertoli's cells; cell-matrix interactions
TAP-1	1.2×10^6	1.8×10^5	CS	Nerve terminals
Brevican	. . .	1.45×10^5	CS	Brain matrix. Interacts with hyaluronate
Neurocan	1.5×10^5	1.2×10^5	CS	Brain. Binds to hyaluronate
Phosphocan	8×10^5	1.7×10^5	CS/KS	Brain
Centoglycan (PG-100)	. . .	7.8×10^4	CS	Bone, skin

*GAG, glycosaminoglycans; CS, chondroitin sulfate; KS, keratan sulfate; HS, heparan sulfate; DS, dermatan sulfate; TAP-1, nerve terminal anchorage protein-1.

During chain elongation, ester sulfate groups are added by the transfer of phosphoadenosinephosphosulfate (PAPS), utilizing two sulfotransferases for sulfation at either the C-4 or C-6 position of the *N*-acetylgalactosamine residues.

Dermatan sulfate subsequently undergoes further modifications, which include the epimerization of glucuronic acid to iduronic acid, and 2-O sulfation of some of the iduronic acid residues. In addition to these modifications, heparan sulfate also undergoes N-deacetylation followed by N-sulfation, as well as occasional additional sulfation of both the glucosamine and uronic acid residues.

The length of the glycosaminoglycan chains is quite variable between various proteoglycans, and even between proteoglycans of the same class but from different tissue compartments. The factors that control chain termination are not yet fully understood.

Proteoglycan Types

Proteoglycans are large, highly anionic glycoproteins ubiquitous to all connective tissues. They are located within the matrix as integral components of the matrix structure, as well as on cell surfaces and within cell organelles. By virtue of their high charge, they have been ascribed a variety of functions including tissue hydration, regulation of collagen fiber formation, growth factor binding, cell adhesion, and cell growth. By definition, a proteoglycan is composed of a single protein core to which one or more glycosaminoglycan side chains are covalently bound. Historically, the classification of proteoglycans has been based on their glycosaminoglycan composition such that proteoglycans were referred to as small dermatan sulfate proteoglycans, or large aggregating chondroitin sulfate proteoglycans (Table 6-2

Table 6-3. Cell Surface Proteoglycans

Name	GAG*	Protein Molecular Mass/kd	Location	Function
Syndecan-1	CS/HS	3×10^4	Epithelial cells, fibroblasts, lymphocytes, embryonic dental mesenchyme, embryonic lung mesenchyme	Cell differentiation, receptor-signal transduction, responsive to growth factors
Syndecan-2 (fibroglycan)	HS	20×10^4	Fibroblast	Cell-cell; cell matrix interactions
Syndecan-3 (N-syndecan)	HS/CS	1.2×10^5	Schwann's cells and cartilage	Nerve cell–matrix (N-syndecan) interactions
Syndecan-4 (ryudocan)	HS	3.0×10^4	Endothelial cells	Cell-matrix interactions
Syndecan-4 (amphiglycan)	HS	3.5×10^4	Fibroblasts and epithelium	Cell-matrix interactions
Thrombomodulin	CS	4×10^4	Vascular endothelium	Thrombin binding
CD44 (Hermes antigen, Hutch-1, GP90, PGp-1, H-CAM)	CS/HS	9×10^4	Surface of hematopoietic cells, epithelial cells, and fibroblasts	Lymphocyte homing and lymphocyte-endothelial interactions
Epican	HS/CS	1.8×10^5	Keratinocytes	Cell-cell interactions
Glypican	HS	$6–8 \times 10^4$	Fibroblast	Cell-cell; cell-matrix interactions
Betaglycan	HS/CS	1×10^5	Widely distributed on many cell types	TGF-β type III receptor
C1q Inhibitor	CS	3×10^4	Lymphocytes	C1q precipitation
Invariant chain	CS	…	Lymphocytes and macrophages	Depress antigen presentation, biosynthesis of Ia antigens
NG2	CS	3.0×10^5	Neural and glioma cells	Associated with response to injury

*GAG, glycosaminoglycans; KS, keratan sulfate; HS, heparan sulfate.

However, in recent years the classification system for proteoglycans has shifted from this simple approach to one more often based on core protein sequence or tissue location. Regardless of the names given to the proteoglycans, they can still be classified into at least three separate groups, namely matrix organizers and tissue space fillers, cell surface proteoglycans, or intracellular proteoglycans of the hematopoietic cells (see Tables 6-2, 6-3, and 6-4). The following is a brief overview of the myriad proteoglycans likely to be of significance in the make up of the periodontal tissues. A more specific discussion of the proteoglycans identified to date in the periodontum will follow later (Chapter 10).

Matrix Organizers and Space Fillers

Large extracellular proteoglycans.

Aggrecan is a large proteoglycan that contains both keratan sulfate and chondroitin sulfate chains and is able to form macromolecular aggregates with hyaluronan. Although not found in the periodontal tissues, aggrecan is worthy of discussion as it is the archetypal proteoglycan. Aggrecan is probably the best studied proteoglycan, and for this reason the model of aggrecan (formerly called *large aggregating chondroitin sulfate proteoglycan*) was considered the benchmark for all proteoglycans. It was not until subsequent studies began to isolate

Table 6-4. Proteoglycans of Hematopoietic Cells

Cells	Proteoglycan	GAG	Location	Function
Mast cells	Serglycin	CS*/heparin	Intracellular granules	Enzyme packaging, protease modulation
T Lymphocytes	Serglycin	CS-4, HS	Intracellular, secreted regulators	Control of B cell maturation
B Lymphocytes	Serglycin Invariant chain Syndecan CD44	CS CS CS/HS CS	Intracellular, secreted	Cell activation, antigen presentation, cell surface, maturation, cell surface homing receptor
NK Cells	Serglycin	CS	Secretory granules	Cell activation, protection
Kurloff cells	CS-PG	CS	Cytoplasmic inclusions	Storage, activation
HL-60 cells	Serglycin	CS	Intracellular, cell surface	Differentiation
Granulocytes	Serglycin	CS-A CS-E	Lysosomes, cell surface	Storage, cell-matrix interaction
Monocytes/macrophages	Serglycin Invariant chain	CS-A CS-E	Storage granules, cell surface	Storage, arterial disease (bind LDL), antigen presentation
Platelets	Serglycin C1q-inhibitor	CS-4 CS	Alpha granules, granules	Storage, PF4 binding, C1q inhibition
Mast cells	Serglycin CS-E	CS-A	Cytoplasmic granules	Packaging, physiologic regulation of activation

*GAG, glycosaminoglycans; CS, chondroitin sulfate; NK, natural killer; CS-PG, chondroitin sulfate proteoglycan.

Table 6-5. Proteoglycans that Bind Growth Factors

Name	Growth Factor Bound	Binding Region
Decorin	TGF-β	Protein core
Betaglycan	TGF-β, FGF	Protein core
Syndecan	TGF-β, αFGF, GMCSF*, CSF, IL-3, IFN-γ	HS
Cell surface HSPGs	FGF	HS
Serglycin	Platelet factor-4	CS

*GMCSF, granulocyte macrophage colony stimulating factor; IL-3, interleukin-3; IFG-gamma, interferon gamma; HSPG, heparan sulfate proteoglycan.

proteoglycans from tissues other than cartilage that this structure was found to be quite unique and specific for cartilage only.

Aggrecan has two extended regions and three globular regions (Fig 6-3). At the amino terminus, the G1 and G2 regions are separated by a short extended domain (E1). Following the G2 portion there is a large extended region (E2), which carries the bulk of the glycosaminoglycan chains, and this is followed at the carboxyl terminus with another globular domain. The E2 domain is further subdivided into a portion that carries mainly keratan sulfate chains close to the G2 domain, and an extended portion rich in serine and glycine repeats that carry the chondroitin sulfate chains (Hardingham and Fosang 1992). The G1 domain shares homology with the link protein sequence, composed of

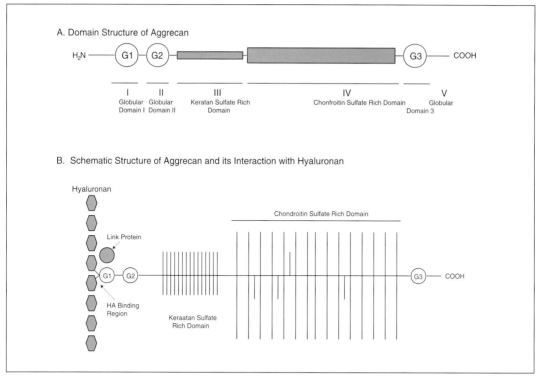

A. Domain Structure of Aggrecan

I	II	III	IV	V
Globular Domain I	Globular Domain II	Keratan Sulfate Rich Domain	Chondroitin Sulfate Rich Domain	Globular Domain 3

B. Schematic Structure of Aggrecan and its Interaction with Hyaluronan

Fig 6-3 Schematic representation of aggrecan. **(a)** shows the various domains of aggrecan and **(b)** shows the likely structure of both the intact molecule as well as some detail of the hyaluronan binding region.

three loop structures containing stabilizing disulfide bonds, and it is intimately associated with hyaluronan aggregation. The G2 domain shares homology with the G1 sequence, but lacks the ability to interact with hyaluronan (to date, the function of G2 is unknown). Within these structures, structural motifs are found that share common sequences found in other proteins. For example, the G1 domain has a β-sheet structure found in immunoglobulins and associated with cell recognition (Perkins et al 1989), while at the carboxy terminus, sequences are present that share homology with type C animal lectins and epidermal growth factor Hardingham & Fosang 1992).

The human aggrecan gene has been mapped to 15q25 through 15q26.2. It contains 19 exons; one is noncoding, and the remaining 18 code for structural and functional modules within the aggrecan core protein (Just et al 1993). In the rat gene there is a minor promoter that initiates transcription and encompasses exon 1, and lacks the TATA and CAAT elements (Doege et al 1994).

Versican was originally isolated from fibroblasts, but has since been found to be present in a wide variety of tissues including aorta, brain, cartilage, placenta, and tendon, as well as skin (Ruoslahti 1989). This large proteoglycan is considered to be the soft connective tissue form of aggrecan due to its ability to aggregate with hyaluronan. Versican is considered a large proteoglycan, as it is composed of a core protein of over 300 kd, to which approximately 12 glycosaminoglycan chains are attached. N- and O-linked oligosaccharides

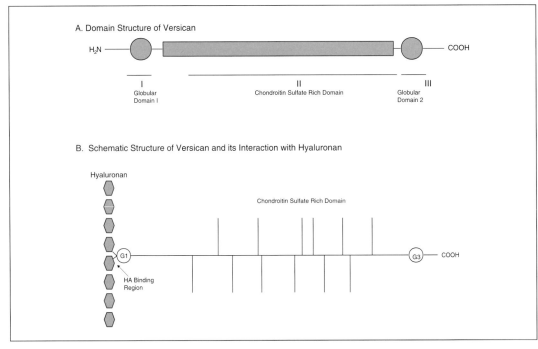

Fig 6-4 Schematic representation of versican. **(a)** shows the various domains of versican and **(b)** shows the likely structure of both the intact molecule as well as some details of the hyaluronan binding region.

also contribute to the composition of this molecule (Zimmerman and Ruoslahti 1989).

Apart from its ability to aggregate with hyaluronan, versican shares several other features in common with aggrecan (Fig 6-4). For example, globular domains are present at both the amino terminus (G1) and the carboxyl terminus (G3), and these have significant homology with the similar regions of the aggrecan core protein. The G1 domain contains the hyaluronan binding region. The portion of the core protein that carries exclusively chondroitin sulfate chains (or dermatan sulfate in some cases) differs significantly from the extended portion of the aggrecan core protein, which carries both chondroitin sulfate and keratan sulfate. At the G3 region, versican core protein carries sequences with homology to EGF, a lectinlike sequence and a complement regulatory protein domain. Ver-

sican also shares similar sequence homology within the amino and carboxyl terminal domains of another large extracellular proteoglycan, neurocan (found in the brain). However, there are sufficient unique sequences within the extended central portion of the core proteins of aggrecan, versican, and neurocan to consider these separate proteoglycans. The gene for human versican has been located to the long arm of chromosome 5 from 5q12 to 5q14, and it contains 15 exons that code for the various domains of the protein core (Iozzo et al 1992). The promoter for versican contains a typical TATA box 16 base pairs upstream of the transcription start site (Naso e al 1994).

Perlecan is another so-called large proteogly can composed of a 466-kd protein core t which approximately three or four hepara

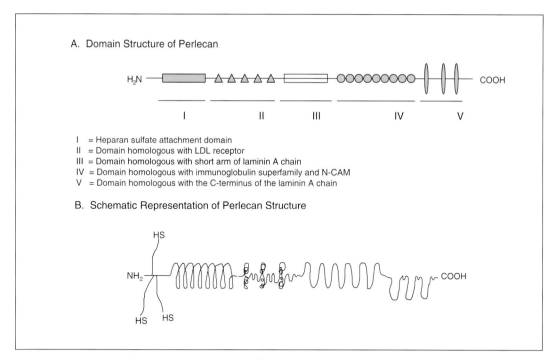

A. Domain Structure of Perlecan

I = Heparan sulfate attachment domain
II = Domain homologous with LDL receptor
III = Domain homologous with short arm of laminin A chain
IV = Domain homologous with immunoglobulin superfamily and N-CAM
V = Domain homologous with the C-terminus of the laminin A chain

B. Schematic Representation of Perlecan Structure

Fig 6-5 Schematic representation of perlecan. **(a)** shows the various domains of perlecan and **(b)** shows the likely structure of the intact molecule. HS, heparan sulfate.

sulfate chains are bound (Fig 6-5). This proteoglycan was originally identified as a basement membrane–specific proteoglycan where it formed aggregates with type IV collagen and laminin (Noonan et al 1991; Noonan and Hassell 1993). Perlecan derives its name from the numerous globular domains within its protein core that give it an appearance similar to a chain of pearls. At least five domains have been recognized within the core protein of perlecan that are associated with cell growth, cell-matrix signaling, and acting as molecular sieves. Domain I is unique to perlecan and provides perlecan with its individual character, domain II has an identity with the low-density lipoprotein receptor, domain III shares homology with the short arm of the laminin A chain, domain IV encodes a sequence with homology to the immunoglobulin superfamily and the neural cell adhesion molecule (N-CAM), and domain V has a sequence similar to the C-terminus of the A chain of laminin. More recently, perlecan has been found to be expressed by a wide variety of epithelial and mesenchymal cells (Iozzo et al 1994). The gene for human perlecan has been located to the telomeric region of chromosome 1 with the primer site most likely at the 1p36.1 band (Iozzo et al 1994). The gene is composed of 94 exons spanning some 120 kb of genomic DNA; it codes for the protein domains described above for the low-density lipoprotein receptor, laminin, epidermal growth factor, and the neural cell adhesion molecule. The gene has several transcription initiation sites, which is consistent with the lack of TATA and CAAT boxes, but several GC boxes with binding sites for the transcription factors SP1 and ETF (Cohen et al 1993).

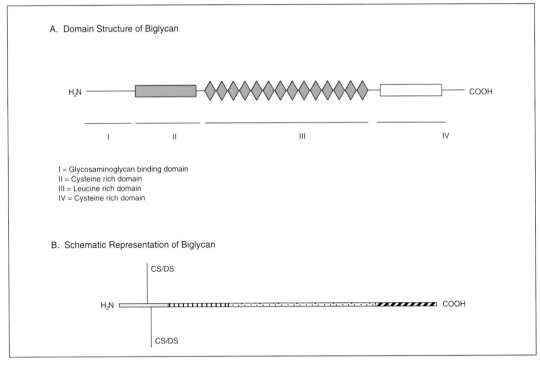

A. Domain Structure of Biglycan

H₂N — COOH

I   II   III   IV

I = Glycosaminoglycan binding domain
II = Cysteine rich domain
III = Leucine rich domain
IV = Cysteine rich domain

B. Schematic Representation of Biglycan

CS/DS

H₂N   COOH

CS/DS

Fig 6-6 Schematic representation of biglycan. **(a)** shows the various domains of biglycan and **(b)** shows the likely structure of the intact molecule. CS, chondroitin sulfate; DS, dermatan sulfate.

Small extracellular proteoglycans.

Leucine-rich interstitial proteoglycans. The leucine-rich interstitial proteoglycans are a group of small proteoglycans with core proteins of around 40 kd that share homologous leucine-rich core proteins. This group includes decorin, biglycan, fibromodulin, and lumican. Decorin and biglycan have relatively wide distributions throughout most tissues, while lumican and fibromodulin, which have similar core proteins but are substituted with keratan sulfate rather than dermatan sulfate, are found mainly in tendon and cartilage (fibromodulin), and in cornea and heart-valve tissues (lumican).

Biglycan (originally known as PGI, PG-S1, or DS-PG-1) has two sites where glycosaminoglycan chains may attach and has a core protein of approximately 45 kd (Fisher et al 1989) (Fig 6-6). This proteoglycan appears to have a propeptide sequence of approximately 18 amino acids that is subsequently cleaved. The glycosaminoglycan attachment site is at the N-terminus, which shows considerable interspecies variability. Following this domain is a small cysteine-rich region, followed by the well-conserved leucine-rich portion of the protein flanked by another cysteine-rich region, and a smaller less-homologous sequence toward the carboxyl terminus, which has a characteristic conserved disulfide loop (Kresse et al 1993). The human biglycan gene has been mapped to the long arm of the X chromosome at the Xq27 to Xq28 region (McBride et al 1990; Traupe et al 1992) and consists of eight exons, one of which encodes the 5′-untranslated region of the mRNA. The

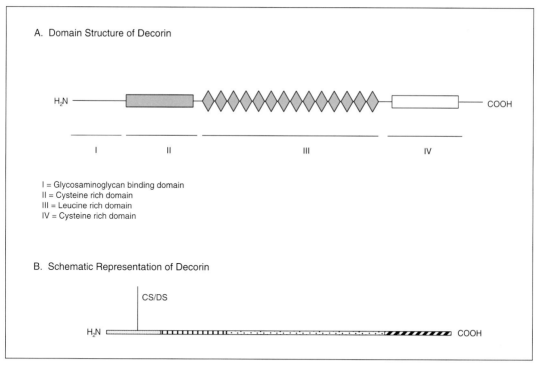

A. Domain Structure of Decorin

H₂N ——— COOH

I II III IV

I = Glycosaminoglycan binding domain
II = Cysteine rich domain
III = Leucine rich domain
IV = Cysteine rich domain

B. Schematic Representation of Decorin

CS/DS

H₂N COOH

Fig 6-7 Schematic representation of decorin. (a) shows the various domains of decorin and (b) shows the likely structure of the intact molecule. CS, chondroitin sulfate; DS, dermatan sulfate.

promoter for the biglycan gene does not have CAAT or TATA sequences, it is rich in GC content and contains five possible pregnancy specific B-1 glycoproteins (SPI) and one activator protein 2 (AP2) *trans*-acting factor–binding site consensus sequences (Fisher et al 1991). Biglycan is generally found in developing bone and cartilage, as well as in close association with cells such as keratinocytes and fibroblasts (Bianco et al 1990; Fisher et al 1991). While biglycan can bind some matrix molecules, it does not appear to bind to collagens; rather it is generally found close to cell surfaces and in the immediate pericellular environment. The expression of biglycan can be modulated by growth factors such as TGF-β1 and growth hormone.

Decorin has a similar size and structure to biglycan, except that it has only one site that can be substituted with a glycosaminoglycan chain (Fisher et al 1989; Fisher et al 1991) (Fig 6-7). Older names for decorin were proteoglycan II, PG-S2, and PG-40. The core protein of decorin is also leucine-rich and of a similar size and domain structure with respect to biglycan. As for biglycan, the protein core of decorin appears to be synthesized with a short (14 amino acids) propeptide sequence, which is subsequently cleaved, and has the glycosaminoglycan attachment site located near its N-terminus (Day et al 1987). The decorin gene appears to be similar to the biglycan gene, spanning more than 38 kb of DNA containing eight exons. Two alternatively spliced leader exons, called Ia and Ib, have been identified within the 5'-untranslated region (Danielson et al 1993; Santra et al 1994). The human decorin gene has been localized to the region of chromosome 12q23 (Danielson et al 1993). Ia contains two GC boxes, while the Ib promoter contains one CAAT and two TATA boxes near the transcription start site. Distinct from biglycan, decorin shows a strong association with collagen type I that appears to be mediated through the core protein rather than the glycosaminoglycan side chain. In soft tissues, decorin is localized to the d- or e-band of type I collagen. This localization is absent in bone and may implicate a role for decorin in the mineralization process. Decorin also interacts with other matrix molecules such as fibronectin and thrombospondin (Schmidt et al 1987; Winnemöller et al 1992).

Fibromodulin is a small, leucine-rich proteoglycan substituted with keratan sulfate chains. The amino acid sequence of bovine fibromodulin shows very close homology with both decorin and biglycan (Oldberg et al 1989). The sequence homology diverges at the amino terminus, which is the region of O-linked chondroitin sulfate or dermatan sulfate chain attachment in decorin and biglycan. In contrast, keratan sulfate chains that are N-linked to the fibromodulin core protein occur in the central, leucine-rich region (Plaas et al 1990). In addition to keratan sulfate chains, fibromodulin core protein may also be substituted with N-linked oligosaccharides. The fibromodulin gene has been localized to chromosome 1q32. As for decorin, fibromodulin binds to collagen types I and II, leading to delayed fibril formation (Hedbom and Heinegard 1989). The binding sites for fibromodulin to collagen differ from those for decorin, and appear to be limited to the a- and c-bands. Since both decorin and fibromodulin bind to collagen, yet have different glycosaminoglycan chains, such binding is mediated through the protein core.

Lumican is another small proteoglycan, originally found in the cornea, substituted with keratan sulfate chains. It has a molecular mass of about 38 kd (Blochberger et al 1992). The lumican gene has been mapped to the distal region of chromosome 10 (Funderburgh et al 1995). The core protein contains 338 amino acids synthesized from a 1.9-kb mRNA, and, compared to other small proteoglycans, shows the most homology with fibromodulin. The primary structure of lumican is similar to the other small leucine-rich proteoglycans decorin, biglycan, and fibromodulin. Lumican contains five potential N-glycosylation sites; four are located in the leucine-rich region. The glycosylation sites need not all be substituted with keratan sulfate, but may be substituted (as is fibromodulin) with N-linked oligosaccharides. As do other small leucine-rich proteoglycans, lumican interacts strongly with collagen.

Centoglycan (PG100) is a small proteoglycan synthesized by osteoblasts and fibroblasts (Bosse et al 1994). It is slightly larger than decorin and biglycan, with a core protein of approximately 78 kd, and substituted with N- and O-linked oligosaccharides as well as with a single chondroitin-6-sulfate chain for a total mass of approximately 100 kd (Bosse et al 1993). The biologic role of this proteoglycan has not been elucidated, although recent reports indicate that PG-100 is the proteoglycan form of the macrophage colony stimulating factor (CSF-1) (Partenheimer et al 1995).

Cell Surface Proteoglycans

Proteoglycans associated with cell membranes form a distinct class of structurally and functionally related molecules. Of these, the heparan sulfate–containing proteoglycans are the most prominent (Gallagher 1989; Yanagashita and Hascall 1992). Proteoglycans may be associated with cell membranes via three separate mechanisms: (1) as an integral membrane protein spanning the lipid bilayer, (2) partial insertion into the lipid bilayer of a phosphatidylinositol component of the proteoglycan, or (3) binding of a glycosaminoglycan side chain to specific plasma membrane

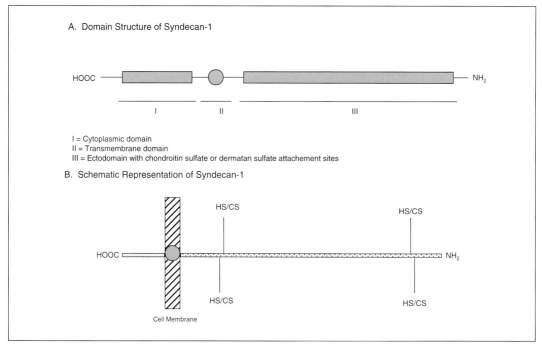

A. Domain Structure of Syndecan-1

I = Cytoplasmic domain
II = Transmembrane domain
III = Ectodomain with chondroitin sulfate or dermatan sulfate attachement sites

B. Schematic Representation of Syndecan-1

Fig 6-8 Schematic representation of syndecan-1. **(a)** shows the various domains of syndecan-1 and **(b)** shows the likely structure of the intact molecule. HS, heparan sulfate; CS, chondroitin sulfate.

receptors (Gallagher 1989). Given their strategic position on cell surfaces, these proteoglycans have been ascribed varied functions, most of which relate to cell-cell and cell-matrix interactions.

Syndecans. The syndecans are a family of related proteoglycans whose protein cores span the plasma membrane of mammalian cells (Bernfield et al 1992). These molecules have a unique protein core composed of both hydrophobic and hydrophilic domains; they may be substituted with heparan sulfate or chondroitin sulfate, or both (Fig 6-8). To date, four syndecans have been identified on the basis of their cDNA-derived amino acid sequence and named according to the order in which they were identified. They appear to come from a common ancestral protein; the location and nature of the GAG binding sites are relatively well-conserved. With respect to size and gly-

cosaminoglycan substitution and protein sequence, syndecan-1 and syndecan-3 show approximately 30% sequence homology, while syndecan-2 and syndecan-4 share around 38% sequence identity. While the transmembrane and cytoplasmic domains of the syndecan proteins are well-conserved across several species (including humans), the extracellular domains appear to show considerable divergence except for the glycosaminoglycan attachment sites (Bernfield et al 1992). In the mouse it appears that the genes for each of the four syndecans are located on different chromosomes (Spring et al 1994). The syndecan genes appear to be encoded by five exons, which are conserved in all family members (Goldberger et al 1993). A signal peptide is encoded by exon 1, exon 2 codes for the N-terminal glycosaminoglycan attachment sites, exon 3 codes for the bulk of the extracellular domain, exon 4 codes for the protease-susceptible sequence, and exon 5 codes for the transmembrane and cytoplasmic domains of the core protein. Three transcription start sites have been identified; the promoter portion contains both TATA and CAAT boxes and other potential binding sites for transcription factors such as SP1, nuclear factor (NF)-kappaB, and MyoD (E Box).

While most cells and tissues express multiple forms of these transmembrane proteoglycans, their expression is selectively regulated in cell-, tissue-, and development-specific manners (Kim et al 1994). The functions of the syndecans are reported to be quite varied. By virtue of their strategic location on the cell surface, many functions are related to cell-cell, cell adhesion, and cell-matrix interactions. Heparan sulfate chains may self aggregate or interact with growth factors, cytokines, extracellular matrix components, or protease inhibitors. In addition to these interactive functions, differential expression of various syndecans has been noted during different stages of development. For example, ryudocan and syndecan 1 are differentially expressed during development as well as during wound healing of blood vessels. The role of syndecanlike molecules in the binding of a variety of growth factors has recently been studied (see later section in this chapter).

Syndecan-1, first identified in mouse mammary epithelial cells (Saunders et al 1989), is considered the archetypal syndecan. Since its isolation, syndecan-1 has been found to be associated with a variety of cells including lymphocytes, embryonic dental mesenchyme, and embryonic lung mesenchyme. This proteoglycan has a core protein of approximately 30 kd with approximately five glycosaminoglycan attachment sites (both heparan sulfate and chondroitin sulfate). The gene for syndecan maps to human chromosome 2p23 (chromosome 12 in mouse) (Ala-Kapee et al 1990; Oettinger et al 1991). Syndecan-1 is both constitutively and developmentally regulated, and this may explain its morphogenetic,

rather than histologic, pattern of distribution during embryogenesis, in which it is closely associated with epithelial-mesenchymal interactions (Vainio 1991).

Syndecan-2 (also known as fibroglycan) was first isolated from the cell surface of fibroblasts and identified as a heparan sulfate–containing proteoglycan with a core protein of approximately 20 kd (Marynen et al 1989; David et al 1990). Almost simultaneously, an identical proteoglycan called fibroglycan was isolated from rat liver and cloned (Pierce et al 1992). Like syndecan-1, syndecan-2 can form large dimers or multimers. The gene for syndecan-2 maps to human chromosome 8q23 (chromosome 15 in the mouse). The cDNA for this proteoglycan encodes a protein of 211 amino acids, of which the deduced sequence indicates a 24–amino acid transmembrane domain, a 33–amino acid cytoplasmic domain, and a larger ectodomain that contains from three to five heparan sulfate chains (Pierce et al 1992). The gene for human fibroglycan appears to be located on chromosome 8q23 (Marynen et al 1989).

Syndecan-3 (also known as N-syndecan) was isolated simultaneously from both neural and cartilage tissues in 1992 (Carey et al 1992; Gould et al 1992) as a heparan sulfate proteoglycan with a 120-kd core protein. Like syndecan-1, this proteoglycan may also carry some chondroitin sulfate chains. Syndecan-3 shares several structural features common to syndecan-1 and fibroglycan, especially within the cytoplasmic and transmembrane domains. The extracellular domain of syndecan-3 differs quite substantially in both amino acid sequence and location of its eight to ten GAG attachment sites. The gene for syndecan-3 has been localized to chromosome 4 in the mouse (Spring et al 1994). Syndecan-3 is expressed in high amounts during chondrogenesis and in neonatal rat brain, heart and Schwann's cells.

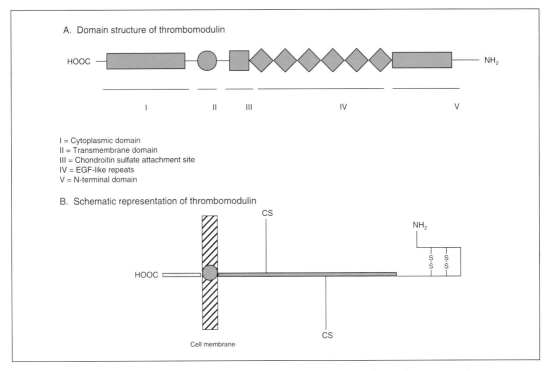

A. Domain structure of thrombomodulin

I = Cytoplasmic domain
II = Transmembrane domain
III = Chondroitin sulfate attachment site
IV = EGF-like repeats
V = N-terminal domain

B. Schematic representation of thrombomodulin

CS

NH₂

HOOC

CS

Cell membrane

Fig 6-9 Schematic representation of thrombomodulin. **(a)** shows the various domains of thrombomodulin and **(b)** shows the likely structure of the intact molecule. EGF, epidermal growth factor; CS, chondroitin sulfate.

Syndecan-4 is also known as ryudocan or amphiglycan. Ryudocan was first isolated from rat microvascular endothelial cells (Kojima et al 1992), and has since been identified as an important component of most endothelial cells. This molecule localizes specifically to the luminal surface of endothelial cells. Amphiglycan has been isolated from both epithelial cells and fibroblasts (David et al 1992), and has an amino acid sequence identical to that of ryudocan. These proteoglycans have three putative glycosaminoglycan (heparan sulfate) attachment sites, and a core protein of approximately 20 kd. The human ryudocan gene has been localized on chromosome 20q12 (Kojima et al 1993).

Thrombomodulin is a transmembrane protein that may be substituted with a single

chondroitin sulfate chain on its extracellular portion (Bourin et al 1990). This molecule has important anticoagulation properties that may be related to the protein core as well as to the single GAG (Bourin et al 1990; Bourin and Lindahl 1990; Bourin 1991). As with other intercalated proteoglycans, thrombomodulin has several domains (Fig 6-9). Its hydrophobic amino terminus forms a disulfide-bonded loop that is followed by a unique sequence of six EGF-like repeat sequences. Adjacent to this sequence there is a short region available for GAG attachment, followed by a transmembrane sequence, and a cytosolic portion at the carboxy terminus.

CD44 is a very broad class of transmembrane glycoproteins expressed on the cell surfaces of epithelial, mesenchymal, and hema-

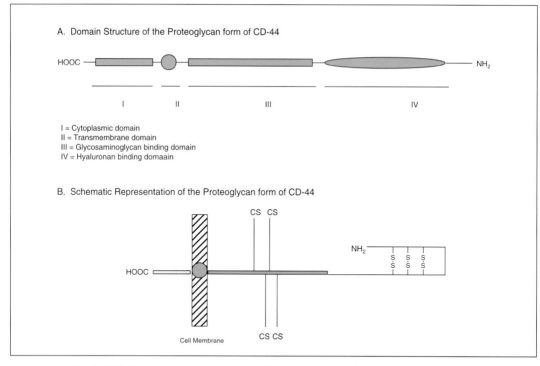

A. Domain Structure of the Proteoglycan form of CD-44

I = Cytoplasmic domain
II = Transmembrane domain
III = Glycosaminoglycan binding domain
IV = Hyaluronan binding domaain

B. Schematic Representation of the Proteoglycan form of CD-44

Fig 6-10 Schematic representation of the proteoglycan form of CD44. **(a)** shows the various domains of the proteoglycan form of CD44 and **(b)** shows the likely structure of the intact molecule. CS, chondroitin sulfate.

topoietic cells and can exist in both a proteoglycan (substituted with chondroitin sulfate, heparan sulfate, or both) or a nonproteoglycan form in which there is no GAG substitution. While CD44 is well recognized as important for lymphocyte homing, its function on epithelial cells and fibroblasts is not as clear, but it is presumed to be associated with cell adhesion and the binding of extracellular matrix components such as fibronectin, laminin, collagen, and hyaluronate. This molecule has several domains (Fig 6-10). A short cytoplasmic portion at the carboxy terminus is followed by a hydrophilic transmembrane domain. The ectodomain contains a region that contains the glycosaminoglycan attachment sites, as well as a domain capable of interacting with hyaluronan at the amino terminus.

Although derived from a single copy gene on chromosome 11, the CD44 family of molecules shows significant heterogeneity. Such heterogeneity is most likely associated with alternative mRNA splicing within the extracellular and cytoplasmic domains. Indeed, the multiple isoforms of CD44 appear to arise from one to ten alternatively spliced exons (v1–v10) inserted within the extracellular domain; the proteoglycan forms of CD44 are alternatively spliced variants containing the v3 exon (Jackson et al 1995). In addition, variable levels of glycosylation with respect to N- and O-linked oligosaccharides, as well as the addition of chondroitin sulfate and heparan sulfate, contribute to the heterogeneity of CD44.

Differences in the amino acid sequence of CD44 molecules associated with different cells have also been noted. For example, in epican, a form of CD44 expressed by keratinocytes, the core protein is approximately 150 kd and, compared to the leukocyte form of CD44, contains an additional novel sequence of between 130 and 339 amino acids inserted in its carboxy terminus in the ectodomain containing both CS and HS glycosaminoglycan chains (Brown et al 1991; Kugelman et al 1992).

Glypicans are a group of glycosylphosphatidylinositol (GPI)-anchored cell surface heparan sulfate proteoglycans (David et al 1990). To date, four members have been identified including glypican, K-glypican, cerebroglycan, and OCI-5 (Watanabe et al 1995). These proteoglycans are widely expressed by many different cells and are characterized by a similar core protein size of around 57.5 kd, potential attachment sites for heparan sulfate chains, and a GPI anchor located at its carboxyl terminal. The core protein of glypicans have highly conserved structural features that distinguish them from other cell surface proteoglycans. The human glypican gene has been located to the region of chromosome 2q35 to 2q37 (Vermeesch et al 1995). The function of these proteoglycans is unclear, but it has been proposed that they may play an important role in neural development and regulation of the cell cycle (Lander et al 1996).

Betaglycan, formerly known as the type III TGF-β receptor, is a membrane-anchored proteoglycan that binds TGF-β via its core protein (Andres et al 1989). This proteoglycan is found in most cells and tissues, but is particularly abundant in bone and osteoblastic cells. Betaglycan may exist in either a cell-membrane form or in a soluble form released into serum and extracellular matrices. Betaglycan has a protein core of around 100 to 120 kd and may be substituted with heparan sulfate, chondroitin sulfate, or both. As deduced from its cDNA sequence, the membrane form of betaglycan has an extracellular domain containing several potential sites for glycosaminoglycan attachment, a hydrophobic portion consistent with membrane intercalation, and a short cytoplasmic portion. The soluble form of betaglycan lacks both the transmembrane and cytoplasmic portions. The cell membrane form of betaglycan binds TGF-β and presents this growth factor directly to the kinase subunit of the signaling receptor (which has a limited ability to bind TGF-β), forming a high-affinity ternary complex and thereby enhancing the cell responsiveness to this growth factor (Lopez-Casillas et al 1993). The presence of glycosaminoglycan chains is not essential for TGF-β binding (Lopez-Casillas et al 1991). Betaglycan can also bind fibroblast growth factor, but this interaction differs from its TGF-β interaction in that this interaction occurs via the glycosaminoglycan chains rather than via the protein core (Andres et al 1992).

Proteoglycans of Hematopoietic Cells

For years it was assumed that only cells of mesenchymal or ectodermal origin had the capacity to synthesize, secrete, and express a variety of proteoglycans. With the development of more refined detection systems, it became apparent that proteoglycans were, indeed, ubiquitous to all mammalian cells (Kolset and Gallagher 1990). Of particular interest was a new breed of proteoglycan identified within hematopoietic cells. It was found in secretory granules and was distinct from those proteoglycans residing in the matrix or cell surface (Kolset and Gallagher 1990). This proteoglycan was subsequently named serglycin.

Serglycin, the major secretory granule proteoglycan identified to date, was first identified in mast cells and so named because of the unique large repeat sequence of serine and glycine residues in its protein core (Stephens 1987). Subsequently, these proteoglycans have been identified in the secretory granules of

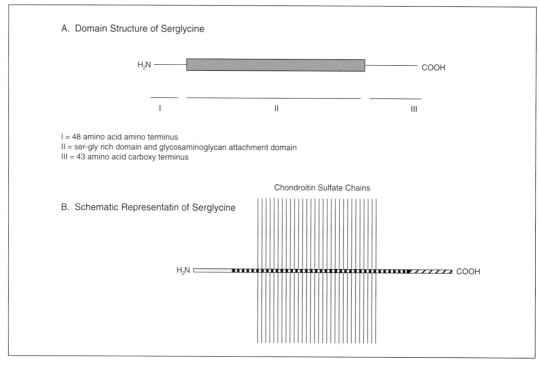

A. Domain Structure of Serglycine

H₂N ——————[   ]—————— COOH

I   II   III

I = 48 amino acid amino terminus
II = ser-gly rich domain and glycosaminoglycan attachment domain
III = 43 amino acid carboxy terminus

Chondroitin Sulfate Chains

B. Schematic Representatin of Serglycine

H₂N ▭ ▪▪▪▪▪▪▪▪▪▪▪▪▪▪▪▪▪▪▪▪▪▪▪▪▪▪▪▪▪▪▪▪▪▪▪▪▪▪ ▨▨▨ COOH

Fig 6-11 Schematic representation of serglycine. **(a)** shows the various domains of the serglycine and **(b)** shows the likely structure of the intact molecule. CS, chondroitin sulfate.

mast cells, basophils, neutrophils, platelets, lymphocytes, and natural killer cells. They are very resistant to protease attack, and are released in response to specific stimuli. The serglycin core protein associated with mucosal mast cells, basophils, natural killer cells, and platelets contains a cluster of chondroitin sulfate chains that often contain more than one ester sulfate per disaccharide. The connective tissue mast cell synthesizes a different form of serglycin in which the chondroitin sulfate chains are replaced with heparin. Therefore, although the protein cores of the secretory granule proteoglycans are well-conserved, the types of glycosaminoglycans attached are often quite divergent, varying in the type of hexosamine, location and amount of sulfation, and degree of iduronate epimerization. This indicates that the primary amino acid sequence of the protein core is not instrumental in determining the type of glycosaminoglycan substitution. The newly synthesized serglycin core protein contains a signal peptide of 25 amino acids that is rapidly removed to leave a nascent peptide chain of 153 amino acids containing a unique domain with 24 serine-glycine repeats between residues 89 and 137 (Avraham et al 1988). The Ser-Gly repeat sequence is the region for attachment of approximately 15 heparin or chondroitin sulfate chains (Fig 6-11). The human gene for serglycin has been characterized and consists of three exons and two introns spanning more than 16.7 kb (Humphries et al 1992). Exon 1, present at the 5′ region, encodes the 25–amino acid signal peptide. The second exon contains the N-terminal domain of 48 amino acids, and the third exon codes for a 79–amino acid sequence, which includes the Ser-Gly repeat sequence and the C-terminal chain of 43 amino acids. Similar to other proteoglycan genes, but unlike most eukaryotic genes, the secretory granule gene does not contain a TATA-box or GC-rich promoter region (Avraham et al 1989). The human gene has been localized to band q22.1 on chromosome 10 (Mattei et al 1989).

Due to the large number of glycosaminoglycan chains on a relatively short protein core, serglycin has the highest concentration of anionic groups of all the proteoglycans studied to date. While the functions of these molecules are still largely unknown, it has been speculated that they may be involved in enzyme packaging, or as mediators of cellular activity. Indeed, because of their high charge concentration, these proteoglycans may serve to interact with various cellular enzymes stored within the cells, and prevent their autolysis prior to release from the cell.

A number of other proteoglycans have been identified to be associated with the cells of the hematopoietic system. As discussed above, syndecans and CD44 form important proteoglycan components of the cell surfaces of all mammalian cells including hematopoietic cells. The invariant chain (Ii) of the Ia antigen on lymphocytes has been shown to be a proteoglycan (Sant et al 1985). This molecule differs significantly from most other plasma membrane proteoglycans. Instead of a carboxyl terminus located in the cytoplasm, the invariant chain has its N-terminus located in the cytoplasm and its glycosaminoglycan chains located extracellularly toward the carboxyl terminus. Another cell surface molecule associated with lymphocytes is the C1q inhibitor of complement (Ghebrehiwet et al 1982). This chondroitin sulfate membrane proteoglycan has properties similar to a proteoglycan (isolated from serum) that can bind the C1q subunit of complement (Silvestri et al 1981). A proteoglycan isolated from platelets also appears to be very similar to the proteoglycan form of the C1q inhibitor, and may be the source of this proteoglycan in serum (Okayama et al 1986).

Proteoglycan Functions

With the identification of numerous proteoglycan types and structures, it has become increasingly apparent that the structure of the proteoglycans is intimately related to their function within the tissues or cellular compartments they comprise. As for the classification of the proteoglycans, it is convenient to consider the functions of proteoglycans not as individual entities, but as groups of functions. For these reasons, the functions can be directly related to their broad classification.

The extracellular matrix proteoglycans and tissue-organizing proteoglycans are principally associated with conferring physicochemical properties to the tissues (Comper and Laurent 1978; Gallagher 1989; Scott 1992; Yanagashita 1993). The large proteoglycans, such as aggrecan and versican, are highly charged due to their high glycosaminoglycan content. This high net charge serves to maintain tissue hydration. In addition, by contributing to the overall structural scaffolding of the extracellular matrix, the glycosaminoglycan chains of the proteoglycans also help to exclude large molecules, yet allow lower molecular weight solutes to easily pass through the matrix. The smaller extracellular matrix proteoglycans, such as decorin and fibromodulin, serve important functions in binding to other matrix molecules such as collagens, serving either to aid fibrillogenesis or to act as bridging molecules between various tissue elements (Scott 1988).

The cell surface proteoglycans, such as the syndecans, thrombomodulin, and CD44, provide the necessary means for cells to attach to their matrix. In doing so, the cells are able to communicate with the matrix, providing important feedback to the cell regarding its immediate milieu (Wight et al 1992).

The intracellular proteoglycans of the hematopoietic cells, as discussed, are believed to be important in enzyme packaging in order to prevent nonspecific enzymatic activity or autolysis of the cell (Kolset and Gallagher 1990). In addition, the secretory granule proteoglycans may act as soluble mediators themselves. For example, a T-cell proteoglycan has been demonstrated to be mitogenic for B cells (Levitt and Olmstead 1986).

In recent years it has been recognized that many proteoglycans have the capacity to bind and regulate growth factor activity (Ruoslahti and Yamaguchi 1991; David et al 1995) (see Table 6-5). This important regulatory function provides an additional mechanism for cells to communicate with their environment, as well as to regulate growth factor and extracellular matrix expression through feedback loops. Of particular interest has been the role that both cell surface proteoglycans such as syndecan, and matrix proteoglycans such as decorin and betaglycan, play in growth factor modulation. All of these proteoglycans have the ability to bind and regulate growth factor activity as well as to act as an extracellular reservoir for these potent polypeptide messengers..

Summary

The proteoglycans form an extremely diverse group of molecules located intracellularly, on cell membranes, and within the extracellular matrix. The many functions of proteoglycans are related not only to their location, but also to their structure, in which both the protein core and glycosaminoglycan side chains play important roles. As the various proteoglycans become cloned and sequenced, further insights into their classifications will be made. In addition, the yet-to-be sequenced gene structures controlling glycosaminoglycan synthesis, chain elongation, and chain termination will provide additional important information regarding this diverse group of molecules. From the diverse functions noted to date, it is apparent that all proteoglycans fulfill a number of critical biologic needs of the cells and tissues in which they reside.

References

Ala-Kapee M, Nevanlinna H, Mali M, Jalkanen M, Schröder J. Localization of gene for human syndecan, an integral membrane proteoglycan and matrix receptor, to chromosome 2. Somat Cell Mol Genet 1990;16:501.

Andres JL, DeFalcis D, Noda M, Massague J. Binding of two growth factor families to separate domains of the proteoglycan betaglycan. J Biol Chem 1992;267:5927.

Andres JL, Stanley K, Cheifetz S, Massague J. Membrane-anchored and soluble forms of betaglycan, a polymorphic proteoglycan that binds transforming growth factor-β. J Cell Biol 1989;109:3137.

Avraham S, Austen KF, Nicodemus CF, Gartner MC, Stevens RL. Cloning and characterization of the mouse gene that encodes the peptide core of secretory granule proteoglycans and expression of this gene in transfected rat-1 fibroblasts. J Biol Chem 1989;264:16719.

Avraham S, Stevens RL, Gartner MC, Austen KF, Lalley PA, Weis JH. Isolation of a cDNA that encodes the peptide core of the secretory granule of rat basophilic leukemia-1 cells and assessment of its homology to the human analogue. J Biol Chem 1988;263:7292.

Baker JR, Cifonelli JA, Roden L. The linkage of corneal keratan sulfate to protein. Connect Tissue Res 1975;3:149.

Balazs EA. Guide to nomenclature. In: Balazs EA, ed. Chemistry and Molecular Biology of the Intercellular Matrix. New York: Academic Press; 1967;1:39.

Bernfield M, Kokenysi R, Kato M, et al. Biology of the syndecans: A family of transmembrane heparan sulfate proteoglycans. Annu Rev Cell Biol 1992;8:365.

Bianco P, Fisher LW, Young MF, Termine JD, Gehron Robey P. Expression of the two small proteoglycans biglycan and decorin in developing human skeletal and non skeletal tissues. J Histochem Cytochem 1990;38:1549.

Blochberger TC, Vergnes J-P, Hempel J, Hassell JR. cDNA to chick lumican (corneal keratan sulfate proteolgycan) reveals homology to the small interstitial proteoglycan gene family and expression in muscle and intestine. J Biol Chem 1992;267:347.

Bosse A, Kresse H, Schwarz K, Muller KM. Immunohistochemical characterization of the small proteoglycans decorin and proteoglycan-100 in heterotypic ossification. Calcif Tissue Int 1994;54:119.

Bosse A, Schwarz K, Vollmer E, Kresse H. Divergent and co-localization of the two small proteoglycans decorin and proteoglycan-100 in human skeletal tissues and tumors. J Histochem Cytochem 1993;41:13.

Bourin MC. Thrombomodulin: a new proteoglycan Structure-function relation. Ann Biol Clin (Paris) 1991 49:199.

Bourin MC, Lindahl U. Functional role of the polysaccharide component of rabbit thrombomodulin proteoglycan. Effects on the inactivatin of thrombin by antithrombin, cleavage of fibrinogen by thrombin and thrombin-catalysed activation of factor V. Biochem J 1990;270:419.

Bourin MC, Lundgren-Akerlund E, Lindahl U. Isolation and characterization of the glycosaminoglycan component of rabbit thrombomodulin proteoglycan. J Biol Chem 1990;265:15424.

Bray BA, Lieberman R, Meyer K. Structure of human skeletal keratosulfate: the linkage region. J Biol Chem 1967;242:3373.

Brown TA, Bouchard T, St John T, Carter WG. Human keratinocytes express a new CD44 core protein (CD44E) as a heparan sulfate intrinsic membrane proteoglycan with additional exons. J Cell Biol 191;113:207.

Carey DJ, Evans DM, Stahl RC, et al. Molecular cloning and characterization of N-syndecan, a novel transmembrane heparan sulafate proteoglycan. J Cell Biol 1992;117:191.

Cohen IR, Grässel S, Murdoch AD, Iozzo RV. Structural characterization of the complete perlecan gene and its promoter. Proc Natl Acad Sci USA 1993;90:10404.

Comper WD, Laurent TC. Physiological function of connective tissue polysaccharides. Physiol Rev 1978;58:255.

Danielson KG, Fazzio A, Cohen I, Cannizzaro LA, Eichstetter I, Iozzo RV. The human decorin gene: Intron-exon organization, discovery of two alternatively spliced exons in the 5' untranslated region, and mapping of the gene to chromosome 12q23. Genomics 1993;15:146.

David G, Daneels A, Duerr J, et al. Heparan sulfate proteoglycans. Essential co-factors in receptor-mediated processes with relevance to the biology of the vascular wall. Atherosclerosis 1995;118:S57.

David G, Lories V, Decock B, Marynen P, Cassiman JJ, Van den Bergh H. Molecular cloning of a phosphatidylinositol-anchored membrane heparan sulfate proteoglycan from human lung fibroblasts. J Cell Biol 1990;111:3165.

David G, van der Schueren B, Marynen P, Cassiman JJ, van den Berghe H. Molecular cloning of amphiglycan, a novel integral membrane heparan sulfate proteoglycan expressed by epithelial and fibroblastic cells. J Cell Biol 1992;118:961.

Day AA, McQuillan CI, Termine JD, Young MF. Molecular cloning and sequence analysis of the cDNA for small proteoglycan II of bovine bone. Biochem J 1987;248:801.

DeLuca S, Lohmander LS, Nilsson B, Hascall VC, Caplan AI. Proteoglycans from chick limb bud chondrocyte cultures. Keratan sulfate and oligosaccharides which contain mannose and sialic acid. J Biol Chem 1980;225:6077.

Doege KF, Garrison K, Coulter SN, Yamada Y. The structure of the rat aggrecan gene and preliminary characterization of its promoter. J Biol Chem 1994;269:29232.

Fisher LW, Heegard AM, Vetter U, et al. Human biglycan gene. Putative promoter, intron-exon junctions and chromosomal localization. J Biol Chem 1991;266:14371.

Fisher LW, Termine JD, Young MF. Deduced-protein sequence of bone small proteoglycan I (biglycan) shows homology with proteoglycan II (decorin) and several non-connective tissue proteins in a variety of species. J Biol Chem 1989;264:4571.

Fransson LA. Mammalian glycosaminoglycans. In: Aspinall GO, ed. The Polysaccharides. New York: Academic Press; 1985;3:337.

Funderburgh JL, Funderburgh ML, Hevelone ND, et al. Sequence, molecular properties and chromosomal mapping of mouse lumican. Invest Ophthalmol Vis Sci 1995;36:2296.

Gallagher JT. The extended family of proteoglycans: social residents of the pericellular zone. Curr Opin Cell Biol 1989;1:1201.

Ghebrehiwet B, Hamburger M. Purification and partial characterization of a C1q inhibitor from the membranes of human peripheral blood lymphocytes. J Immunol 1982;129:157.

Goldberger OA, Neumann PE, Kokenyesi R, Bernfield M. Organization and promoter activity of the mouse syndecan-1 gene. J Biol Chem 1993;268:11440.

Gould SE, Upholt WB, Kosher RA. Syndecan 3: A member of the syndecan family of membrane intercalated proteoglycans that is expressed in high amounts at the onset of chicken limb cartilage differentiation. Proc Natl Acad Sci USA 1992;89:3271.

Hardingham TE, Fosang AJ. Proteoglycans: many forms and many functions. FASEB J 1992;6:861.

Hascall VC. Proteoglycans: The chondroitin sulfate/keratan sulfate proteoglycan of cartilage. ISI Atlas of Science Biochemistry 1988;1:189.

Hascall VC, Heinegard DK, Wight TN. Proteoglycans: metabolism and pathology. In: Hay ED, ed. Cell Biology of the Extracellular Matrix. New York: Plenum Press; 1992;149.

Hassel JR, Kimura JH, Hascall VC. Proteoglycan core protein families. Annu Rev Biochem 1986;55:4920.

Hedbom E, Heinegard D. Interaction of a 59-kDa connective tissue matrix protein with collagen I and collagen II. J Biol Chem 1989;264:6898.

Hopwood JJ, Robinson HC. The alkali labile linkage between keratan sulphate and protein. Biochem J 1974;141:57.

Humphries DE, Nicodemus CF, Schiller V, Stevens RL. The human serglycin gene. Nucleotide sequence and methylation pattern in human promyelocytic leukemia HL-60 cells and T-lymphoblast Molt-4 cells. J Biol Chem 1992;267:13558.

Iozzo RV, Cohen IR, Grässel S, Murdoch AD. The biology of perlecan: the multifaceted heparan sulfate proteoglycan of basement membranes and pericellular matrices. Biochem J 1994;302:625.

Iozzo RV, Naso MF, Cannizzaro LA, Wasmuth JJ, McPherson JD. Mapping of the versican proteoglycan gene (CSPG2) to the long arm of human chromosome 5 (5q12-5q14). Genomics 1992;14:845.

Jackson DG, Bell JI, Dickinson R, Timans J, Shields J, Whittle N. Proteoglycan forms of the lymphocyte homing receptor CD44 are alternatively spliced variants containing the v3 exon. J Cell Biol 1995;128:673.

Jackson RL, Busch SJ, Cardin AD. Glycosaminoglycans: Molecular properties, protein interactions and role in physiological processes. Physiol Rev 1991;71:481.

Jeanloz RW. The nomenclature of mucopolysaccharides. Arthritis Rheum 1960;3:233

Just W, Klett C, Vetter U, Vogel W. Assignment of the human aggrecan gene AGC1 to 15q25–q 26.2 by in situ hybridization. Hum Genet 1993;92:516.

Kim CW, Goldberger OA, Gallo RL, Bernfield M. Members of the syndecan family of heparan sulfate proteoglycans are expressed in distinct cell-, tissue-, and development-specific patterns. Mol Biol Cell 1994;5:797.

Kojima T, Inazawa J, Takamatsu J, Rosenberg RD, Saito H. Human ryudocan core protein: Molecular cloning and characterization of the cDNA and chromosomal localization in the gene. Biochem Biophys Res Commun 1993;190:814.

Kojima T, Schworak NW, Rosenberg RD. Molecular cloning and expression of two distinct cDNA-encoding heparan sulfate proteoglycan core proteins from a rat endothelial cell line. J Biol Chem 1992;267:4870.

Kolset SO, Gallagher JT. Proteoglycans in haemopoietic cells. Biochim Biophys Acta 1990;1032:191.

Kresse H, Hausser H, Schönherr E. Small proteoglycans. Experientia 1993;49:403.

Kuettner KE, Kimura JH. Proteoglycans: An overview. J Cell Biochem 1985;27:327.

Kugelman LC, Ganguly S, Haggerty JG, Weissman SM, Milstone LM. The core protein of epican, a heparan sulfate proteoglycan on keratinocytes, is an alternative form of CD44. J Invest Dermatol 1992;99:381.

Lander AD, Stipp CS, Ivins JK. The glypican family of heparan sulfate proteoglycans—major cell surface proteoglycans of the developing nervous system. Perspect Dev Neurobiol 1996;3:347.

Laurent TC, Fraser JRE. Hyaluronan. FASEB J 1992; 6:2397.

Levitt D, Olmstead L. Stimulation of mouse B cells by a factor that coisolates with T-cell proteoglycan. Cell Immunol 1986;98:78.

Lindahl U, Roden L. Carbohydrate-peptide linkages in proteoglycans of animal, plant and bacterial origin. In: Gottschalk A, ed. Glycoproteins. Amsterdam: Elsevier; 1972:491.

Lohmander LS, DeLuca S, Nilsson B, et al. Oligosaccharides on proteoglycans from the Swarm rat chondrosarcoma. J Biol Chem 1980;255:6084.

Lopez-Casillas F, Cheifetz S, Doody J, Andres JL, Lane WS, Massague J. Structure and expression of the membrane proteoglycan betaglycan, a component of the TGF-β receptor system. Cell 1991;67:785.

Lopez-Casillas F, Wrana JL, Massague J. Betaglycan presents ligand to the TGFβ signalling receptor. Cell 1993; 73:1435.

Marynen P, Zhang J, Cassiman JJ, van den Berghe, David G. Partial primary structure of the 48- and 90-kilodalton core proteins of cell surface-associated heparan sulfate proteoglycans of lung fibroblasts. Prediction of an integral membrane domain and evidence for multiple distinct core proteins at the cell surface of human lung fibroblasts. J Biol Chem 1989;264:7017.

Mathews MB, Lozaityte I. Sodium chondroitin sulfate-protein complexes of cartilage. I. Molecular weight and shape. Arch Biochem Biophys 1958;74:158.

Mattei MG, Perin JP, Alliel PM, et al. Localization of human platelet proteoglycan gene to chromosome 10, band q22.1, by in situ hybridization. Hum Genet 1989; 82:87.

McBride OW, Fisher LW, Young MF. Localization of PG1 (biglycan BGN) and PGII (decorin DCN, PG-40) genes on human chromosomes Xq13-qter and 12q, respectively. Genomics 1990;6:219.

Meyer K. The chemistry and biology of mucopolysaccharides and glycoproteins. Cold Spring Harb Symp Quant Biol 1958;6:91.

Naso MF, Zimmermann DR, Iozzo RV. Characterization of the complete genomic structure of the human versican gene and functional analysis of its promoter. J Biol Chem 1994;269;1994.

Nilsson B, Nakazawa K, Hassell JR, Newsome DA, Hascall VC. Structure of oligosaccharides and the linkage region between keratan sulfate and the core protein on proteoglycans from monkey cornea. J Biol Chem 1983;258:6056.

Noonan DM, Fulle A, Valente P, et al. The complete sequence of perlecan, a basement membrane heparan sulfate proteoglycan reveals extensive similarity with laminin A chain, low density lipoprotein-receptor and the neural cell adhesion molecule. J Biol Chem 1991;266:22939.

Noonan DM, Hassell JR. Perlecan, the large low-density proteoglycan of basement membranes: Structure and variant forms. Kidney Int 1993;43:53.

Oettinger HF, Streeter H, Lose E, et al. Chromosome mapping of the murine mouse syndecan gene. Genomics 1991;11:334.

Okayama M, Oguri K, Fujiwara Y, et al. Purification and characterization of human platelet proteoglycan. Biochem J 1986;233:73.

Oldberg A, Antonsson P, Lindblom K, Heinegard D. A collagen-binding 59-kd protein (fibromodulin) is structurally related to the small interstitial proteoglycans PG-S1 and PG-S2 (decorin). EMBO J 1989;8:2601.

Partenheimer A, Schwarz K, Wrocklage C, Kolsch E, Kresse H. Proteoglycan form of colony-stimulating factor-1 (proteoglycan-100)—stimulation of activity by glycosaminoglycan removal and proteolytic processing. J Immunol 1995;155:5557.

Partridge SM, Davis HF, Adair GS. The constitution of the chondroitin sulphate-protein complex in cartilage. Biochem J 1961;79:15.

Perkins SJ, Nealis A, Dudhia J, Hardingham TE. Immunoglobulin fold and tandem repeat structures in proteoglycan N-terminal domains and link protein. J Mol Biol 1989;206:737.

Pierce A, Lyon M, Hampson IN, Cowling GJ, Gallagher JY. Molecular cloning of the major cell surface heparan sulfate proteoglycan from rat liver. J Biol Chem 1992; 267:3894.

Plass AHK, Neame PJ, Nivens CM, Reiss L. Identification of the keratan sulfate attachment sites on bovine fibromodulin. J Biol Chem 1990;265:20643.

Prehm P. Identification and regulation of the eucaryotic hyaluronate synthetase. In: The Biology of Hyaluronan, Ciba Foundation Symp 143. Chicester, England: Wiley; 1989;21.

Roden L. Structure and metabolism of connective tissue proteoglycans. In: Lennarz W, ed. The Biochemistry of Glycoproteins and Proteoglycans. New York: Plenum; 1980;267.

Ruoslahti E. Proteoglycans in cell recognition. J Biol Chem 1989;264:13369.

Ruoslahti E, Yamaguchi Y. Proteoglycans as modulators of growth factor activities. Cell 1991;64:867.

Sant AJ, Schwartz BD, Cullen SE. Cellular distribution of the Ia-associated chondroitin sulfate proteoglycan. J Immunol 1985;135:408.

Santra M, Danielson KG, Iozzo RV. Structural and functional characterization of the human decorin gene promoter. A homopurine-homopyrimidine S1 nuclease-sensitive region is involved in transcriptional control. J Biol Chem 1994;269:579.

Saunders S, Jalkanen M, O'Farrell S, Bernfield M. Molecular cloning of syndecan, an integral membrane proteoglycan. J Cell Biol 1989;108:1547.

Schmidt G, Robenek H, Harrach B, et al. Interaction of small dermatan sulfate proteoglycan from fibroblasts with fibronectin. J Cell Biol 1987;104:1683.

Scott JE. Proteoglycan fibrillar collagen interactions. Biochem J 1988;252:313.

Scott JE. Supramolecular organization of extracellular matrix glycosaminoglycans, in vitro and in the tissues. FASEB J 1992;6:2639.

Silvestri L, Baker JR, Roden L, Stroud RM. The C1q inhibitor in serum is a chondroitin 4-sulfate proteoglycan. J Biol Chem 1981;256:7383.

Spring J, Goldberger OA, Jenkins NA, Gilbert DJ, Copeland NG, Bernfield M. Mapping of the syndecan genes in the mouse: linkage with members of the myc gene family. Genomics 1994;21:597.

Stephens RL. Intracellular proteoglycans in cells of the immune system. In: Wight TN, Mecham R, eds. Biology of Proteoglycans. New York: Academic Press; 1987:367.

Thonar EJMA, Sweet MBE. An oligosaccharide component in proteoglycans of articular cartilage. Biochim Biophys Acta 1977;584:353.

Traupe H, van den Ouweland AMW, van Oost BA, et al. Fine mapping of the human biglycan (BGN) gene within the Xq28 region employing a hybrid cell panel. Genomics 1992;13:481.

Vainio S, Jalkanen M, Vaahtokari A, et al. Expression of syndecan gene is induced early, is transient, and correlates with changes in mesenchymal cell proliferation during tooth organogenesis. Dev Biol 1991;147:322.

Vermeesch JR, Mertens G, David G, Marynen P. Assignment of the human glypican gene (GPC1) to 2q35-q37 by fluorescence in situ hybridization. Genomics 1995;25:327.

Watanabe K, Yamada H, Yamaguchi Y. K-glypican—A novel GPI-anchored heparan sulfate proteoglycan that is highly expressed in developing brain and kidney. J Cell Biol 1995;130:1207.

Wight TN, Kinsella MG, Qwarnstrom EE. The role of proteoglycans in cell adhesion, migration and proliferation. Curr Opin Cell Biol 1992;4:793.

Winnemöller M, Schön P, Vischer P, Kresse H. Interactions between thrombospondin and the small proteoglycan decorin: interference with cell attachment. Eur J Cell Biol 1992;59:47.

Yanagashita M. Function of proteoglycans in the extracellular matarix. Acta Pathol Jpn 1993;43:283.

Yanagashita M, Hascall VC. Cell surface heparan sulfate proteoglycans. J Biol Chem 1992;267:9451.

Zimmermann DR, Ruoslahti E. Multiple domains of the large fibroblast proteoglycan, versican. EMBO J 1989; 8:2975.

Part III

Periodontal Connective Tissues

Developmental Aspects
of the Periodontium

Introduction

The periodontium is composed of four distinct tissues: gingiva, periodontal ligament, cementum, and bone. Together, these tissues are responsible for holding the tooth within its bony socket, and protecting the tooth root and adjacent structures from the external environment. No consideration of these tissues would be complete without discussion of their formation and development. Indeed, through understanding the development of tissues, the mechanisms required for inducing repair and regeneration of damaged tissues become better understood.

Development of Components of the Periodontium

General Concepts

Neural crest development. Tooth development is a very complex yet well-defined series of morphologic events driven by molecular processes that are only just beginning to be unraveled (Schroeder 1991; Ten Cate 1994; Marks 1995; Moxham and Berkovitz 1995). During the first 3 weeks of embryonic development there is rapid cell proliferation and migration. By about 8 days, cell differentiation has occurred and two distinct cell types are present, called endoderm and ectoderm, which form a bilaminar disc. By the third week, this bilaminar arrangement separates with the development of the mesoderm, which forms between the endoderm and ectoderm layers. During the next few weeks, the ectoderm thickens and forms raised margins to eventually form the neural folds, and ultimately the neural tube. As the neural crest develops, an important group of cells can be seen to differentiate at the lateral borders of the crest; these are neural crest cells. The neural crest cells are responsible for a large proportion of the embryonic connective tissues of the facial region. Indeed, most of the dental structures (dentin and cementum, but not enamel) and their supporting tissues (periodontal ligament and alveolar bone) are produced by cells originating in the neural crest. The enamel is produced from cells originating in the ectoderm.

Dental lamina. In humans, structures identifiable as the developing maxilla and mandible can be seen between the 28th and 40th days of gestation. These processes are lined with an epithelium consisting of a superficial layer of flattened cells and a basal layer of columnar cells that overlie a basement membrane. During the 6th week of embryogenesis, tooth development begins with a thickening of the oral epithelium lining the future dental arches to form the dental lamina. The dental lamina contains the immediate precursor of the ectodermal portion of teeth. Following development of the dental lamina, small areas of cellular coalescence occur that begin to invaginate into the underlying mesenchymal tissues to establish the earliest form of the future primary teeth. The initiation of such tooth de-

velopment appears to be directed by the subepithelial ectomesenchyme, which originates from the neural crest. The coordination of odontogenesis, morphogenesis, and differentiation of the various odontogenic cells occurs via well-controlled inductive molecular interactions that have their origins in the ectoderm (enamel organ) and ectomesenchyme (dental papilla and dental follicle).

The development of permanent teeth follows essentially the same pattern, originating from the dental lamina. For the incisors, canines, and premolars, the dental lamina is located on the lingual aspects of the developing deciduous teeth, whereas the permanent molars develop from the dental lamina forming from the lining epithelium in the posterior portion of the developing maxilla and mandible.

The early series of events for tooth development are usually divided into three identifiable morphologic stages called the bud, cap, and bell stages (Fig 7-1).

Bud stage. The bud stage of tooth development is the stage at which portions of the epithelium in the dental lamina first begin to aggregate and form an invagination into the underlying connective tissue.

Cap stage. With time, the epithelium continues to proliferate forming a parabolic- or cap-like structure. By this stage, the enamel organ is in its earliest stage of development. Immediately underneath the epithelial cap, the mesenchymal cells begin to proliferate and form the dental papilla, which will ultimately give rise to the dentin and dental pulp. The cells from the dental papilla continue to proliferate and begin to encapsulate the enamel organ to form the dental follicle from which the root cementum, periodontal ligament, and alveolar bone will eventually develop.

Bell stage. Following the cap stage of development, the enamel organ continues to enlarge and takes on a bell-shaped appearance

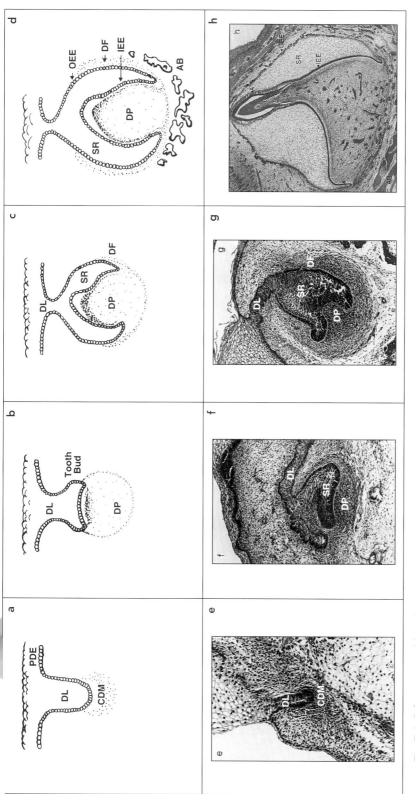

Fig 7-1 Schematic and histologic representation of the stages of tooth development. (**a** and **b**) Dental lamina stage of development shows that initiation of tooth development is characterized by thickening of the presumptive dental epithelium and subsequent condensation of the underlying mesenchyme. The histologic section (e) was stained with hematoxylin and eosin (original magnification 200×). (**c** and **d**) Bud stage of development is characterized by the identification of a tooth bud and underlying dental papilla. The histologic section (f) was stained with hematoxylin and eosin (original magnification 100×). (**e** and **f**) Cap stage demonstrates that the shape of the crown is now being determined. The histologic section (g) was stained with hematoxylin and eosin (original magnification 100×). (**g** and **h**) Bell stage demonstrates that crown formation continues during this stage. The histologic section (h) was stained with hematoxylin and eosin (original magnification 40×). PDE, presumptive dental epithelium; CDM, condensed dental mesenchyme; SR, stellate reticulum; DP, dental papilla; DF, dental follicle; DL, dental lamina; IEE, inner enamel epithelium; OEE, outer enamel epithelium: AB, alveolar bone.

By this stage, the enamel organ contains four types of cells. These are the outer enamel epithelium, which forms the outermost portion of the enamel organ; the inner enamel epithelium, which lines the innermost portion of the enamel organ and will eventually differentiate into the enamel, forming cells known as ameloblasts; the stratum intermedium, which is adjacent to the inner enamel epithelium; and the stellate reticulum, which lies between the stratum intermedium and the outer enamel epithelium. At the bell stage, the cells that comprise the dental lamina and form the link between the oral epithelium and the developing tooth bud begin to desegregate and this leads to the developing tooth being fully submerged below the oral epithelium.

Crown formation commences once the bell stage of development has been completed. Dentin is deposited by odontoblasts and provides a matrix for ameloblasts to further differentiate into secretory cells capable of producing the enamel matrix. Once the formation of enamel and dentin has neared completion at the site of the future cementoenamel junction, root formation commences with the continuing downward proliferation of epithelial cells of the enamel organ to form the Hertwig's epithelial root sheath (Thomas 1995). As for enamel formation, it seems that dentin deposition precedes cementum deposition.

Cementum Development

Cementum is the hard tissue that covers the root surface and serves two important functions. Through the insertion of Sharpey's fibers, cementum provides an anchorage mechanism between the tooth root and periodontal ligament. In addition, the thin cementum coating of root surfaces serves to protect the pulp by providing a surface covering the relatively porous dentin structures.

After completion of crown formation, the cells of the inner and outer enamel epithelium form the bilayer of cells known as Hertwig's

epithelial root sheath (Fig 7-2). This band of cells serves to separate the cells comprising the dental papilla and dental follicle. The cells of the inner enamel epithelium induce adjacent cells in the dental papilla to differentiate into odontoblasts and subsequently deposit the root dentin.

The genesis of cementum varies between rodents and humans. In rats, Hertwig's epithelial root sheath covers newly formed predentin, and this must first be fragmented before the surrounding connective tissue cells can penetrate the sheath and differentiate into cementoblasts (Cho and Garant 1989; Yamomoto and Wakita 1990). In humans, however, the Hertwig's sheath, which consists of former inner and outer layers of enamel epithelium, is disintegrated, and it does not cover much of the external surface of newly formed predentin. Therefore, the advancing root edge in humans is accessible to cementum-forming (dental follicle) cells from the beginning of root formation (Schroeder 1992).

Despite these differences, in both primates and rodents, a fine layer of epithelial matrix (hyaline layer) is deposited upon the newly formed dentin surface by the overlying epithelial cells (Lindskog 1982; Slavkin et al 1988). Following the fragmentation of the Hertwig's epithelial root sheath, cells from the dental follicle can be seen to attach and align onto the matrix coating the dentin surface, and these subsequently differentiate into cementoblasts and form the root cementum (Hammarström et al 1996). In rats, dental follicle cells are believed to form the cementum, and dentin mineralization appears to influence the formation of acellular cementum in these animals (Alatli-Burt et al 1994). These cells first form compartments with cellular processes that demarcate intrinsic collagen fibers that are parallel to the long axis of the root surface. Extrinsic fibers are formed later. The extracellular compartments appear to regulate the architecture of the principal fibers, and they are also necessary for the formation of intrinsic-extrinsic fiber structure

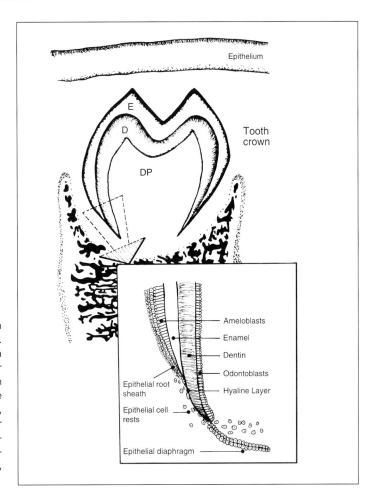

Fig 7-2 Schematic representation of root and cementum formation. Following completion of crown formation, the cells of the outer and inner enamel epithelium form the bilayer of cells known as the Hertwig's epithelial root sheath, which lays down the precursor matrix necessary for root formation via dentin and cementum deposition. E, enamel; D, dentin; DP, dental papilla.

(Yamomoto et al 1994; Yamamoto and Hinrichsen 1993). Once cementum is formed, the cells retract their processes and form intrinsic fibers around the principal fibers (Yamamoto and Hinrichsen 1993).

The fragmented epithelial cells of the Hertwig's epithelial root sheath never completely disappear from the periodontal environment and persist in small clusters known as epithelial cell rests of Malassez; the function of these cells is, at present, still speculative.

Cementum may be deposited on the root surface either during tooth development, or subsequent to eruption of the tooth during normal function. The cells responsible for cementum formation may be cementoblasts, ce-

mentocytes, or fibroblasts located within the periodontal ligament—all of these cells have their origin in the cells of the dental follicle. Cementoblasts are the primary source of cementum during both development and later posteruption function (Schroeder 1992, Bosshardt and Schroeder 1996). These cells are located in close apposition to the cementum surface, they have an appearance typical of a cell active in matrix production, and they strongly resemble osteoblasts. Cementocytes (like osteocytes) are located within the mineralized matrix of cementum, and, like their counterpart in bone (osteocytes), have a slightly lower level of matrix synthesis. The role of fibroblasts in cementogenesis is less clear.

Nonetheless, populations of mesenchymal cells within the periodontal ligament form a pool of cells that have the potential to differentiate into either periodontal ligament fibroblasts or cementoblasts, depending upon their location and exposure to inductive agents.

To date, five major types of cementum have been identified and classified according to their cellular and fiber content (Schroeder 1992). These classes of cementum include acellular afibrillar cementum (AAC), acellular extrinsic fiber cementum (AEFC), cellular intrinsic fiber cementum (CIFC), acellular intrinsic fiber cementum (AIFC), and cellular mixed stratified cementum (CMSC) (see also Chapter 8).

Acellular afibrillar cementum (AAC) is generally found deposited on mature enamel surfaces. It may be deposited during tooth formation, during tooth eruption, or possibly after tooth eruption, and can only be distinguished by its electron-microscopic appearance. At the light-microscopic level, AAC cannot be distinguished from other forms of cementum that might contain collagenous fibers. Acellular afibrillar cementum classically appears as cementum spurs or cementum islands on the crowns of erupted teeth. While uncommon in humans, AAC deposition on enamel surfaces is normal in many herbivores. This type of cementum is probably of little functional significance because it is not involved in fiber insertion and tooth anchorage. Rather, it most likely represents an aberration of the development process in which part of the reduced enamel epithelium disaggregates and allows cells from the dental follicle to interact with the exposed enamel matrix, leading to cementum deposition. Interestingly, this process lends additional support to the thesis that enamel matrix components are important in the induction of cementum.

Acellular extrinsic fiber cementum (AEFC) contains densely packed collagen fibers that project in a perpendicular manner from the cementum matrix into the periodontal ligament. This type of cementum forms on newly synthesized dentin surfaces after dissolution of the Hertwig's epithelial root sheath and subsequent exposure of the root surface to cells of the dental follicle. It is made by a particular class of fibroblasts that are alkaline phosphatase positive (Groeneveld et al 1994). These cells produce the first AEFC matrix as small bundles of collagen fibrils that increase in length and density in the apicocoronal direction. The fibers eventually are parallel to each other and perpendicular to the root surface, forming a fiber fringe. These fibers terminate and intermingle with the fibers of the dentinal matrix. As the density and diameter of the fiber bundles increase, cytoplasmic extensions that surround the fibers retract and the fiber bundles coalesce to form thicker fibers. In this type of cementum, mineralization starts as isolated patches. As soon as the first fiber fringe reaches maximum density, the external mineralization front approaches the zone of interdigitation of the fringe fibers and the dentin matrix, and the base of the fiber fringe begins to mineralize. The fiber fringe elongates along with the advancement of the mineralization front, which eventually becomes smooth and stabilized. The fiber fringe later becomes connected to the principal fibers. The AEFC fibers increase in thickness with age, and the rate and extent of thickening vary in different teeth (Sequeira et al 1992), and new fibril segments are added to preexisting collagen fibers (Bosshardt and Schroeder 1993). This type of cementum is usually located on the coronal one third of the root surface.

Cellular mixed fiber cementum (CMFC) contains both collagen fibers and calcified matrix and appears to be synthesized solely by cementoblasts. As its name suggests, this type of cementum contains a mixture of collagen fibers. A distinct feature is the presence of intrinsic collagen fibers produced by the cementoblasts that run parallel to the root surface. In addition to these intrinsic fibers, some extrinsic Sharpey's fibers may be seen in this type of cementum. Thus, cellular mixed fiber cementum consists of AEFC and CIFC that alternate and appear to be deposited in irregular sequence upon one another (Schroeder 1993). The CIFC frequently appears as the first layer of CMSC, and it forms first on newly produced dentin when the advancing root edge reaches the apical region. CIFC forms faster than AEFC, and its formation, matrix production, and attachment to dentin occur along a very short zone extending coronally from the advancing root edge. It is produced by cementoblasts. First, basophilic RER-rich (pre)cementoblasts form numerous, randomly oriented, fingerlike cytoplasmic processes extending into the matrix (Bosshardt and Schroeder 1992). The collagen fibers in the matrix gradually thicken in a coronal direction and the cementoblasts withdraw. Coronal to the precementoblasts is a region of rapid matrix production, and mature cementoblasts become embedded in this CIFC matrix and compartmentalize the collagen fibrils. The CIFC rapidly increases in thickness and cementoblasts may become cementocytes; human CIFC formation involves multipolar and unipolar cementoblasts responsible for rapid and slow matrix development. These cells do not form Sharpey's fibers. AEFC may also be formed on top of already laid CIFC/AIFC. In both AEFC and CIFC, newly formed cementum matrix attaches to the outer layer of still-nonmineralized dentin as the tooth erupts and attachment progresses in the coronal direction. Attachment involves interdigitation of collagen fibrils with those of the dentin matrix, and the attachment is secured by mineralization. In contrast to humans, in rodents, CIFC cells are the Hertwig's epithelial root sheath trapped between dentin and new cementum, and cementum and Sharpey's fibers are formed simultaneously (Yamamoto and Wakita 1991). This cementum is usually deposited on the root surfaces lining furcations, and eventually extends to cover most of the apical portion of the roots.

Cellular intrinsic fiber cementum (CIFC) is, in addition to being a component of cellular mixed stratified cementum, also considered to be a form of reparative cementum. This type of cementum is commonly associated with the repair of resorptive defects and the healing of root fractures. The principal cell involved in the synthesis of this type of cementum is the cementoblast, which produces both a fibrous and mineralized matrix, and does not demonstrate any evidence of extrinsic fiber insertion in the form of Sharpey's fibers.

Acellular intrinsic fiber cementum (AIFC) is an acellular variant of cellular intrinsic fiber cementum that is also deposited during adaptive responses to external forces, and that forms without leaving cells behind (Bosshardt and Schroeder 1990).

The identification of different types of cementum has significant ramifications with respect to periodontal regeneration because the ultimate goal of regenerative procedures is to induce the production of both acellular extrinsic fiber cementum and cellular mixed fiber cementum (Schroeder 1992). In many instances, attempts at periodontal regeneration have resulted in the formation of cellular intrinsic fiber cementum (reparative cementum), which does not have the functional integrity of cementum containing the extrinsic Sharpey's fibers.

During cementogenesis, cementum contains abundant osteopontin, bone sialoprotein, and osteocalcin as prominent noncollagenous proteins in the acellular and cellular cementum, as well as the Sharpey's fibers. Osteopontin is also found in the lacunae of cementoblasts and cementocytes. In acellular cementum, osteopontin is present throughout the granular matrix. It is dispersed among collagen fibrils, present at mineralization fronts, and it appears to coat collagen fibers of the periodontal ligament and those on the cement line. In cellular cementum, osteopontin is present amongst the collagen fibers and mineralized regions of Sharpey's fibers. Osteopontin is prominent in intrinsic fiber cementum and at ligament insertion sites. Bone sialoprotein is also associated with Sharpey's fibers; it is present at sites of calcification, including the cementum matrix along the mineralization front (McKee et al 1996; McKee and Nanci 1996).

Periodontal Ligament Development

The periodontal ligament spans the space between the root surface and alveolar bone. It is a fibrous connective tissue produced mainly by fibroblasts, with minor contributions from vascular and neurologic components. Periodontal ligament fibroblasts have their origins in the dental follicle and begin to differentiate during root development (Ten Cate et al 1971). With continuing apical development of the root, the cells of the dental follicle differentiate into cementoblasts to form the cementum lining of the root surface, and this subsequently leads to the appearance of periodontal ligament fibroblasts and the formation of the periodontal ligament (see Fig 7-2). All of these developmental processes occur prior to eruption of the tooth (Grant and Bernick 1972).

While the gross developmental aspects of the periodontal ligament are similar for most teeth, subtle differences do exist between primary teeth and teeth that do not have primary precursors, such as permanent molars in the marmoset and in human dentition (Grant et al 1972). These differences are due largely to the stage at which alveolar bone is formed. In the development of primary teeth and permanent molars, the tooth crown emerges through the alveolar bone. For secondary teeth, which develop within a bony crypt lingual to the primary teeth, alveolar bone must first be deposited on the crypt lining prior to development of the periodontal ligament fibers. Once the alveolar bone is deposited, then ligament formation may proceed during the pre-eruptive and eruptive phases in a manner similar to primary teeth and to permanent teeth that have no precursor. However, some exceptions to this generalization are evident for different species, as well as for different teeth within the same species. For example, the timing at which the fibers appear to completely span the ligament space from cementum to bone surface is variable. Such inconsistencies highlight the complexity of the development process and indicate the need for further detailed studies.

The orientation of the early periodontal ligament formed prior to eruption is dramatically different from its final form (Fig 7-3) (Levy and Bernick 1968). Initially, the fibers become embedded in the cementum as Sharpey's fibers and are laid down in a coronal direction within the region identified as the developing periodontal ligament, giving them an orientation almost parallel to the root surface. Fiber formation and deposition occur sequentially from the newly forming cementoenamel junction (CEJ) to the apex of the tooth root. The first fibers to be deposited ultimately become the dentogingival and transseptal fibers of the gingiva, while those fibers deposited apical to the CEJ ultimately form the fibers of the periodontal ligament. By the time approximately one third of the root formation is complete, fibers are inserted within a cementum matrix from the CEJ and traverse in a coronal direction, following the outline of the newly formed crown. At this early stage, no insertion of collagen fibers into the bone adjacent to the CEJ is noted. Fiber deposition and insertion continue along the developing root surface in a loosely arranged fashion, initially oriented parallel to the root surface. Fiber insertion also occurs along the lining of the bony socket wall opposite the developing root surface. These fibers traverse the ligament space in a similar superior oblique arrangement to the fibers originating from the root surface. Both the root surface–derived and bone-derived fibers ultimately coalesce in the middle third of the ligament space to form the intermediate plexus.

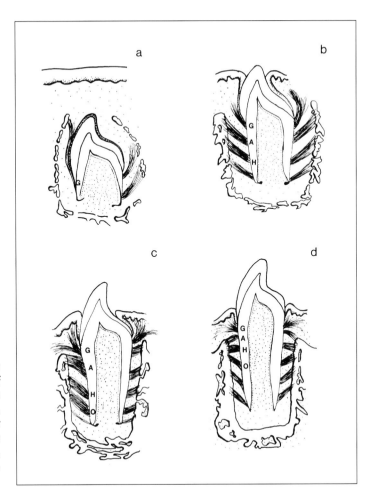

Fig 7-3 Schematic representation of the sequential organization of the periodontal ligament fibers in developing marmoset teeth. G, free gingival fibers; A, alveolar crest fibers; H, horizontal fibers; O, oblique fibers. (From: Levy BM, Bernick S. J Dent Res 1968;47:27. Reproduced with permission.)

As the teeth begin to erupt, the orientation of the ligament fibers changes according to the stage of eruption (Grant and Bernick 1972). It is also possible that fiber orientation is influenced by the positional relationship of the erupting tooth to the adjacent teeth. The dentogingival fibers continue to align from the CEJ in an occlusal direction, terminating in the connective tissue of the gingiva. The transseptal fibers extend from the root surface in an oblique direction, over the alveolar crest toward the surface of the adjacent developing tooth root. In the cervical one third of the root surface of an emerging tooth, the fibers are arranged in an oblique manner running in an apico-occlusal direction from the cementum to the alveolar bone. Fibers in the middle third become more defined, although no direct connection can be seen between fibers originating from the bone and those originating from cementum surfaces. In the apical portion, where root formation is still being completed, the fiber arrangement is still poorly developed and similar to the arrangement in the pre-eruptive phase of tooth development.

Once the tooth is fully erupted, and in functional occlusal contact, the ligament fibers adopt their final arrangements. The dentogingival, transseptal, and alveolar crest fibers emanate from the CEJ. Below the crestal fibers, and within the coronal one third of the root surface, the fibers have a horizontal orientation. In the middle third of the root, the fibers have an oblique orientation, running in an occlusal direction from the cementum surface to the alveolar bone. While in the apical third, the fiber arrangement remains oblique but runs in an apical direction from the cementum surface to the alveolar bone.

Alveolar Bone Development

Teeth are located within bony sockets in the alveolar processes of the maxilla and mandible. The alveolar process consists of several different compartments that make the unit functional. The thin lamella of bone that lines the tooth socket wall and contains inserting Sharpey's fibers is known as the alveolar bone. A thicker outer layer of bone, lining the lingual and labial surfaces of the alveolar process, surrounds the alveolar bone and comprises cortical plates and spongy bone, which is located in the region between the labial and lingual cortical plates. The alveolar bone has been defined as bundle bone (Schroeder 1992). This type of bone contains several layers of bone deposited in an orientation parallel to the tooth socket wall, which has bundles of collagen (Sharpey's fibers) emanating from it at right angles.

The alveolar bone (ie, the portion of the alveolar process that lines the tooth socket) is formed during root development and is derived from cells (osteoblasts) originating in the dental follicle. Its development is independent of other portions of the alveolar process and is intimately associated with the presence and development of teeth, and the subsequent development of the periodontal attachment apparatus. Primary teeth, and permanent teeth that do not have any precursor tooth, develop alveolar bone around their roots during development and subsequent eruption (Fig 7-4). Initially, the succedaneous tooth germs are located within the same osseous cavity as their deciduous precursors. However, as the deciduous teeth erupt, alveo-

lar bone is deposited around the developing roots and serves to separate the erupting deciduous tooth from the crown of the underlying developing succedaneous tooth. Thus, the developing succedaneous teeth become encased within their own bony crypt, located lingual and apical to the primary tooth in the basal bone of the alveolar process. During the eruption of a succedaneous tooth, the walls of the bony crypt, the roots of the superficial primary tooth, and the alveolar bone housing the primary tooth are all resorbed. With the loss of the primary tooth, the succedaneous tooth moves into the vacated area, and only then is new alveolar bone deposited around the erupting succedaneous tooth to accommodate its new position and anatomy. With the emergence of succedaneous teeth, the alveolar bone of the maxilla and mandible also remodel, leading to increases in facial length. Hence, with the emergence of succedaneous teeth, there is a complete deposition of new alveolar bone and significant remodeling of the whole alveolar process.

Development of Gingival Tissues

The gingival tissues are composed of a superficial epithelium of ectodermal origin and an underlying connective tissue of mesodermal origin. Both of these tissues appear to have components that derive from both the oral mucosa and from the developing tooth germ (Listgarten 1972; Mackenzie 1988).

The epithelium of the gingival tissues is composed of the nonkeratinized junctional epithelium, which originates from the enamel organ, together with the nonkeratinized sulcular epithelium and the keratinized gingival epithelium, which originates from the oral mucosa. The gingival connective tissue is largely a fibrous connective tissue that has elements originating directly from the oral mucosa connective tissues, as well as some fibers (dentogingival) that originate from the developing dental follicle (Fig 7-5).

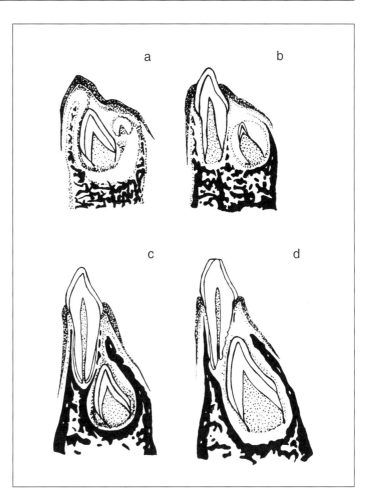

Fig 7-4 Schematic representation of the relationship between a deciduous tooth and its accompanying succedaneous tooth detailing the formation of the alveolar bone portion of the periodontium (adapted from Scott and Symons 1974). **a** At birth, both the deciduous incisor and the tooth germ for its permanent successor share the same alveolus and follicle. **b** At about 7 months, the deciduous incisor erupts into the oral cavity and a separate follicle begins to form around the associated permanent successor. **c** By 2½ years, the incisor is fully erupted and is encased in its own bony socket. The forming permanent successor is contained in a fully formed crypt. **d** By 7 years, the permanent successor begins to erupt and is accompanied by resorption of the bone forming the roof of its crypt and the root of the deciduous incisor.

The gingival tissues (both epithelial and connective tissue) associate with the tooth via separate mechanisms. The epithelial tissues interface with the tooth via an epithelial attachment called the junctional epithelium, which, in health, is usually located at, or coronal to, the CEJ. The gingival tissues attach to the root surface at or below the CEJ via fiber insertion into the cementum of the root surface, which lies coronal to the alveolar crest.

The development of the epithelial attachment to teeth follows a well-defined series of events (see Fig 7-5). Prior to eruption of the tooth, the enamel of the fully formed crown is covered with a few layers of flattened cuboidal cells (originating from ameloblasts and cells of the stratum intermedium of the enamel organ), called the reduced enamel epithelium. The reduced enamel epithelium completely encapsulates the newly formed crown and terminates (usually) at the CEJ. At this early stage, the epithelial attachment to the crown surface is via hemidesmosomes. As the tooth begins to erupt, the reduced enamel epithelium covering the tip of the crown or cusp fuses with the oral epithelium, and shortly afterward, degenerates to result in the first exposure of the crown to the oral cavity. The first evidence of the junctional epithelium is seen upon crown exposure. This epithelium extends a short way apically along the crown surface and then merges into the reduced

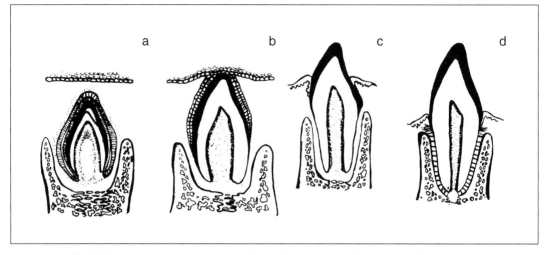

Fig 7-5 Schematic representation of the development of the gingival tissues. **(a)** The developing crown is submerged underneath the oral epithelium. **(b)** With the commencement of root formation, tooth eruption commences. Early fusion between the reduced enamel epithelium and the oral epithelium is seen. **(c)** Root formation and eruption continue with clear fusion between the reduced enamel epithelium and the oral epithelium. **(d)** The tooth is now fully erupted with root formation completed. The gingival tissues seem to have arisen from the oral epithelium, while the junctional epithelium seems to have been derived from the reduced enamel epithelium.

enamel epithelium covering the bulk of the submerged crown surface. As the tooth continues to erupt, the conversion of the reduced enamel epithelium into junctional epithelium continues. The conversion process involves the cells derived from both the ameloblasts and the stratum intermedium. Once enamel formation is complete, the reduced ameloblasts attach via hemidesmosomes to a basal lamina that covers the crown surface, referred to as the internal basal lamina of the reduced enamel epithelium. This basal lamina extends apically to the CEJ, where it then loops back to form an interface (external basal lamina) between the reduced enamel epithelium and the connective tissue of the mucosa that surrounds the entire crown. The cuboidal cells derived from the ameloblasts begin to flatten and elongate, aligning themselves parallel to the crown surface, and begin to take on an appearance similar to that of junctional epithelial cells. These cells (postsecretory ameloblasts) have lost all capacity to divide, and, thus, are eventually exfoliated at the bottom of the developing gingival sulcus. The gingival sulcus begins to form as the tooth erupts, and a separation occurs between the attached epithelium and the tooth surface. Simultaneously, the epithelial cells derived from the stratum intermedium (which are adjacent to the basement membrane) also begin to transform into cells with the appearance of junctional epithelium. However, distinct from the cells derived from the ameloblasts, the cells originating from the stratum intermedium resume their proliferative activity. The future basal cells of the junctional epithelium arise through the proliferative activity of these cells. The newly formed daughter cells migrate coronally toward the base of the gingival sulcus where they are eventually exfoliated, and thus allow the junctional epithelium to maintain its structure via a constant renewal process.

Epithelial-Mesenchymal Tissue Interactions

General Features

Both tissue morphology and phenotype are controlled by a complex interplay between tissues of ectodermal and mesodermal origin. For example, many organs arise from an initial condensation or clustering of epithelial cells, with subsequent branching or budding occurring over a specialized area of mesenchymal cell condensation. Such processes have strongly implicated a role for some form of communication between tissues of ectodermal and mesenchymal origins. The interactions are controlled through secreted products released from cells residing within both of these tissues, and these are regulated via the genetic code of these cells. The implications for these interactions lie not only in understanding the developmental aspects of normal growth and development, but also in understanding the mechanisms involved in the maintenance of tissue phenotype in adult life, as well as the regulation of tissue regeneration following damage or injury.

Developmental Aspects

During embryonic development of all organs, an intricate and functional relationship exists between the epithelial and mesenchymal tissues. The relationship of this interaction has been the subject of great interest and research, and, in recent years, significant insights have been gained into this complex issue. The early studies of Spemann (1938) demonstrated that in order for organogenesis to proceed, some form of communication between the epithelial and mesenchymal tissue was required. Subsequently, this interaction was called secondary embryonic induction and was shown to regulate not only morphogenesis, but also cell differentiation.

While odontogenesis is of prime interest and importance to dentists and dental scientists, it has provided an excellent model system for studying epithelium–mesenchymal tissue interactions, and has attracted a great deal of interest from all individuals interested in the fundamental aspects of developmental biology. Signaling between the epithelium and underlying mesenchymal tissues operates from the earliest induction of odontogenesis and is inextricably connected to both morphogenesis and cell differentiation. In order to try to understand whether specific tissues assume ultimate control of the differentiation process, numerous tissue recombination experiments between differing tissues of ectodermal and mesodermal origins have been carried out (Kollar and Baird 1970; Ruch 1987; Mina and Kollar 1987).

Thus, experiments in which various epithelia and connective tissues have been separated and recombined in various permutations have provided useful insights into the development of teeth, their supporting periodontal structures, and the surrounding mucosal tissues. For example, if epithelium from a developing tooth bud site is placed onto mesenchyme distant from the dental arch, no tooth formation results. However, if epithelium from a site that does not normally produce teeth is layered over mesenchyme from the dental arch, then normal tooth bud formation occurs. Furthermore, if epithelium from a developing tooth bud site is placed over connective tissue derived from the neural crest, then tooth development progresses. These findings indicate that in undifferentiated tissues (such as neural crest tissue), the epithelium has an instructive component leading to the development of the ectomesenchyme. Indeed, the ectomesenchyme cells are believed to originate from the neural crest under inductive influences from the overlying oral ectoderm (Lumsden 1988). Once this differentiation process has been initiated, the ectomesenchyme adopts the dominant role in epithelial-mesenchymal interactions.

Although there are many examples of the inductive influence of the mesenchyme on ectodermal tissues, it should be remembered that the process can be reciprocal. For example, once the enamel organ has formed during tooth development, the cells of the inner enamel epithelium appear to induce the adjacent cells in the dental papilla to differentiate into odontoblasts. This is an example of the epithelium exerting an influence over the mesenchyme. However, enamel formation by ameloblasts cannot proceed until the odontoblasts have begun to secrete dentin. Such an interaction between the two tissues and cell types illustrates the concept of reciprocal induction, in which the future development of each tissue is dependent upon the other.

Therefore, it is apparent that the messages flow freely in both directions between the epithelium and mesenchyme such that, depending on the stage of development, the epithelial tissue may govern one phase of mesenchymal development followed by mesenchymal tissue influencing epithelial activity. For example, during odontogenesis, at 10 sites, each in the developing maxilla and mandible, foci of mesenchyme induce the overlying epithelium to proliferate and form the earliest vestiges of a tooth bud. Subsequently in tooth development, the epithelial tissues dictate further mesenchymal differentiation and development. Thus, the tissue interactions occurring during odontogenesis are both sequential in their timing and reciprocal in their effect.

Genetic Features

The development of organs is highly ordered following a pathway of initiation, morphogenesis, and differentiation (Fig 7-6). Each of these stages involves the production of numerous molecular signals via the initiation of gene expression. At the earliest initiation stage, when organogenesis is determined and commenced, there is no visible evidence of organ development. Nonetheless, encrypted within the genetic architectural plans for development are codes for the signaling mechanisms that will instruct the cells to pursue activities that will ultimately lead to organ development. Among the earliest of these signaling mechanisms to be expressed are the transcription factors (see Chapter 1). These are nuclear proteins that bind to DNA and control the expression of other genes.

One group of transcription factors that bind to DNA via the homeodomain in target genes is contained within the so-called homeobox (*Hox*), a 180-bp sequence (Scott 1992). Other transcription factors bind to DNA sequences through well-conserved sequences such as paired boxes and zinc finger encoding motifs. The homeobox genes appear to have a significant role in development, being involved in the regulation of positional information (Fig 7-7). Thus, during development, each of the branchial arches expresses a unique combination of the *Hox* genes that encodes specific positional and morphogenic instructions (Hunt and Krumlauf 1991). By extension, homeobox genes could be involved in specifying the spatial location of future tooth germs (Thesleff 1995). The expression of other transcription factors such as *Dlx-1* and *Dlx-2* has been noted in areas of epithelial thickening where tooth development is presumed to proceed (Sharpe 1995). It has been suggested that the expression of these transcription factors are downstream targets for the earlier expression of homeobox genes dictating the location of such tooth development sites. Other evidence to suggest a role for transcription factors comes from experiments with transgenic animals in which the genes *LEF-1, Msx-1,* and *Msx-2* have been deleted and do not develop any teeth (along with other organs such as hair and mammary glands, which have a similar epithelial-mesenchymal developmental pattern) (Satokata and Maas 1994).

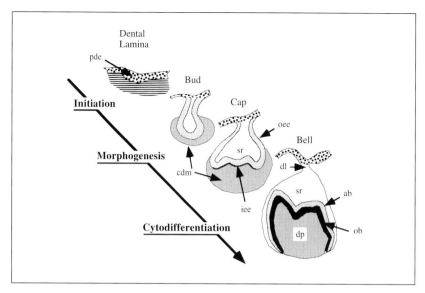

Fig 7-6 Schematic representation of tooth morphogenesis. Initiation of tooth development is characterized by thickening of the presumptive dental epithelium and subsequent condensation of the neural crest–derived mesenchymal cells around the epithelial bud. As a result of epithelial morphogenesis, the shape of the tooth crown is determined during the cap and bell stages. ab, ameloblasts; cdm, condensed dental mesenchyme; dl, dental lamina; dp, dental papilla; iee, inner enamel epithelium; oee, outer enamel epithelium; ob, odontoblasts; pde, presumptive dental epithelium; sr, stellate reticulum. (Reproduced with permission from Thesleff et al 1996.)

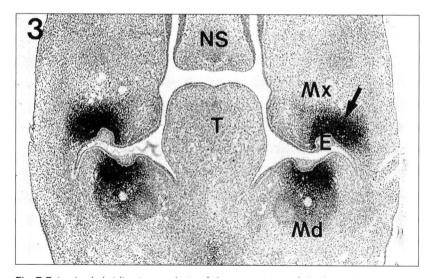

Fig 7-7 In situ hybridization analysis of the expression of the homeobox-containing transcription factor *Msx-1* during early tooth development. A frontal section through the molar tooth germ of an E12 mouse embryo. Intense expression (arrow) is restricted to the presumptive dental mesenchymal cells around the forming epithelial tooth buds. E, epithelial tooth buds; T, tongue; NS, nasal septum; Mx, maxilla; Md, mandible. (Reproduced with permission from Thesleff et al 1995.)

Molecular Features

Following gene expression, cell differentiation and organ development continue to be controlled by locally secreted molecules that provide a specific instructional signal to target cells. Among these signals, growth factors, cell surface glycoproteins, and components of the extracellular matrix appear to be prime candidates for governing developmental processes.

Growth factors are soluble polypeptides, secreted by cells, that act within the local environment, either on other cells in a paracrine function, or by feedback upon themselves in an autocrine manner. The growth factors that have been identified to date form a long and formidable list, and as such, it is not possible to discuss all the growth factors considered to be involved in epithelial-mesenchymal interactions. Growth factors (and other signaling molecules) exert their influence on cells via specific cell surface receptors. Often these are specific for a given growth factor or more generic for a group or family of growth factors. The mechanisms of cell surface signaling are covered in more detail in Chapter 2. Nonetheless, it is important to note that, following receptor-mediated binding of growth factors, a cascade of intracellular events is activated that ultimately leads to altered cellular activity, usually through altered gene expression of other molecular regulatory systems, adhesive properties, or proliferative responses of the target cell.

The presence of numerous growth factors has been reported at specific stages of growth and development (Fig 7-8). During odontogenesis, the bone morphogenetic proteins (BMPs) transforming growth factor-β (TGF-β) and fibroblast growth factor (FGF) have been studied in some detail and found to be differentially expressed according to the stage of development, morphogenesis, and cell differentiation. However, other growth factors, including platelet-derived growth factor (PDGF), epidermal growth factor (EGF), and growth hormone have been associated with different stages of tooth development (Young 1995; Zhang et al 1997).

During odontogenesis, TGF-β1 is first seen in the epithelial thickenings that dictate the sites of developing teeth. Shortly after its expression in this odontogenic epithelium, TGF-β1 is expressed in the underlying mesenchyme. This observation implies some form of communication between these two tissues and that this growth factor probably acts in some form of paracrine function (Thesleff et al 1995b).

The bone morphogenetic proteins (BMPs) are a group of 20 to 30 related differentiation factors of the TGF-β superfamily that appear to be intimately associated with epithelial-mesenchymal signaling. BMP-2 and BMP-4 are expressed within the thickened layers of the budding odontogenic epithelium and, later, these two molecules are expressed by the underlying mesenchyme, again illustrating the inductive effect of growth factors on different tissues.

The fibroblast growth factors (FGFs) also comprise a group of growth factors that have a variety of roles. FGF-3 appears in the mesenchyme of developing teeth at the late bud stage and persists through to the late bell stage (Wilkinson et al 1989). While FGF-3 appears to be restricted to expression by mesenchymal cells, the expression of another member of the family, FGF-4, is restricted to cells of epithelial origin (Jernvall et al 1994).

In light of the above, a unifying series of events for growth factor expression and regulation of tissue development during odontogenesis has been proposed by Thesleff et al (1995a). In this scheme, numerous growth factors are sequentially expressed during the initiation, morphogenesis, and differentiation stages of tooth development (Fig 7-9). For example, BMP-2 and BMP-4 are expressed very early during initiation of tooth development in the odontogenic epithelium, which leads to subsequent expression in the underlying mesenchyme. The mesenchyme then expresses both TGF-β1 and FGFs, which in

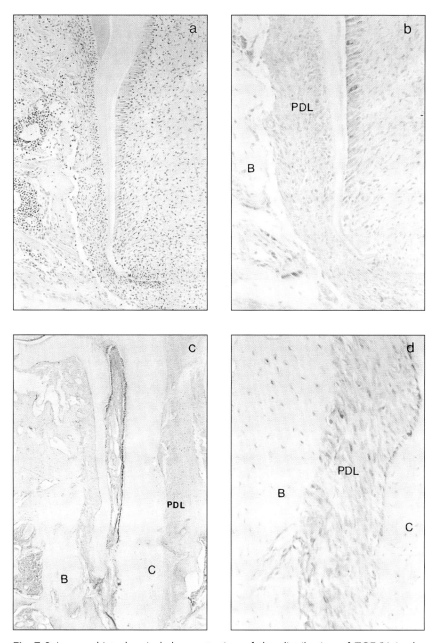

Fig 7-8 Immunohistochemical demonstration of the distribution of TGF-β1 in the developing periodontal ligament. **(a)** Control section demonstrating no reactivity towards the antibody. **(b)** TGF-β1 distribution in 2-week-old rat developing periodontal ligament (low power, × 100); **(c)** TGF-β1 distribution in 11-week-old rat developing periodontal ligament (low power, × 100); **(d)** TGF-β1 distribution in 11-week-old rat developing periodontal ligament (high power, × 200). Reactions positive for TGF-β1 are stained light brown. B, alveolar bone; C, cementum; PDL, periodontal ligament. (Figures kindly provided by Dr J Gao, University of Queensland.)

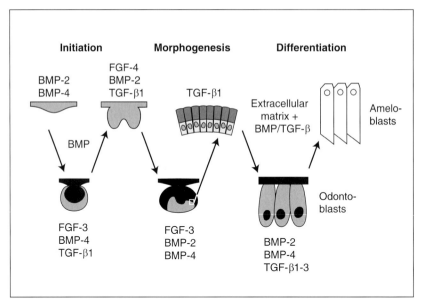

Fig 7-9 A model, proposed by Thesleff et al, suggesting roles for growth factors in reciprocal epithelial-mesenchymal signaling during advancing tooth morphogenesis. Growth factors that have been localized in the epithelial (upper) and mesenchymal tissues are indicated. The arrows represent the sequential and reciprocal inductive interactions between the epithelium and mesenchyme. BMPs may be early epithelial signals specifying dental mesenchymal determination, whereas FGFs and TGF-βs may participate in subsequent signaling between tissues. During odontoblast and ameloblast differentiation, BMPs and TGF-βs may also act as epithelial and mesenchymal inductors, but in these interactions cell-matrix contacts also influence differentiation. BMP, bone morphogenetic protein; FGF, fibroblast growth factor; TGF, transforming growth factor. (Reproduced with permission from Thesleff et al 1995a.)

turn leads to up-regulation of the expression of TGF-β1, FGFs, and BMP-2 by the epithelial cells of the developing tooth germ. The expression of growth factors continues in a stepwise fashion, alternating between the epithelial tissues and mesenchyme, ultimately leading to the differentiation of some epithelial cells into ameloblasts. The cells of the mesenchyme, immediately adjacent to the newly differentiated ameloblasts, appear to respond to the BMPs and TGF-β1 released by the ameloblasts, and are instructed to differentiate odontoblasts. Subsequent expression of the dentin matrix and release of BMP-2, BMP-4, and TGF-β1 by the odontoblasts then leads to enamel matrix deposition by the ameloblasts.

Such interactions of growth factors elaborated by epithelial and mesenchymal tissues clearly illustrate the concepts of reciprocal signaling and induction in odontogenesis.

Role of the Extracellular Matrix

Apart from secreted growth factors, other components that reside in the extracellular matrix and cell surface may also have an instructional effect upon cells. In general, these interactions are initiated from the mesenchymal cells and influence the activity of the overlying ectodermal tissues. Several components of the extracellular matrix have been studied during odontogenesis, including type

III collagen, fibronectin, and tenascin (Thesleff et al 1991). Of these, collagen does not appear to be specifically associated with tooth development. However, tenascin, which is known to interact with a number of cell surface and matrix molecules (Erickson 1993), accumulates in the condensing mesenchyme of the dental papilla at the bud stage and may be involved in early mesenchymal-epithelial interactions. Recent experimental evidence indicates that tenascin expression in the mesenchymal tissues of developing teeth is under direct epithelial cell control (Vainio et al 1989; Vainio and Thesleff 1992). During the cap stage there is little specific deposition of matrix-specific molecules. As development progresses into the bell stage, both tenascin and fibronectin begin to accumulate in the basement membrane and may be involved in subsequent odontoblast differentiation, since experiments in which fibronectin deposition is depleted demonstrated a retardation in odontoblast differentiation (Thesleff and Pratt 1980). With continuing tooth development, both dentin matrix and enamel matrix are deposited through a series of intricate epithelial-mesenchymal cell-matrix interactions. The precise molecular events associated with the deposition of these two mineralized matrices are still unclear. Nonetheless, it is likely that some matrix components of the predentin and dentin, such as various proteoglycans, phosphoproteins, γ-carboxyglutamate–containing proteins, and other acidic noncollagenous proteins will play some regulatory role in matrix deposition and tissue development (Zhang et al 1995).

As discussed above, cell surface components will be intimately associated with the regulatory mechanisms of cell function. Apart from the various receptors for growth factors, other cell surface components, including an array of proteoglycans and other glycoproteins, have been noted to be associated at various stages of tooth development, and as such, implicated in the interactions between epithelium and mesenchyme. Syndecan-1 is a cell surface proteoglycan that has been implicated in the interactive processes between developing mesenchymal and ectodermal tissues. In the early bud stage of development, syndecan-1 is strongly expressed in the condensing mesenchyme of the dental papilla under the control of the overlying dental epithelium (Vainio et al 1989; Vainio and Thesleff 1992). Syndecan-1 continues to be strongly expressed in the dental mesenchyme through to the cap stage of tooth development, and is almost nonexistent in the mesenchyme of the surrounding developing jaw. During the transition from the cap to the bell stage of development, the expression of syndecan-1 decreases significantly.

The pattern of expression of EGF receptors during tooth development is interesting, in that it is expressed highly in the epithelium during the bud stage, and this distribution shifts to the underlying mesenchyme in the bell stage. With the transition to the bell stage of development, EGF receptor expression diminishes in a manner similar to syndecan-1 (Thesleff et al 1991).

Role of Epithelial-Mesenchymal Tissue Interactions in Maintaining Tissue Phenotype

Apart from tooth formation, epithelial-mesenchymal tissue interactions are also important with respect to maintenance of epithelial phenotype in the periodontal tissues. The junctional epithelium is initially derived from the reduced enamel epithelium, whereas the gingival epithelium originates from the ectodermal tissues covering the maxillary and mandibular arches. Thus, these two tissues are considered to have distinct origins, phenotypes, and, possibly, function. The role that the underlying connective tissue plays in maintaining these phenotypes is important. Moreover, the fact that junctional epithelium can reappear despite its complete excision during periodontal surgery indicates that factors other than a tissue's embryonal genesis are important for its appearance. The controlling influence of connective tissue substrate on epithelial phenotype has been recognized for some time. For example, if whole skin is grafted onto a prepared bed of oral mucosal connective tissue, then skin development progresses normally, complete with maturation of hair follicles. However if skin epidermis is grafted onto a mucosal connective tissue bed, the epidermis reverts to express the phenotype of oral mucosa. Similarly, if components of palatal and buccal mucosa are cross-grafted, the pattern of epithelial differentiation is controlled by the underlying connective tissue (Ten Cate 1994).

Since the connective tissues of the periodontal ligament and the gingival connective tissue have different embryonal origins, as do the gingival epithelium and the junctional epithelium, it is not surprising that instructive and permissive influences of these two different connective tissues are considered to play an important role in regulating the adjacent epithelial phenotype. Indeed, periodontal ligament connective tissue has been suggested to be nonpermissive for epithelial growth and differentiation (Mackenzie 1988, 1990). This could explain the inability of junctional epithelium to extend apically beyond its periodontal connective tissue interface with the tooth, as well as the relative lack of proliferation of the epithelial cell rests of Mallasez. On the other hand, the connective tissue of the gingival tissues does permit epithelial growth and proliferation, which lead to expression of the gingival epithelial phenotype in the gingivae and the gingival sulcus.

Summary

The development of teeth is a well coordinated but complex process. The development of the periodontal tissues involves both ectodermal and mesenchymal tissues. A good un-

derstanding of the principals of tooth formation, and, in particular, formation of the periodontal structures, is essential for unraveling the mechanisms associated with tissue regeneration. The interactions between epithelial and connective tissues are regulated via a large number of soluble mediators, including transcription factors, growth factors, and their respective receptors. While these interactions are of undoubted importance for normal development, the clinical ramifications lie in the regulatory mechanisms governing the correct expression of epithelial and connective tissue components during wound repair and regeneration.

References

Alatli-Burt I, Hultenby K, Hammarstrom L. Disturbances of cementum formation induced by single injection of 1-hydroxyethylidene-1,1-bisphosphonate (HEBP) in rats: light and scanning electron microscopic studies. Scand J Dent Res 1994;102:260.

Bosshardt D, Schroeder HE. Evidence for rapid multipolar and slow multipolar production of human cellular and acellular cementum matrix with intrinsic fibers. J Clin Periodontol 1990;17:663.

Bosshardt DD, Schroeder HE. Evidence for rapid multipolar and slow unipolar production of cellular and acellular cementum matrix with intrinsic fibers. J Clin Periodontol 1990;17:663.

Bosshardt DD, Schroeder HE. Initial formation of cellular intrinsic fiber cementum in developing human teeth. A light- and electron-microscopic study. Cell Tissue Res 1992;267:321.

Bosshardt DD, Schroeder HE. Attempts to label matrix synthesis of human root cementum in vitro. Cell Tissue Res 1993;274:343.

Bosshardt DD, Schroeder HE. Cementogenesis reviewed: A comparison between human premolars and rodent molars. Anat Rec 1996;245:287.

Cho MI, Garant PR. Radioautographic study of [^{3}H]mannose utilization during cementoblast differentiation, formation of acellular cementum and development of periodontal ligament principal fibers. Anat Rec 1989;223:209.

Erickson H. Tenascin-C, tenascin-R and tenascin-X: a family of talented proteins in search of functions. Curr Opin Cell Biol 1993;5:869.

Grant DA, Bernick S. The formation of the periodontal ligament. J Periodontol 1972;43:17.

Grant DA, Bernick S, Levy BM, Dreizin S. A comparative study of the periodontal ligament development in teeth with and without predecessors in marmosets. J Periodontol 1972;43:162.

Groeneveld MC, Everts V, Beertsen W. Formation of afibrillar acellular cementum-like layers induced by alkaline phosphatase activity form periodontal ligament explants maintained in vitro. J Dent Res 1994;73:1588.

Hammarström L, Atali I, Fong CD. Origins of cementum. Oral Diseases 1996:2:63.

Hunt P, Krumlauf R. Deciphering the hox code: clues to patterning branchial regions of the head. Cell 1991; 66:1075.

Jernvall J, Kettunen P, Karanova I, Martin LB, Thesleff I. Evidence for the role of the enamel knot as a control center in mammalian tooth cusp formation, non-dividing cells express growth stimulating Fgf-4 gene. Int J Dev Biol 1994; 38:463.

Kollar EJ, Baird GR. Tissue interactions in embryonic mouse tooth germs: II. The inductive role of the dental papilla. J Embryol Exp Morphol 1970;24:173.

Levy BM, Bernick S. Studies on the biology of the periodontium in marmosets: II. Development and organization of the periodontal ligament of deciduous teeth in marmosets (*Callithrax jaccus*). J Dent Res 1968;47:27.

Lindskog S. Formation of intermediate cementum I. Early mineralization of aprismatic enamel and intermediate cementum in monkey. J Craniofac Genet Dev Biol 1982; 2:147.

Listgarten MA. Normal development, structure, physiology and repair of gingival epithelium. Oral Sci Rev 1972;1:3.

Lumsden AGS. Spatial organization of the epithelium and the role of neural crest cell in the initiation of mammalian tooth germ. Development 1988;103:155.

Mackenzie IA. Factors influencing the stability of the gingival sulcus. In: Guggenheim B, ed. Periodontology Today. Basel: Karger; 1988:41.

Mackenzie IC. Formation and subsequent changes of the periodontium. In: Genco RJ, Goldman HM, Cohen WD, eds. Contemporary Periodontics. St Louis: Mosby; 1990:55.

Marks SC. The basic and applied biology of tooth eruption. Connect Tissue Res 1995;32:149.

McKee MD, Nanci A. Osteopontin at mineralized tissue interfaces in bone, teeth, and osseointegrated implants: ultrastructural distribution and implications for mineralized tissue formation, turnover and repair. Microsc Res Tech 1996;33:141.

McKee MD, Zalzal S, Nanci A. Extracellular matrix in tooth cementum and mantle dentin: Localization of osteopontin and other noncollagenous proteins, plasma proteins, and glycoconjugates by electron microscopy. Anat Rec 1996;245:293.

Mina M, Kollar EJ. The induction of odontogenesis in non-dental mesenchyme combined with early murine mandibular arch epithelium. Arch Oral Biol 1987;32:123.

Moxham BJ, Berkovitz BKB. Development of the periodontal ligament. In: Berkovitz BKB, Moxham BJ, Newman HE, eds. The Periodontal Ligament in Health and Disease. London: Mosby-Wolfe; 1995;161.

Ruch JV. Determinations of odontogenesis. Cell Biol Rev 1987;14:1.

Satokata I, Maas R. Msx1 deficient mice exhibit cleft palate and abnormalities of craniofacial and tooth development. Nat Genet 1994;6:348.

Schroeder HE, ed. Oral Structural Biology. New York: Thieme; 1991.

Schroeder HE. Biological problems of regenerative cementogenesis: synthesis and attachment of collagenous matrices on growing and established root surfaces. Int Rev Cytol 1992;142:1.

Schroeder HE. Human cellular mixed stratified cementum: A tissue with alternating layers of acellular extrinsic- and cellular intrinsic fiber cementum. Schweiz Monatsschr Zahnmed 1993;103:550.

Scott JH, Symons NBB. Introduction to Dental Anatomy. 7th ed. Edinburgh: Churchill Livingstone; 1974.

Scott MP. Vertebrate homeobox gene nomenclature. Cell 1992;71:551.

Sequeira P, Bosshardt DD, Schroeder HE. Growth of acellular extrinsic fiber cementum (AEFC) and density of inserting fibers in human premolars of adolescents. J Periodont Res 1992;27:134.

Sharpe PT. Homeobox genes and orofacial development. Connect Tissue Res 1995;32:17.

Slavkin HC, Bringas P, Bessem C, et al. Hertwig's epithelial root sheath differentiation and initial cementum and bone formation during long-term organ culture of mouse mandibular first molars using serumless, chemically defined medium. J Periodont Res 1988;23:28.

Spemann H. Embryonic Development and Induction. New Haven: Yale University Press; 1938.

Ten Cate AR. Epithelial-mesenchymal relations. In: Ten Cate AR, ed. Oral Histology. Development, Structure and Function. 4th ed. St Louis: Mosby; 1994:100.

Ten Cate AR, Mills GC, Solomon G. The development of the periodontium. A transplantation and autoradiographic study. Anat Rec 1971;170:365.

Thesleff I. Homeobox genes and growth factors in regulation of craniofacial and tooth morphogenesis. Acta Odontol Scand 1995;53:129.

Thesleff I, Partanen A-M, Vainio S. Epithelial-mesenchymal interactions in tooth morphogenesis: The roles of extracellular matrix, growth factors and cell surface receptors. J Craniofac Genet Dev Biol 1991;11:229.

Thesleff I, Pratt RM. Tunicamycin-induced alterations in basement membrane formation during odontoblast differentiation of mouse tooth germ. Dev Biol 1980;80:175.

Thesleff I, Vaahtokari A, Kettunen P, Aberg T. Epithelial-mesenchymal signalling during tooth development. Connect Tissue Res 1995a;32:9.

Thesleff I, Vaahtokari A, Partanen A-M. Regulation of organogenesis. Common molecular mechanisms regulating the development of teeth and other organs. Int J Dev Biol 1995b;39:35.

Thesleff I, Vaahtokari A, Vainio S, Jowett A. Molecular mechanisms of cell and tissue interactions during early tooth development. Anat Record 1996;245:151.

Thomas HF. Root formation. Int J Dev Biol 1995;39:231.

Vainio S, Jalkanen M, Thesleff I. Syndecan and tenascin expression is induced by epithelial-mesenchymal interactions in embryonic tooth mesenchyme. J Cell Biol 1989;108:1945.

Vainio S, Thesleff I. Sequential induction of syndecan, tenascin and cell proliferation associated with mesenchymal cell condensation during early tooth development. Differentiation 1992;50:97.

Wilkinson DG, Bhatt S, Mcmahon AP. Expression pattern of the FGF-related proto-oncogene *int*-2 suggests multiple roles in fetal development. Development 1989;105:131.

Yamamoto T, Damon T, Takahashi S, Wakita M. Comparative study of the initial genesis of acellular and cellular cementum in rat molars. Anat Embryol (Berl) 1994;190:521.

Yamamoto T, Hinrichsen KV. The development of cellular cementum in rat molars with special reference to the fiber arrangement. Anat Embryol (Berl) 1993;188:537.

Yamamoto T, Wakita M. Initial attachment of principal fibers to root dentin surface in rat molars. J Periodont Res 1990;25:113.

Yamamoto T, Wakita M. The development and structure of principal fibers and cellular cementum in rat molars. J Periodont Res 1991;26:129.

Young WG. Growth hormone and insulin-like growth factor-1 in odontogenesis. Int J Dev Biol 1995;39:263.

Zhang CZ, Li H, Bartold PM, Young WG, Waters MJ. Effect of growth hormone on the distribution of decorin and biglycan during odontogenesis in the rat incisor. J Dent Res 1995;74:1636.

Zhang CZ, Li H, Young WG, Bartold PM, Chen C, Waters MJ. Evidence for a local action of growth hormone in embryonic tooth development in the rat. Growth Factors 1997;14:131.

Biochemistry of Normal Periodontal Connective Tissues

Gingiva
  Gingival Epithelium
  Gingival Connective Tissue

Periodontal Ligament

Cementum

Alveolar Bone

Introduction

The tissues that support and invest the teeth are collectively referred to as the periodontium. The periodontium includes two soft connective tissues (gingiva and periodontal ligament) and two hard connective tissues (alveolar bone and cementum). Each of these periodontal components has a distinct biochemical composition and connective tissue architecture; yet they function as one integrated unit. The biochemical constituents of one periodontal component can influence the cellular activities of other structures. The major functions of the periodontium are anchoring the teeth and responding to masticatory forces (Schluger et al 1990).

The periodontium is constantly subjected to mechanical and bacterial stresses, yet it efficiently retains its structural composition and functional integrity because it can react to these stresses and continuously remodel its connective tissue components. The periodontal connective tissues are made up of biochemical constituents commonly found in other connective tissues, however, they manifest several unique features. Extensive studies over the

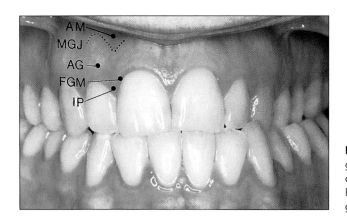

Fig 8-1 Clinical appearance of healthy gingiva. AG, attached gingiva; AM, alveolar mucosa; IP, interdental papilla; FGM, free gingival margin; MGJ, mucogingival junction.

past two decades have provided information about the types and properties of the periodontal connective tissue constituents, while ultrastructural studies have revealed how various structural macromolecules are distributed and organized into distinct architectural patterns in each periodontal component.

In this chapter we review the biochemical composition and structure of healthy periodontal tissues and how they are regulated. How they are affected in the diseased periodontium is outlined in the next chapter.

Gingiva

The gingiva is the oral mucosa encircling the necks of the teeth and, in health, it fully covers the root surface and supporting alveolar bone (Fig 8-1). The gingival tissues are subclassified as free marginal gingiva, interdental gingiva, or attached gingiva, based on the anatomical location (Schluger et al 1990). All these structures consist of an epithelium that overlays the deeper connective tissue of the lamina propria to which it is intimately attached. Both tissues have extracellular matrices, but due to their vastly different structures and functions, these matrices differ quite significantly.

Gingival Epithelium

Although the gingival epithelium is not strictly a connective tissue, due to its relationship to the underlying connective tissue and functional demands it must be considered as an essential periodontal component. Indeed, the gingival epithelium is a strategic component of the host defense against bacterial assault on the periodontal tissues.

Gingival epithelium adopts morphologically variant forms at different locations, and these forms can be distinguished by differentiation markers. These are known as junctional, oral, or sulcular epithelium, and as pocket epithelium in periodontally diseased gingiva. These epithelial structures vary in their degree of keratinization, number of cells, and presence of rete pegs (Fig 8-2a). There are no fibrous protein components of the epithelial extracellular matrix, and the nonfibrous epithelial components include water and a variety of glycoproteins, lipids, and proteoglycans, and extensions of intercalated cell surface molecules (Bartold 1987).

Early studies using histochemical techniques failed to indicate whether epithelial cells had the ability to produce extracellular products such as proteoglycans and other glycoproteins (Fig 8-2b) (Braun-Faulco 1959; Thonard and Scherp 1962; Pedlar 1979)

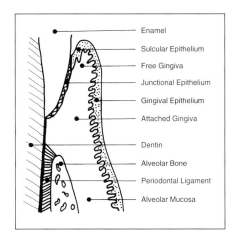

a

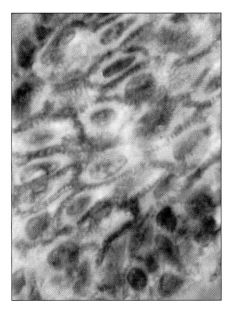

b

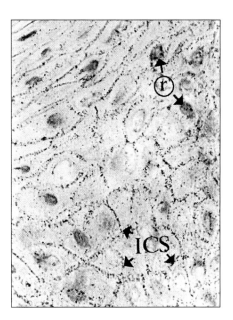

c

Fig 8-2 Human gingival epithelium.

(a) Schematic representation of the architecture of healthy gingival tissues indicating the relationships of the different epithelia including junctional epithelium, sulcular epithelium, and free gingival epithelium.

(b) Histochemical localization of glycosaminoglycans in human gingival epithelium (Hale's iron stain, original magnification × 1000). (Reproduced with permission from Thonard and Scherp 1962.)

(c) Autoradiographic demonstration of sulfated glycosaminoglycans in human gingival epithelium. r, retention of silver grains; ICS, intercellular staining. (Reproduced with permission from Wiebkin and Thonard 1981.)

However, following the development of autoradiographic methods (Fig 8-2c), it has been demonstrated that gingival epithelial cells can synthesize and secrete sulfated molecules that contribute to the makeup of the intercellular cementing substance of gingival epithelium (Wiebkin and Thonard 1981). With the development of highly specific immunohistochemical and histochemical probes, more precise identification of the proteoglycan content of epithelium has been possible. For example, hyaluronan, decorin, syndecan, and CD44 have all been identified in human gingival epithelial intercellular spaces (Häkkinen et al 1993; Tammi et al 1990). Some variation in the distribution of the extracellular macromolecules has been noted, but their significance is unclear (Kogaya et al 1989; Oyarzún-Droguett 1992).

Until recently, culturing of oral epithelial cells (and in particular gingival, sulcular and junctional epithelium) had been elusive.

However, recent developments resulting in improved methods of culturing oral keratinocytes (Willie et al 1990) have helped to characterize the synthesis and secretion by gingival keratinocytes of several proteoglycans containing heparan sulfate and other molecular species (Potter-Perigo et al 1993). These in vitro studies have confirmed the results obtained for whole extracts of human gingival epithelium; however, the molecular identities of the proteoglycans synthesized by gingival epithelial cell cultures have not yet been precisely determined.

Gingival Connective Tissue

Underlying the gingival epithelium is the lamina propria of the gingiva, the gingival connective tissue (Fig 8-3). The gingiva is attached to tooth surfaces and alveolar bone through fibrous attachments of the connective tissues. Approximately one tenth of the gingival connective tissue volume is occupied predominantly by fibroblasts (Schluger et al 1990). These cells are responsible for producing connective tissue elements in both normal and diseased gingivae (Fig 8-4) (Narayanan and Page 1983). Besides the fibroblasts, most other cells present in the gingival connective tissue are largely derived from blood vessels and the blood itself. These cells include endothelial cells, polymorphonuclear leukocytes, macrophages, lymphocytes, plasma cells, and mast cells. In normal gingival connective tissues, inflammatory cells are present in relatively small numbers. These cells increase in number during inflammation, however, their proportions differ from one site to another according to the type and severity of the inflammatory reaction. One of the most distinguishing features of the gingival connective tissue is its rapid remodeling and high turnover rate. Indeed, the turnover rates of gingival and periodontal ligament collagens are higher than those of most other connective tissues, including skin. This very high turnover rate of ma-

trix components does not appear to decrease greatly with age (Page and Ammons 1974; Sodek 1976; Sodek and Ferrier 1988).

The various collagen fibers of the gingival connective tissue provide a rigid structural framework in the gingiva. Collagens are the most abundant biochemical components in the gingival connective tissue, where they provide greater than 60% of the total tissue protein. These fibers are organized into several characteristic and architecturally distinct units that are classified into various groups based on their location, origin, and insertion (Schluger et al 1990). The fibers that arise from the cementum immediately apical to the base of the epithelial attachment and splay out into the gingiva are called dentogingival fibers (Fig 8-5a). Those that bend apically over the alveolar crest and insert into the buccal and lingual periosteum are classified as dentoperiosteal fibers. The alveologingival fibers originate from the alveolar crest, traverse coronally, and terminate in the free and papillary gingiva, whereas those fibers that pass circumferentially around the cervical region of teeth in the free gingiva are classified as circular fibers. Other fibers, called semicircular fibers, traverse from the cementum at the proximal root surface, extend into the free marginal gingiva, and insert into a corresponding position on the opposite site of the tooth (see Fig 8-5b). The fibers traversing from the cementoenamel junction to the free marginal gingiva of the adjacent tooth are transgingival fibers, while the intergingival fibers extend along facial and lingual marginal gingiva from tooth to tooth. Other fibers arise from the cemental surface just apical to the base of the epithelial attachment, traverse the interdental bone, and insert into a comparable position on the opposite tooth; these are transseptal fibers. The transseptal fibers form a ligament between teeth and connect all the teeth in the arch, and are important for the structural integrity of the gingival tissues. The various gingival fiber groups mentioned above are interdependent for function and differ in

Fig 8-3 Histologic appearance of gingival connective tissue elements.

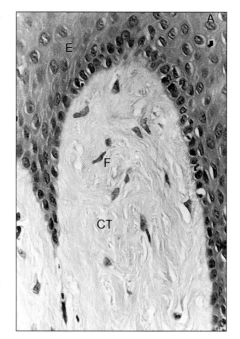

(a) Section of human gingiva stained with hematoxylin and eosin. E, epithelium; CT, connective tissue; F, fibroblasts. Original magnification 250×.

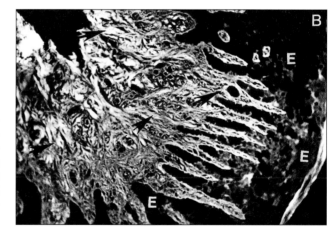

(b) Collagen fibers of gingival connective tissue as revealed by immunostaining with an anti–type I collagen antibody. Collagen fibers (arrows) are distributed throughout the connective tissue, however, they are not present in the epithelium (E). Original magnification 100×.

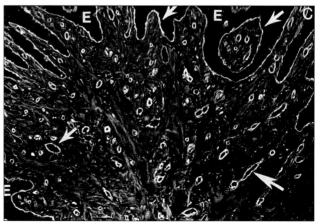

c) Demonstration of basement membrane structures in human gingiva using anti–type IV collagen antibody. This collagen is present in basement membranes at the epithelium–connective tissue interface, in rete pegs, and around blood vessels and nerves (arrows). Original magnification 160×.

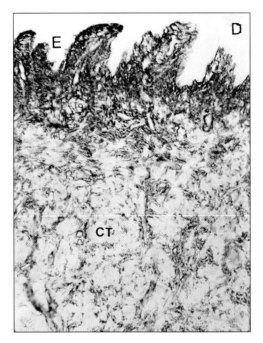

(d) Immunohistochemical demonstration of dermatan sulfate. Sections were reacted with a monoclonal antibody (9-A-2) to chondroitinase ABC-digested tissues, and dermatan sulfate was visualized using immunoperoxidase immunohistochemistry. Dermatan sulfate appears to localize strongly to the connective tissue (CT) immediately subjacent to the epithelium (E). Original magnification 75×. (Reproduced with permission from Bartold 1991.)

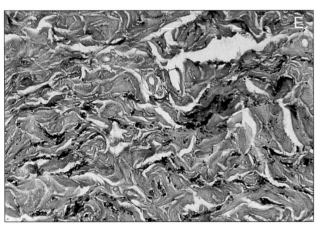

(e) Immunohistochemical demonstration of elastin in human alveolar mucosa. Note the heavy deposits (black amorphous material between collagen fibers) within the connective tissue. Elastin was detected using a polyclonal antibody to tropoelastin and visualized by silver-intensified protein A–gold immunohistochemistry. Original magnification 100×. (Reproduced with permission from Bartold 1991.)

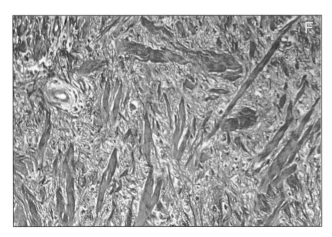

(f) Immunohistochemical demonstration of elastin in human gingiva. Note virtual absence of stained material (compared to Fig 8-3e). Elastin was detected using a polyclonal antibody to tropoelastin and visualized by silver-intensified protein A–gold immunohistochemistry. Original magnification 100×. (Reproduced with permission from Bartold 1991.)

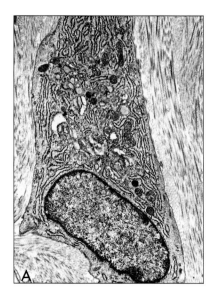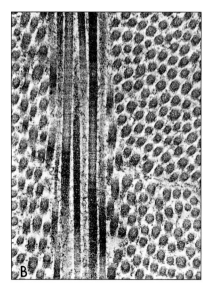

Fig 8-4 Electron micrograph of a resident fibroblast and collagen fibers in normal gingiva. **(a)** A typical fibroblast containing lamallae of RER and Golgi and surrounded by collagen fibers. **(b)** Collagen fiber bundles at higher magnification showing characteristic 640-nm periodicity. Fibers are seen longitudinally and in cross section (× 6860). (Reproduced with permission from Schluger et al 1990.)

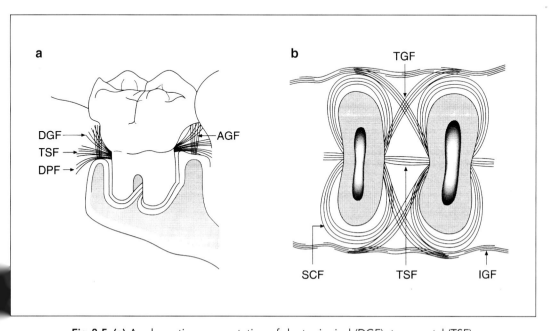

Fig 8-5 (a) A schematic representation of dentogingival (DGF), transseptal (TSF), dentoperiosteal (DPF), and alveologingival (AGF) collagen fibers. **(b)** Transgingival fibers (TGF), semicircular fibers (SCF), transseptal fibers (TSF), and intergingival fibers (IGF) are shown (adapted from Schluger et al 1990).

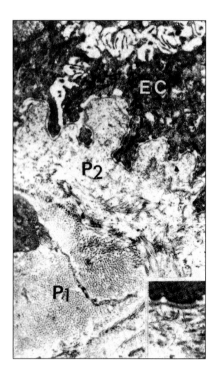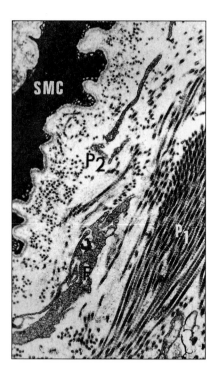

Fig 8-6 Distribution of dense (60–70 nm, P1) and thinner (40–60 nm, P2) collagen fibers at the gingival lamina propria **(a)** and near a blood vessel **(b)**, respectively, viewed by electron microscopy (× 10,000). The P2 is a loose pattern of organization mixed with nonstriated fibrillar material, and it is found near basement membranes. EC, epithelial cell; SMC, smooth muscle cell; F, fibroblast. The inset at the lower right of Fig 8-6a shows P2 magnified × 20,000. (Reproduced with permission from Chavrier et al 1984.)

how they are affected during inflammatory periodontal diseases. For example, portions of transseptal fibers remain unaffected even in advanced stages of periodontitis, and those that are destroyed appear to reform at a more apical level.

The gingival collagen fibers, like those fibers of other connective tissue, are made up of a heterotypic mixtures of collagen types, of which type I collagen is the major species (Bartold and Narayanan 1996; Narayanan and Page 1983; Narayanan and Bartold 1996). Ultrastructural studies using collagen type specific antibodies and electron mi-

croscopy have shown that these fibers are arranged in two patterns of organization, either as large, dense bundles of thick fibers, or in a loose pattern of short thin fibers mixed with a fine reticular network (Fig 8-6) (Chavrier et al 1984; Narayanan et al 1985; Rao et al 1979). They contain principally type I and III collagen; type I collagen is preferentially organized into denser fibrils within the lamina propria. Although it is not restricted to any particular region, type III collagen appears to be localized mostly as thinner fibers and distributed in a reticular pattern near the basement membrane adjacent to the epithelia junction (Fig 8-7) (Chavrier et al 1984; Narayanan et al 1985; Romanos et al 1992; Wang et al 1980). Gingival connective tissue contains only small quantities of type V collagen, which, in healthy gingiva, accounts for less than 1% of the total collagen (Narayanan and Page 1983). Immunostaining studies have revealed that this collagen distributes throughout the tissues in a parallel filamentous pattern and appears to coat denser fibers composed of type I and III collagens (Narayanan et al 1985; Romanos et al 1991a, 1991b). The gingival connective tissue also contains the beaded fibril-forming collagen, type VI, which is present as diffuse microfibrils throughout the lamina propria (Romanos et al 1991a, 1991b). Type VI collagen is also present near basement membranes around blood vessels, and near the epithelial basement membrane and nerves in rats, but not in marmosets.

In the gingiva, basement membrane structures separate underlying connective tissues from the gingival epithelium, from endothelial cells in blood vessels, and from surrounding nerves (see Fig 8-3c). Between the epithelium and tooth surface, an internal basal lamina serves as the interface through which junctional epithelium is attached to the root surface. These basement membranes are similar in biochemical composition to other basement membrane structures, and immunolocalization studies have revealed that type IV collagen and laminin are two major constituents (Chavrier et al 1984; Graner et al 1995; Narayanan et al 1985; Romanos et al 1991a, 1991b; Sawada et al 1990). However, while both of these molecules are present in the external basal lamina, the internal basal lamina appears to contain only laminin, at least in rats (Graner et al 1995). The basal lamina of the epithelium is invested into the underlying connective tissue through anchoring fibrils containing type VII collagen. The attachment of epithelial cells to basement membranes and to the tooth surface is mediated via hemidesmosomes. The hemidesmosomes contain type XVII collagen (also called

bullous pemphigoid antigen-2, BAPG-2) and at least two other proteins, BAPG-1, a 230-kd noncollagenous protein, and the integrin $\alpha6\beta4$ (Uitto et al 1996).

The distribution of integrins in the gingiva has been examined by immunocytochemistry. The β_1 integrin subunit, which associates with several α subunits and serves as a receptor for many matrix proteins, is mainly located in the membranes of cells at the basal layer of keratinized epithelium, on fibroblasts in the connective tissues, and in blood vessel walls. The integrin subunit α_4 is found on inflammatory cells, while the α_5 species is located mainly in connective tissue cells (Hormia et al 1990; Larjava et al 1992b). One of the major components of hemidesmosomes is the integrin $\alpha_6\beta_4$; this integrin is localized in the basal layer forming the basement membrane and at the tooth gingival interface in junctional epithelium (Hormia et al 1990; Hormia et al 1992; Larjava et al 1992b). The α_6 integrin is expressed throughout the junctional epithelium and located on cell membranes, whereas β_4 integrin is found on cells facing internal and external basal lamina (Hormia et al 1992). The $\alpha_2\beta_1$ and $\alpha_3\beta_1$ integrins are present on basal keratinocytes in the epithelium. Examples of integrin distribution in human gingival tissues are shown in Fig 8-8.

The gingiva contains several noncollagenous proteins. One of these is fibronectin, which is localized throughout the connective tissue and codistributed with collagens (Narayanan et al 1985; Pitaru et al 1987). Another gingival noncollagenous protein is tenascin, which is present diffusely in the connective tissue and prominently near subepithelial basement membrane in the upper connective tissue and capillary blood vessels (Steffensen et al 1992; Lukinmaa et al 1991). Elastin is a minor component of the gingival connective tissue; it is relatively more prominent in the submucosal tissues of the more movable and flexible alveolar mucosa (Bartold 1991). In addition to these proteins, osteonectin has also been detected in gingival con-

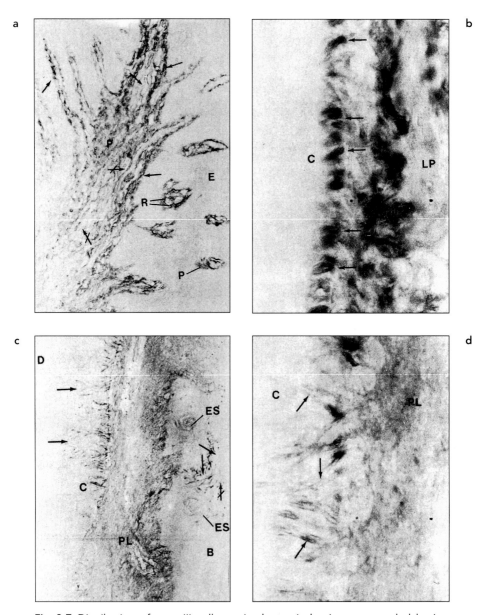

Fig 8-7 Distribution of type III collagen in the periodontium as revealed by immunostaining with anti–type III collagen antibody. **(a)** Section of gingival papilla in which the antibody strongly stains areas adjacent to epithelium (arrows) and rete peg junctions, and blood vessel wall (crossed arrows). E, epithelium that is unstained; P, papilla; R, reticular pattern of staining. Original magnification 845×.**(b)** Junction between cementum (C) and lamina propria (LP) of gingiva; cementum is unstained and strongly staining material (arrows) is Sharpey's fibers. Original magnification 3450×.**(c)** Alveolar bone and periodontal ligament. B, alveolar bone; PL, periodontal ligament; C, cementum; D, dentin; ES, endosteal spaces. Cementum and alveolar bone are largely unstained except at Sharpey's fibers (arrows). Original magnification 540×.**(d)** Higher magnification of Sharpey's fibers (arrows). Original magnification 1370×.(Reproduced with permission from Wang et al 1980.)

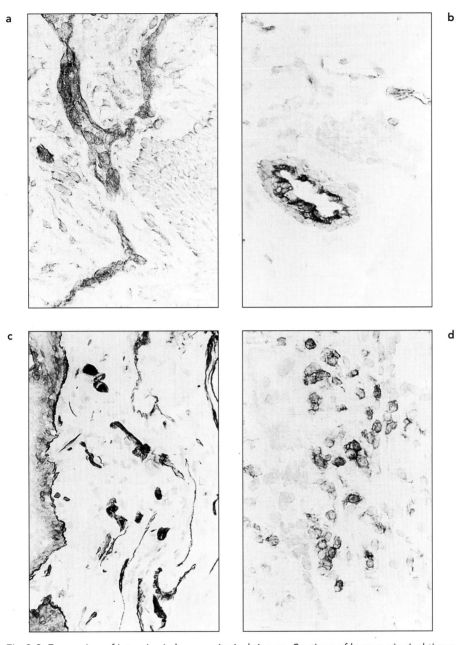

Fig 8-8 Expression of integrins in human gingival tissues. Sections of human gingival tissue were reacted with antibodies against a variety of integrins and visualized by immunohisto-chemistry. **(a)** CD49e (VLA-5), a subunit of the major fibronectin integrin receptor, is present on endothelium and also weakly expressed by mononuclear cells and basal keratinocytes. Original magnification 200×. **(b)** CD61, the β3 subunit of the major vitronectin receptor, is expressed on postcapillary venule endothelium at sites of inflammation. Original magnification 400×. **(c)** CD49f (VLA-6), a component of the major integrin receptor for laminin, is expressed strongly on basal keratinocytes, endothelium, and nerve fibers. Original magnification 200×. **(d)** CD49d (VLA-4), the ligand for vascular cell adhesion molecule (VCAM)-1, is expressed on a subpopulation of T lymphocytes. Original magnification 400×. (Photographs provided courtesy of Dr LJ Walsh, University of Queensland.)

nective tissue by immunocytochemistry (Salonen et al 1990; Tung et al 1985).

With respect to proteoglycan content, uronic acid accounts for 0.3% of the dry weight of the gingiva (Bartold et al 1981). The major glycosaminoglycan of the gingival connective tissue is dermatan sulfate, which accounts for 60% of the total gingival glycosaminoglycans, whereas heparan sulfate accounts for approximately 5%. Within the gingival epithelium, heparan sulfate is the predominant glycosaminoglycan. Hyaluronan and chondroitin sulfate are the other major glycosaminoglycans present in the gingiva. The molecular masses of the sulfated gingival glycosaminoglycans range from 15 kd (heparan sulfate) to 27 kd (dermatan sulfate), though hyaluronan, with a molecular mass of 340 kd, is the largest species (Bartold et al 1982). These glycosaminoglycan components are localized widely in the gingiva, the supraalveolar fiber apparatus, and in loose connective tissues, as well as near the basement membranes. Dermatan sulfate is widespread in the gingival connective tissues; however, it shows a predilection to stain intensely in the tissues immediately subjacent to the epithelium (see Fig 8-3d). There it is associated with the d-band of collagen fibers, and it is believed to provide stability to the collagen fibers (Erlinger et al 1995). In deeper connective tissues of the gingivae, dermatan sulfate is present on collagen fibers along with chondroitin sulfate (Bartold 1992), and it is also located in the perivascular areas associated with most blood vessels (Shibutani et al 1989). Chondroitin sulfate is also widely distributed in the gingival connective tissue, although it is present less prominently than the dermatan sulfate. Like dermatan sulfate, chondroitin sulfate also locates strongly to the perivascular tissues (Bartold 1992; Shibutani et al 1989). In contrast to these glycosaminoglycan species, heparan sulfate is largely found within the basement membranes, on cell surfaces, and in capillary endothelium, where it forms a network (Shibutani et al 1989).

Proteoglycan species identified in the gingiva so far include decorin, biglycan, versican, and syndecan (Bratt et al 1992; Larjava et al 1992a). Decorin is a major proteoglycan localized on collagen fiber bundles, and it appears to be prominently localized in the subepithelial region (Häkkinen et al 1993). Oral epithelium contains biglycan, which forms fine filamentlike structures in the epithelium and underlying connective tissue. In addition to these proteoglycans, a high molecular weight proteoglycan is concentrated at deeper gingival connective tissues, but is sparsely distributed near the epithelium. Another proteoglycan, CD44, is a cell surface proteoglycan located on fibroblasts, and at cell-to-cell contact areas at basal and spinous areas of the oral epithelium (Häkkinen et al 1993).

The cells that synthesize collagens, proteoglycans, and other connective tissue elements are predominantly the fibroblasts in the gingival connective tissue, and epithelial and endothelial cells in the epithelium and blood vessels, respectively (Narayanan and Page 1983). It is possible to culture these cells either by explant technique or after enzyme digestion of the tissue (Fig 8-9). Cultured gingival fibroblasts have provided important information concerning the biosynthesis and regulation of collagens and other matrix components in healthy and diseased periodontal tissues (Narayanan and Page 1983; Narayanan and Bartold 1996). The type and proportion of collagens produced by these cells roughly parallel those present in tissues. Gingival fibroblasts may synthesize up to six different proteoglycans including decorin, biglycan, versican, and syndecan (Bartold and Page 1987; Larjava et al 1992a). The spectrum of the proteoglycan molecules synthesized by gingival fibroblasts resembles that identified in gingival tissues (Bartold et al 1981). In vitro experiments using these cells have offered tremendous insight into how cells in the tissues respond to various growth factors, cytokines, and lymphokines, and how the expression and production of collagens and pro-

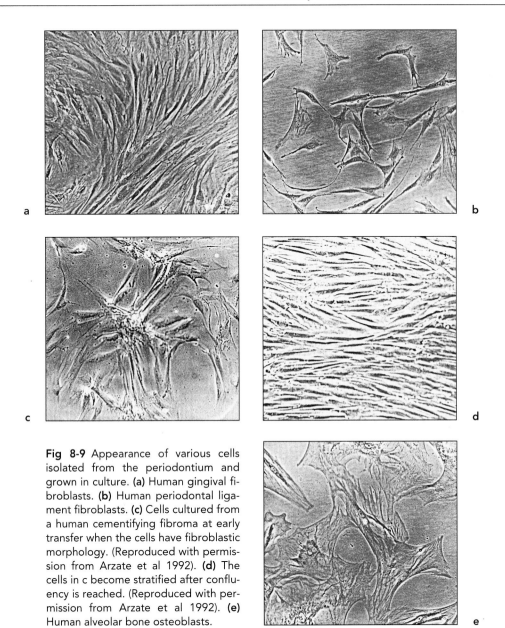

Fig 8-9 Appearance of various cells isolated from the periodontium and grown in culture. **(a)** Human gingival fibroblasts. **(b)** Human periodontal ligament fibroblasts. **(c)** Cells cultured from a human cementifying fibroma at early transfer when the cells have fibroblastic morphology. (Reproduced with permission from Arzate et al 1992). **(d)** The cells in c become stratified after confluency is reached. (Reproduced with permission from Arzate et al 1992). **(e)** Human alveolar bone osteoblasts.

teoglycans are affected by these molecules (Narayanan and Bartold 1996). Gingival fibroblasts and epithelial cells (keratinocytes) have been extensively characterized as sources of collagenase and other metalloproteinases, and significant information has been obtained about their regulation by cytokines, growth factors, and bacterial products, and about how they contribute to normal tissue remodeling and pathologic tissue destruction. These results have recently been reviewed by Birkedal-Hansen (1993) and are discussed in the next chapter.

Periodontal Ligament

The anchorage function of the periodontal ligament is provided by collagen fibers. In mature periodontal ligament, collagen fibers are organized into distinct structural forms. These are classified broadly into two groups, principal fibers and secondary fibers. The principal fibers are dense collagenous bundles traversing the periodontal space between tooth roots and the alveolar wall. They can be subdivided into different groups, based on their location and insertion, as alveolar crest, oblique, transseptal, horizontal, interradicular, or apical fibers (Holmstrup 1996). Those collagen fibers inserting into the cementum of the teeth, and those embedded from the periosteum into the outer circumferential and interstitial lamellae of bone are called Sharpey's fibers. In contrast to the principal fibers, secondary fibers are randomly oriented fibrils located between the principal fibers and investing nerves and blood vessels. These fibers do not attach to cementum or bone.

As in the gingival connective tissue, the major collagen of the periodontal ligament extracellular matrix is type I. Anti–collagen type I antibodies localize this collagen uniformly throughout the tissue on collagen fibrils, especially in major cross-striated Sharpey's fibers that enter cementum. These fibers are

codistributed with type III, V, and VI collagens. While type III collagen is predominantly localized on major fibrils, type V collagen has a more limited distribution (Becker et al 1991; Lukinmaa and Waltimo 1992; Romanos et al 1991b; Tung et al 1985; Wang et al 1980). Type VI collagen is present in the periodontal ligament as fine microfibrils appearing to interconnect cross-striated fibrils (Becker et al 1991; Lukinmaa and Waltimo 1992; Sloan et al 1993); however this collagen and type V collagen, which is located pericellularly, do not appear to be present in the Sharpey's fibers. Interestingly, during connective tissue remodeling in the rat, the type VI collagen appears to be lost as a prelude to degradation of banded collagen fibers (Sloan et al 1993). One of the novel collagen components of the periodontal ligament is type XII collagen, which is believed to be involved in the three-dimensional organization of the extracellular matrix. This collagen is restricted to mature tissues and is not expressed during development (Dublet et al 1988; Karimbux et al 1992), but it is expressed during tooth movement (Karimbux and Nishimura 1995). Type XIV collagen is a molecule that is similar in structure to type XIV (see Chapter 4); it is a variant of undulin. In the periodontal ligament, this collagen is associated with major collagen fibrils, but not with microfibrils (Zhang et al 1993).

The periodontal ligament contains fibronectin and small quantities of many other noncollagenous proteins. The fibronectin is widely distributed between cross-striated collagen fibrils, surrounding these fibrils in the microfibrillar network, and in the pericellular matrix of vascular elements in the blood (Pitaru et al 1987; Zhang et al 1993). The periodontal ligament contains tenascin between densely packed collagen fibrils, particularly in attachment zones near the cementum and bone surfaces (Zhang et al 1993). Elastin is present within the periodontal ligament as a meshwork made up of elastic lamillae, which consists of elastin fibers surrounded by microfibrils (Johnson and Pylypas 1992). A few elastic fibers are incorporated into arterial blood vessel walls. In addition to the above proteins, the periodontal ligament also contains osteonectin and other nonmatrix components such as vitronectin (Tung et al 1985). Periodontal ligament also contains osteopontin. It is produced during alveolar bone regeneration in the periodontal ligament and localized at the border with regenerating bone (Lekic et al 1996a, 1996b). Integrin subunits located in periodontal ligament include α_5, α_v, and β_1 (Uitto et al 1992).

The glycosaminoglycan (GAG) components found in the periodontal ligament include hyaluronate, heparan sulfate, dermatan sulfate, and chondroitin sulfate, of which dermatan sulfate is the principal species (Gibson and Pearson 1992). Periodontal ligament glycosaminoglycans have molecular masses of about 18 to 20 kd, making them slightly smaller than their counterparts in the gingival connective tissue. Versican and decorin are the two principal proteoglycans identified in periodontal ligament, and these probably correspond to the dermatan sulfate and chondroitin sulfate proteoglycans identified in cells cultured from this tissue (Häkkinen et al 1993; Pearson and Pringle 1986).

The major cell in the periodontal ligament is the fibroblast, which is responsible for producing the collagens, noncollagenous proteins, and proteoglycans of this tissue (Ramakrishnan et al 1995; Smalley et al 1984). These cells rest with their long axes parallel to the collagen fibers, and synthesize and degrade collagen. Cell culture experiments have provided a considerable amount of information regarding the production and turnover of the extracellular matrix of the periodontal ligament. These cells have been studied extensively for the production and regulation of collagen, proteoglycans, and integrins (Hou et al 1993; Limeback et al 1983; Ramakrishnan et al 1995; Smalley et al 1984). Interestingly, the fibroblasts of this tissue are unlike the cells of other soft connective tissues and appear to consist of subtypes with distinct phenotype. One of these types is the classic, soft tissue–like fibroblasts similar to those of dermis and gingiva, and the second population is characterized by osteoblast-like cells with high alkaline-phosphatase content. The latter cell type is capable of forming mineralized tissue in culture (Cho et al 1992; Nojima et al 1990; Somerman et al 1988). The cells that possess the osteoblastic phenotype are of particular importance since they are believed to differentiate into cementoblasts and to produce Sharpey's fibers of the cementum (Pitaru et al 1994; Schroeder 1992). The periodontal ligament also contains a few remnants of the Hertwig's epithelial root sheath cells, called cell rests of Malassez. There are very few inflammatory cells in the healthy periodontal ligament.

Cementum

Cementum is the calcified connective tissue that covers the root surfaces of teeth from the cementoenamel junction to the apex, and also lines the apex of the root canal. It is one of the most important components of the attachment apparatus because it is the site through which the connective tissues of the periodontal ligament are inserted into the teeth. Histologically, cementum is very similar to bone and dentin; however, chemical and physical analyses of cementum have indicated it to be softer than dentin (Selvig and Selvig 1962).

Cementum has been classified as primary cementum, a term used to describe the structure that is devoid of cells and contains fine, randomly oriented collagen fibrils embedded in a granular matrix. Secondary cementum contains cells and coarse collagen fibrils oriented parallel to the root surface, and Sharpey's fibers at right angles. In recent years, this classification has been modified to include more specific characteristics to distinguish cementum subtypes. This classification is based on the presence of cells and organization of collagen fibers (Jones 1981; Schroeder 1992, 1993) and it recognizes five subtypes of cementum (Fig 8-10). These are:

1. Acellular afibrillar cementum, located at the dentinoenamel junction; this structure consists of a homogenous matrix without cellular components or collagen fibrils.
2. Acellular extrinsic fiber cementum, located in the cervical to middle root region; this structure also has no cells, but it contains Sharpey's fibers involved in tooth anchorage.
3. Cellular intrinsic fiber cementum, which covers apical and interradicular root surfaces, and is found at resorption lacunae and at fracture sites; cementocytes are present along with intrinsic collagen fibers, and this cementum appears to be involved in repair and adaptation.
4. Acellular intrinsic fiber cementum, similar to the cellular intrinsic fiber cementum, but without cells. This cementum type occupies apical and interradicular root surfaces.
5. Cellular mixed stratified cementum, consisting of intrinsic and extrinsic collagen fibers and containing cementocytes; this is involved in root anchorage and adaptation.

The intrinsic and extrinsic fibers represent two fiber systems in cementum with entirely different functions. Intrinsic fibers lie parallel to the root surface and are believed to be primarily repair components produced by cementocytes. In contrast, the Sharpey's, or extrinsic, fibers are embedded at right angles into the root surfaces and are responsible for tooth anchorage. The extrinsic fibers are believed to be produced initially by cells of the dental follicle during development and later by periodontal ligament fibroblasts (Schroeder 1992).

Biochemically, the cementum is made up of an inorganic matrix, approximately 50% of which is hydroxyapatite, and an organic matrix composed of predominantly type I and III collagens (Birkedal-Hansen et al 1977).

Immunocytochemical studies have shown that the collagen fibers, including the Sharpey's fibers, are type I collagen. The cementum remains largely unstained with antibodies to type III collagen, except on Sharpey's fibers and some new collagen fibrils, where the type III collagen appears to coat these fibers (Rao et al 1979; Wang et al 1980). Based on immunostaining, the cementum does not appear to have either type V or type VI collagen (Becker et al 1991; Romanos et al 1991b), but it does contain type XIV. The organic matrix also contains a variety of nonfibrous proteins; prominent and biologically important among these are bone sialoprotein, osteopontin, tenascin, fibronectin, osteonectin, and proteoglycans (Bronckers et al 1994; MacNeil and Somerman 1993; MacNeil et al 1995; McKee et al 1996).

Bone sialoprotein, an RGD-containing protein with cell adhesion properties, appears to be associated with mineralization during cementogenesis (Bronckers et al 1994; Chen et al 1992; MacNeil et al 1995; McKee et al 1996). Osteopontin is another adhesion protein present in cementum that is associated with acellular cementum in developing mouse incisors (Bronckers et al 1994; McKee et al 1996; MacNeil et al 1995; Chen et al 1992; Somerman et al 1990). The cementum sequesters several growth factors including FGF-1 and 2, bone-morphogenetic protein, TGF-β, and an IGF-I–like molecule and growth factor receptors (Cho and Garant 1988, 1996; Kawai and Urist 1989; MacNeil and Somerman 1993; Nakae et al 1991; Wu et al 1996). Cementoblasts of the cellular cementum appear to produce these proteins along with TGF-β and IGF-I (Bronckers et al 1994; Tenorio et al 1993).

In cementum, glycosaminoglycan components hyaluronan, dermatan sulfate, and chondroitin sulfate have been identified biochemically and immunohistochemically as the predominant species. These components are closely associated with cementoblasts, and they are lightly distributed throughout the

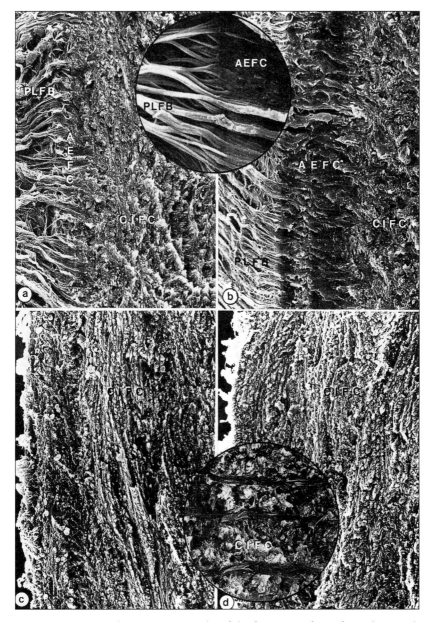

Fig 8-10 Scanning electron micrographs of the fracture surface of a molar root illustrating cellular mixed stratified cementum. Acellular extrinsic fiber cementum (AEFC) is present in **(a)** and **(b)**, but not in **(c)** and **(d)**. The extrinsic fiber bundles are attached perpendicularly to the surface of the cellular intrinsic fiber cementum (CIFC) and insert into it **(a)**. This is shown in higher magnification in the inset in **(a)** and **(b)**, where PLFB indicates periodontal ligament fiber bundles. Intrinsic fibers, on the other hand, run parallel to the CIFC, where a few Sharpey's fibers (SF) are embedded (inset in **c** and **d**). Magnifications: **a**, **b**: ×720; **c**, **d**: ×470; inset in **a** and **b**: ×9400; inset in **c** and **d**: ×1800. (Reproduced with permission from Schroeder 1993.)

matrix (Bartold et al 1988; Bartold et al 1990). Recently, keratan sulfate–containing proteoglycans (lumican and fibroglycan) have been identified in bovine cementum and these are found to localize almost exclusively in precementum and around precementocyte lacunae (Cheng et al 1996). These findings suggest a role for proteoglycans in the formation of the mineralized matrix of cementum.

The identity of the cells responsible for producing the above matrix components in cementum has not been determined. Current evidence indicates that the extrinsic fiber system is produced by fibroblasts from the periodontal ligament, while the intrinsic fibers may be made by cementocytes originating from the bone (Pitaru et al 1994; Schroeder 1992). To date, it has been difficult to culture cementoblasts or cementocytes, although these cells are believed to derive from progenitors in vascular spaces of the periodontal ligament or endosteal spaces of bone (Pitaru et al 1994). Nevertheless, cementoblastlike cells, which produce cementum proteins in culture, can be isolated and grown from cementum tumors (Arzate et al 1992).

Alveolar Bone

The major organic constituent of the alveolar bone matrix is type I collagen, which, like in the periodontal ligament, makes up the bulk of the Sharpey's fibers (Rao et al 1979; Wang et al 1980). In these fibers, the type I collagen is codistributed with type III (Huang et al 1991). The type I collagen is prominently expressed by the osteoblasts, and by osteocytes in areas of remodeling alveolar bone (Helder et al 1993). Periosteal and endosteal layers express fibronectin, its receptors, and tenascin (Pitaru et al 1987). Alveolar bone also contains other bone-specific noncollagenous proteins such as osteocalcin and bone sialoprotein, and nonspecific components such as osteopontin and osteonectin (Bronckers et al 1994; Chen et al

1993; Lekic et al 1996a, 1996b; Helder et al 1993; Maeno et al 1992; McKee et al 1996).

Within the extracellular matrix of the alveolar bone, fibronectin, bone sialoprotein, osteopontin, and several other cell adhesion molecules are stored, along with growth factors including fibroblast growth factor (FGF)-1 and 2, platelet-derived growth factor (PDGF), IGF-I, TGF-β, and bone morphogenetic proteins (Nakae et al 1991). The distribution of integrins in alveolar bone has also been studied; osteoclasts were found to express integrin subunit α_v strongly, and α_5 to a lesser extent. Osteoblasts appear to express the α_5 and α_2 subunits (Steffensen et al 1992). The major alveolar bone glycosaminoglycan species identified in human alveolar bone is chondroitin sulfate. This glycosaminoglycan component is present along with heparan sulfate, dermatan sulfate, and hyaluronate (Bartold 1990; Waddington and Embery 1991). Immunohistochemical localization studies have shown that these molecules are distributed on cells in their lacunae and in the mineralized matrix. Analyses of the alveolar bone proteoglycans have identified a chondroitin sulfate–rich proteoglycan, with a core protein rich in glycine, leucine, glutamate, and aspartate, as the major species (Bartold 1990; Waddington and Embery 1991); this is likely to be a mixture of decorin and biglycan.

The constituent collagen and proteoglycan types and their locations in various periodontal components are summarized in Tables 8-1 and 8-2.

Summary

The extracellular matrices of the tissues that comprise the periodontium are composed of a number of fibrous and nonfibrous proteins. The molecular makeup of each compartment of the periodontium is somewhat similar, however the organization into three-dimensional architecture is specific for each com-

Table 8-1. Distribution of Collagen Types in the Periodontium

Tissue	Collagen Type*	Location
Healthy gingiva	I	Lamina propria
	III	Lamina propria
	IV	Basement membranes
	V	Collagen fibers, blood vessels
	VI	Microfibrils
Periodontal ligament	I	Principal, secondary fibers
	III	Same as type I
	V	Collagen fibers
Cementum	I	Sharpey's fibers, fibrillar cementum
	III	Sharpey's fibers
	V	Sharpey's fibers
Alveolar bone	I	Bone matrix, Sharpey's fibers
	III	Sharpey's fibers
Inflamed gingiva	I	Same as healthy gingiva
	III	Same as healthy gingiva
	V	Same as healthy gingiva
	IV, V, VI	Same as healthy gingiva
	$[\alpha 1(I)_3]$	Lamina propria

*In all structures, type I is the major species of collagen, accounting for 80%–85% in the gingiva, and 99% in bone. Type III is the second most predominant collagen in gingiva and periodontal ligament forming ~15% of the total. In alveolar bone and cementum, type III is restricted to Sharpey's fibers. The total content of all other collagens in healthy tissues is <1%.

Table 8-2. Glycosaminoglycans and Proteoglycans in the Periodontium

Tissue	GAG*	Proteoglycans†
Gingiva	DS‡, HA, CS, HS§ biglycan, versican, CD44	CS-PG, DS-PG, decorin
Periodontal ligament	DS‡, CS, HA, HS	CS-PG, DS-PG
Alveolar bone	CS‡, DS, HA, HS	CS-PG
Cementum	CS‡, DS, HA	CS-PG

* GAG, glycosaminoglycans; DS, dermatan sulfate; CS, chondroitin sulfate; HS, heparan sulfate; PG, proteoglycan.
† The localization of proteoglycans is as follows: CS-PG, general matrix in soft tissues and matrix and lacunae of bone and cementum. DS-PG and decorin, subepithelial matrix in the gingiva. Decorin, predominantly at the subepithelial matrix. HA, mostly in the epithelium. CD44, on epithelial cells. See text for references.
‡ Major species. DS is the major species in gingival connective tissues.
§ HS is the major GAG species in the gingival epithelium.

partment's own particular structure and function. One unique feature of the periodontium is that, although each component is separate structurally, they function together as one unit and the components of one structure affect the cellular activities of others. The production and maintenance of connective tissue components are critical for the overall physiologic well-being of each tissue. Thus, while the tissues of the periodontium undergo very rapid turnover, this process is an important compensatory mechanism to overcome some of the large mechanical and chemical stresses to which the tissues are subjected. An understanding of the molecular composition of the normal tissues is essential for recognizing the requirements for tissue repair and regeneration, as well as for recognizing the effects of tissue degradation. If the delicate molecular architecture of these tissues is destroyed, as seen in the development of periodontal inflammation, the integrity of the tissues is compromised with subsequent loss of function.

References

Arzate H, Olson SW, Page RC, Narayanan AS. Isolation of human tumor cells that produce cementum proteins in culture. Bone Miner 1992;18:15.

Bartold PM. Proteoglycans of the periodontium: Structure, role and functions. J Periodont Res 1987;22:431.

Bartold PM. A biochemical and immunohistochemical study of the proteoglycans of alveolar bone. J Dent Res 1990;69:7.

Bartold PM. Connective tissue of the periodontium. Research and clinical implications. Aust Dent J 1991;36;255.

Bartold PM. Distribution of chondroitin sulfate and dermatan sulfate in normal and inflamed human gingiva. J Dent Res 1992;71:1587.

Bartold PM, Miki Y, McAllister B, Narayanan AS, Page RC. Glycosaminoglycans of human cementum. J Periodont Res 1988;23:13.

Bartold PM, Narayanan AS. The biochemistry and physiology of the periodontium. In: Wilson TG, Kornman KS, eds. Fundamentals of Periodontics. Chicago: Quintessence; 1996:27.

Bartold PM, Page RC. Isolation and characterization of proteoglycans synthesized by adult human gingival fibroblasts *in vitro*. Arch Biochem Biophys 1987;253:399.

Bartold PM, Reinboth B, Nakae H, Narayanan AS, Page RC. Proteoglycans of bovine cementum: Isolation and characterization. Matrix 1990;10:10.

Bartold PM, Wiebkin OW, Thonard JC. Glycosaminoglycans of human gingival epithelium and connective tissue. Connect Tissue Res 1981;9:99.

Bartold PM, Wiebkin OW, Thonard JC. Proteoglycans in human gingiva: molecular size distribution in epithelium and in connective tissue. Arch Oral Biol 1982;27:1.

Becker J, Schuppan D, Rabanus JP, Rauch H, Niechoy U, Gelderblom HR. Immunoelectron microscopic localization of collagens type I, V and VI and procollagen type III in human periodontal ligament and cementum. J Histochem Cytochem 1991;39:103.

Birkedal-Hansen H. Role of matrix metalloproteinases in human periodontal diseases. J Periodontol 1993;64:474.

Birkedal-Hansen H, Butler WT, Taylor RE. Proteins of the periodontium. Characterization of the insoluble collagens of bovine dental cementum. Calc Tissue Res 1977;23:39.

Bratt P, Anderson MM, Mansson-Rahemtulla B, Stevens JW, Zhou C, Rahemtulla F. Isolation and characterization of bovine gingival proteoglycans versican and decorin. Int J Biochem 1992;24:1573.

Braun-Faulco O. The histochemistry of psoriasis. Ann NYork Acad Sci 1959;73:936.

Bronckers AL, Farach-Carlson MC, Van Waveren E, Butler WT. Immunolocalization of osteopontin, osteocalcin, and dentin sialoprotein during dental root formation and early cementogenesis in the rat. J Bone Miner Res 1994;9:833.

Chavrier C, Couble ML, Magloire H, Grimaud JA. Connective tissue organization of healthy human gingiva. Ultrastructural localization of collagen types I-III-IV. J Periodont Res 1984;19:221.

Chen J, McCulloch CA, Sodek J. Bone sialoprotein in developing porcine dental tissues: cellular expression and comparison of tissue localization with osteopontin and osteonectin. Arch Oral Biol 1993;38:241.

Chen J, Shapiro HS, Sodek H. Development expression of bone sialoprotein mRNA in rat mineralized connective tissues. J Bone Miner Res 1992;7:987.

Cheng H, Caterson B, Neame PJ, Lester G, Yamauchi M. Differential distribution of lumican and fibromodulin in tooth cementum. Connect Tissue Res 1996;34:87.

Cho MI, Garant PR, Lee Y-L. Periodontal ligament fibroblasts, preosteoblasts, and prechondrocytes express receptors for epidermal growth factor in vivo: a comparative radioautographic study. J Periodont Res 1988;23:287.

Cho MI, Garant PR. Expression and role of epidermal growth factor receptors during differentiation of cementoblasts, osteoblasts, and periodontal ligament fibroblasts in the rat. Anat Rec 1996;245:342.

Cho MI, Matsuda N, Lin WL, Moshier A. In vitro formation of mineralized nodules by periodontal ligament cells from the rat. Calcif Tissue Int 1992;50:459.

Dublet B, Dixon E, de Miguel E, van der Rest M. Bovine type XII collagen: amino acid sequence of a 10 kDa pepsin fragment for periodontal ligament reveals high degree of homology with the chicken α1 XII sequence. FEBS Lett 1988;233:177.

Erlinger T, Willershausen-Zonnchan B, Welsch U. Ultrastructural localization of glycosaminoglycans in human gingival connective tissue using cupromeronic blue. J Periodont Res 1995;30:108.

Gibson GJ, Pearson CH. Sulfated galactosaminoglycans of bovine periodontal ligament. Evidence for the presence of two major types of hybrids but no chondroitin sulfate. Connect Tissue Res 1992;10:161.

Graner E, Line SR, Jorge J Jr, Lopes MA, Almeida OF. Laminin and collagen IV distribution and ultrastructure of the basement membrane of the gingiva of the rat incisor. J Periodont Res 1995;30:349.

Häkkinen L, Oksala O, Salo T, Rahemtulla F, Larjarva H. Immunohistochemical localization of proteoglycans in human periodontium. J Histochem Cytochem 1993; 41:1689.

Holmstrup P. The microanatomy of the periodontium. In: Wilson TG, Kornman KS, eds. Fundamentals of Periodontics. Chicago: Quintessence; 1996:27.

Helder MN, Bronchers AL, Woltgens JH. Dissimilar expression of osteopontin (OPN) and collagen type I in dental tissues and alveolar bone of the neonatal rat. Matrix 1993;13:415.

Hormia M, Virtanen I, Quaranta V. Immunolocalization of integrin α6, β4 in mouse junctional epithelium suggests an anchoring function to both the internal and the external basal lamina. J Dent Res 1992;71:1503.

Hormia M, Ylänne J, Virtanen I. Expression of integrins in human gingiva. J Dent Res 1990;69:1817.

Hou LT, Yaeger JA. Cloning and characterization of human gingival and periodontal ligament fibroblasts. J Periodontol 1993;64:1209.

Huang YH, Ohsaki Y, Kurisu K. Distribution of type I and III collagen in the developing periodontal ligament of mice. Matrix 1991;11:25.

Johnson RB, Pylypas SP. A re-evaluation of the elastic meshwork within the periodontal ligament of the mouse. J Periodont Res 1992;27:239.

Jones SJ. Dental Anatomy and Embryology. Oxford: Blackwell Scientific; 1981:193–294.

Karimbux NY, Nishimura I. Temporal and spatial expressions of type XII collagen in the remodeling of periodontal ligament during experimental tooth movement. J Dent Res 1995;74:313.

Karimbux NY, Rosenblum ND, Nishimura I. Site-specific expression of collagen I and XII mRNAs in the rat periodontal ligament at two developmental stages. J Dent Res 1992;71;1355.

Kawai T, Urist MR. Bovine tooth-derived bone morphogenetic protein. J Dent Res 1989;68:1069.

Kogaya Y, Haruna S, Vojinovic J, Iwayama Y, Akisaka T. Histochemical localization at the electron microscopic level of sulfated glycosaminoglycans in the rat gingiva. J Periodont Res 1989;24:199.

Larjava H, Hakkinen L, Rahemtulla F. A biochemical analysis of human periodontal tissue proteoglycans. Biochem J 1992a;284:267.

Larjava H, Zhou C, Larjava I, Rahemtulla F. Immunolocalization of β1 integrins in human gingival epithelium and cultured keratinocytes. Scand J Dent Res 1992b; 100:266.

Lekic P, Sodek J, McCulloch CA. Osteopontin and bone sialoprotein expression in regenerating rat periodontal ligament and alveolar bone. Anat Rec 1996a;244:50.

Lekic P, Sodek J, McCulloch CA. Relationship of cellular proliferation to expression of osteopontin and bone sialoprotein in regenerating rat periodontium. Cell Tissue Res 1996b;285:491.

Limeback H, Sodek J, Aubin JE. Variation in collagen expression by cloned periodontal ligament cells. J Periodont Res 1983;18:242.

Lukinmaa PL, Mackie EJ, Thesleff I. Immunohistochemical localization of the matrix glycoproteins—tenascin and the ED-sequence containing form of cellular fibronectin—in human permanent teeth and periodontal ligament. J Dent Res 1991;70:19.

Lukinmaa PL, Waltimo J. Immunohistochemical localization of types I, V and VI collagen in human permanent teeth and periodontal ligament. J Dent Res 1992;71:391.

MacNeil RL, Berry J, D'Errico J, Strayhorn C, Piotrowski B, Somerman MJ. Role of two mineral-associated adhesion molecules osteopontin and bone sialoprotein during cementogenesis. Connect Tissue Res 1995;33:1.

MacNeil RL, Somerman MJ. Factors regulating development and regeneration of cementum. J Periodont Res 1993;28:550.

Maeno M, Taguchi M, Suzuki N, et al. Characterization of mineral-binding 40-kDa glycoprotein extracted from young adult rabbit alveolar bone. J Nihon Univ Sch Dent 1992;34:77.

McKee MD, Zalzal S, Nanci A. Extracellular matrix in root cementum and mantle dentis: localization of osteopontin and other noncollagenous proteins, plasma proteins and glycoconjugates by electron microscopy. Anat Rec 1996;245:293.

Nakae H, Narayanan AS, Raines E, Page RC. Isolation and partial characterization of mitogenic factors from cementum. Biochemistry 1991;30:7047.

Narayanan AS, Bartold PM. Biochemistry of periodontal connective tissues and their regeneration. A current perspective. Connect Tissue Res 1996;34:191.

Narayanan AS, Clagett JA, Page RC. Effect of inflammation on the distribution of collagen types, I, III, IV, and V and type I trimer and fibronectin in human gingivae. J Dent Res 1985;64:1111.

Narayanan AS, Page RC. Connective tissues of the periodontium: A summary of current work. Coll Relat Res 1983;3:33.

Nojima N, Kobayashi M, Shionome M, Takahashi N, Suda T, Hasegawa K. Fibroblastic cells derived from bovine periodontal ligaments have the phenotypes of osteoblasts. J Periodont Res 1990;25:179.

Oyarzún-Droguett A. Ultracytochemical localization of basal lamina anionic sites in the rat epithelial attachment apparatus. J Periodont Res 1992;27:256.

Page RC, Ammons WF. Collagen turnover in the gingival and other mature connective tissues of the marmoset Saguinus oedipus. Arch Oral Biol 1974;19:651.

Pearson CH, Pringle GA. Chemical and immunochemical characteristics of proteoglycans in bovine gingiva and dental pulp. Arch Oral Biol 1986;31:541.

Pedlar J. Histochemistry of glycosaminoglycans in the skin and oral mucosa of the rat. Arch Oral Biol 1979;24 777.

Pitaru S, Aubin JE, Bhargava U, Melcher AH. Immuno-electron microscopic studies on the distributions of fibronectin and actin in a cellular dense connective tissue: the periodontal ligament of the rat. J Periodont Res 1987; 22:64.

Pitaru S, McCulloch CAG, Narayanan AS. Cellular origins and differentiation control mechanisms during periodontal development and wound healing. J Periodont Res 1994; 29:81.

Potter-Perigo S, Prather P, Baker C, Altman LC, Wight TN. Partial characterization of proteoglycans synthesized by human gingival epithelial cells in culture. J Periodont Res 1993;28:81.

Ramakrishnan PR, Lin WL, Sodek J, Cho MI. Synthesis of noncollagenous extracellular matrix proteins during development of mineralized nodules by rat periodontal ligament cells in vitro. Calcif Tissue Int 1995;57:52.

Rao LG, Wang HM, Kalliecharan R, Heersche JN, Sodek J. Specific immunohistochemical localization of type I collagen in porcine periodontal tissues using the peroxidase-labelled antibody technique. Histochem J 1979;11:73.

Romanos G, Schröter-Kermani C, Hinz N, Bernimoulin JP. Immunohistochemical distribution of the collagen types IV, V, VI and glycoprotein laminin in the healthy rat, marmoset (Callithrix jacchus) and human gingivae. Matrix 1991a;11:125.

Romanos GE, Schröter-Kermani C, Hinz N, Wachtel HC, Bernimoulin JP. Immunohistochemical localization of collagenous components in healthy periodontal tissues of the rat and marmoset (Callithrix jacchus) II. Distribution of collagen types IV, V, and VI. J Periodont Res 1991b; 26:323.

Romanos GE, Schröter-Kermani C, Hinz N, Wachtel HC, Bernimoulin JP. Immunohistochemical localization of collagenous components in periodontal tissues of the rat and marmoset (Callithrix jacchus) I. Distribution of collagen types I and III. J Periodont Res 1992;27:101.

Salonen J, Domenicucci C, Goldberg HA, Sodek J. Immunohistochemical localization of SPARC (Osteonectin) and denatured collagen and their relationship to remodeling in rat dental tissues. Arch Oral Biol 1990;35:337.

Sawada T, Yamamoto T, Yanagisawa T, Takuma S, Hasegawa H, Watanabe K. Electron-immunocytochemistry of laminin and type IV collagen in the junctional epithelium of rat molar gingiva. J Periodont Res 1990;25:372.

Schluger S, Yuodelis RA, Page RC. In: Periodontal Diseases. 3rd ed. Philadelphia: Lea & Febiger; 1990.

Schroeder HE. Biological problems of regenerative cementogenesis: Synthesis and attachment of collagenous matrices on growing and established root surfaces. Int Rev Cytol 1992;142:1.

Schroeder HE. Human cellular mixed stratified cementum: a tissue with alternating layers of acellular extrinsic- and cellular intrinsic fiber cementum. Schweiz Monatsshr Zahnmed 1993;103:550.

Selvig KA, Selvig SK. Mineral content of human and seal cementum. J Dent Res 1962;41:624.

Shibutani T, Murahashi Y, Iwayama Y. Immunohistochemical localization of chondroitin sulfate and dermatan sulfate proteoglycan in human gingival connective tissue. J Periodont Res 1989;24:310.

Sloan P, Carter DH, Kielty CM, Shuttleworth CA. An immunochemical study examining the role of collagen type VI in the rodent periodontal ligament. Histochem J 1993; 25:523.

Smalley JW, Shuttleworth CA, Grant ME. Synthesis and secretion of sulfated glycosaminoglycans by bovine periodontal ligament fibroblast cultures. Arch Oral Biol 1984;29:107.

Sodek J. A new approach to assessing collagen turnover by using a micro-assay. A highly efficient and rapid turnover of collagen in rat periodontal tissues. Biochem J 1976: 160:243.

Sodek J, Ferrier JM. Collagen remodelling in rat periodontal tissues: compensation for precursor reutilization confirms rapid turnover of collagen. Coll Relat Res 1988;8:11.

Somerman MJ, Archer SY, Imm GR, Foster RA. A comparative study of human periodontal ligament cells and gingival fibroblasts in vitro. J Dent Res 1988;67:66.

Somerman MJ, Shroff B, Agraves WS, et al. Expression of attachment proteins during cementogenesis. J Biol Buccale 1990;18:207.

Steffensen B, Duong AH, Milam SB, et al. Immunohistological localization of cell adhesion proteins and integrins in the periodontium. J Periodontol 1992;63:584.

Tammi R, Tammi M, Häkkinen L, Lajarva H. Histochemical localization of hyaluronate in human oral epithelium using a specific hyaluronate-binding probe. Arch Oral Biol 1990;35:219.

Tenorio D, Cruchley A, Hughes FJ. Immunocytochemical investigation of the rat cementoblast phenotype. J Periodont Res 1993;28:411.

Thonard JC, Scherp HW. Histochemical demonstration of acid mucopolysaccharides in human gingival intracellular spaces. Arch Oral Biol 1962;7:125–136.

Tung TS, Domenicucci C, Wasi S, Sodek J. Specific immunolocalization of osteonectin and collagen types I and III in fetal and adult porcine dental tissues. J Histochem Cytochem 1985;33:531.

Uitto J, Mauviel A, McGrath J. The dermal-epidermal basement membrane zone in cutaneous wound healing. In: Clark RAF, ed. The Molecular and Cellular Biology of Wound Repair. 2nd ed. New York: Plenum; 1996:513.

Uitto J, Larjava H, Peltonen J, Brunette DM. Expression of fibronectin and integrins in cultured periodontal ligament epithelial cells. J Dent Res 1992;71:1203.

Waddington RJ, Embery G. Structural characterization of human alveolar bone proteoglycans. Arch Oral Biol 1991; 36:859.

Wang H-M, Nanda V, Rao LG, Melcher AH, Heersche JN, Sodek J. Specific immunohistochemical localization of type III collagen in porcine periodontal tissues using the peroxidase-antiperoxidase method. J Histochem Cytochem 1980;28:1215.

Wiebkin OW, Thonard JC. Mucopolysaccharide localization in gingival epithelium. J Periodont Res 1981;16:600.

Willie JJ, Månsson-Rahemtulla B, Rahemtulla F. Characterization of human gingival keratinocytes cultured in serum-free medium. Arch Oral Biol 1990;35:967.

Wu D, Ikezawa K, Parker T, Saito S, Narayanan AS. Characterization of a collagenous cementum-derived attachment protein. J Bone Miner Res 1996;11:686.

Zhang X, Schuppan D, Becker J, Reichart P, Gelderblom HR. Distribution of undulin, tenascin, and fibronectin in human periodontal ligament and cementum. Comparative electron microscopy with ultra-thin cryosections. J Histochem Cytochem 1993;41:245.

Diseased Periodontium

Introduction

Although the periodontium meets the challenges of mechanical and microbial stresses remarkably well and maintains its function, there are numerous situations where the tissue structure and function are severely affected. For example, both acute and chronic inflammatory responses within the gingival connective tissues can lead to significant matrix degradation, impacting not only the gingival connective tissues, but also the periodontal ligament and alveolar bone. Many systemic and drug-induced diseases also affect the periodontal tissues, especially the gingiva.

The diseases affecting the periodontium can be classified broadly into two groups. The first group includes inherited diseases that arise from defects in the gene structure of proteins; these are caused by mutations, deletions, or insertions in the gene. The second group of diseases are acquired, and include those, such as inflammatory diseases, that affect the periodontium directly, and those that are secondary to other diseases, such as diabetes. The acquired diseases may have a genetic component, but they are precipitated by factors other than a defect in molecular structure. Although it is not truly a disease, aging also generates connective tissue changes that are associated with the impairment of periodontal function. This chapter discusses various inherited diseases that have associated periodontal complications. In addition, the biochemical alterations occurring in the extracellular matrix of the periodontium in acquired diseases, especially periodontitis and drug-induced hyperplasias, are outlined. Possible mechanisms that are likely to contribute to these alterations are also discussed.

Periodontal Connective Tissues and Inherited Diseases

There are many inherited diseases and syndromes in which periodontal disease of one form or another is a clinical feature (Table 9-1). These conditions affect a broad range of tissues, cells, biochemical processes, and host defense processes. Significantly, the genes responsible for all of these conditions do not appear to cluster on one particular chromosome; this highlights the multifactorial and polydisperse nature of the periodontal diseases. As such, these conditions need to be recognized and warrant brief discussion.

Connective Tissue Disorders

Conditions affecting the composition of matrix proteins have almost universal effects on the molecular architecture of all connective tissues, including the periodontium. Ehlers-Danlos syndrome is a group of conditions that collectively demonstrate mutations in human procollagen genes (Byers 1995; Hartsfield and Kouseff 1990). Various forms of Ehlers-Danlos syndrome have an associated cementum defect as well as marked periodontal destruction (Barabas 1969; Stewart et al

1977). Mucopolysaccharidoses and mannosidosis are characterized by defects in the enzymes associated with glycosaminoglycan and glycoprotein synthesis. The periodontal implications associated with these conditions are generally restricted to gingival overgrowth with little evidence of significant periodontal destruction (Cawson 1962; Bartold 1992).

Inherited hyperplasias of periodontal tissues include generalized gingival hyperplasia, as well as dental and oral fibromatoses that occur spontaneously. Gingival overgrowth is the major feature in these lesions, which resemble drug-induced gingival overgrowth. Cells derived from these lesions have been noted to differ from cells of normal tissues in their proliferation rates, collagen production, and response to cytokines (Nakao et al 1995). In general, the familial fibromatoses do not tend to demonstrate any association with destructive periodontal disease (Wynne et al 1995).

Metabolic Disorders

Takahara's disease (acatalasia) is a monogenetic condition affecting the production of catalase, an enzyme important in removing the hydrogen peroxide generated during normal cell metabolism. Since hydrogen peroxide can be toxic and leads to generation of superoxide radicals, tissue destruction is a common sequela to its accumulation. These patients are predisposed to bacterial infections of tissues that develop into fulminating areas of excessive tissue destruction (Eaton and Ma 1995). Both gingival necrosis and severe alveolar bone destruction have been noted in these patients (Delgado and Calderon 1979).

Hypophosphatasia represents a group of monogenetic conditions that do not all follow the same inheritance pattern. This condition is characterized by reduced levels of serum alkaline phosphatase, increased urinary phosphoethanolamine, and hypo-osteogenesis leading to significant skeletal abnormalities. In many cases, hypocementosis and prema-

Table 9-1. Monogenetic and Chromosomal Defects Associated with Periodontal Defects

Condition	Tissue/Cell/ Biochemical Defect	Periodontal Condition	Mode of Inheritance
Connective tissue disorders			
Ehlers-Danlos Syndrome			
Type IV	Collagen type III	Fragile tissues and EOP	AR or AD
Type VII	Procollagen peptidase	Fragile tissues and EOP	AR or AD
Type IX	Collagen	Fragile tissues and EOP	X-Linked
Mucopolysaccharidoses	Proteoglycans	Gingival overgrowth	. . .
Mannosidosis	Mannose	Gingival overgrowth	. . .
Familial fibromatoses	Collagen	Gingival overgrowth	Variable
Metabolic disorders			
Acatalasia	Catalase	Gingival necrosis and EOP	AR
Hypophosphatasia	Alkaline phosphatase	Poorly mineralized bone and cementum and EOP	AR (?AD)
Leukocyte defects			
Chédiak-Higashi syndrome	Neutrophil	EOP	AR
Chronic neutropenia	Neutrophil	EOP	AD
Cyclic neutropenia	Neutrophil	EOP	AD
Leukocyte adhesion defect	Neutrophil	EOP	AD
Dermatologic defects			
Papillon-Lefèvre syndrome	Keratin/epithelium	EOP	AR
Chromosomal disorders			
Trisomy 21	Multiple biochemical	CIPD, EOP	. . .

AD, autosomal dominant; AR, autosomal recessive; CIPD, chronic inflammatory periodontal disease; EOP, early-onset periodontitis.

ture loss of deciduous teeth in children are common findings (Whyte 1995). Hypophosphatasia and its associated cementum defect have been implicated in forms of early-onset periodontitis (Page and Baab 1985; Plagmann et al 1994).

Acromegaly and Paget's disease may be associated with hypercementosis, in which the apical third of the root is affected. This does not appear to be associated with any form of periodontal disease.

Leukocyte Defects

Defects in immune cell function lead to inadequate host defense and uncontrolled tissue destruction when challenged by bacterial infections. In patients suffering from various forms of neutropenia, there is a significant reduction in the number of neutrophils, which leads to recurrent bacterial infections of which severe periodontitis is a common feature (Deasy et al 1980; Kirstilia et al 1993). While some forms of neutropenia occur spontaneously, others appear to be of a familial nature and may be autosomal dominant. Qualitative defects in neutrophil function also contribute to severe periodontal destruction. For example, Chédiak-Higashi syndrome is a genetically transmitted disease characterized by reduced neutrophil function and susceptibility to recurrent bacterial infections. Rapidly progressing early-onset periodontitis is a characteristic feature of this disease (Temple et al 1972; Hamilton et al 1974). Leukocyte adhesion deficiency (LAD) is associated with a defect in either the *Mac-1* gene (LAD I) or absence of the membrane glycoprotein, CD15s (LAD II). These conditions, which have strong familial distributions, lead to impairment of leukocyte adhesion and are associated with severe early-onset forms of periodontal disease (Page et al 1983; Waldrop et al 1995). In general, defects in polymorphonuclear leukocyte chemotaxis and adhesion have been noted in approximately 75% of patients with early-onset forms of periodontitis (Altman et al 1985; Van Dyke et al 1980). In some of these individuals, the reduction in expression of cell surface attachment proteins is inherited in an X-linked fashion (Crowley et al 1980). In other forms of early-onset periodontitis, where high levels of immunoglobulin G2 have been noted, the mode of inheritance seems to be autosomal dominant (Marazita et al 1996).

Dermatologic Disorders

Papillon-Lefèvre syndrome is a monogenetic condition characterized by hyperkeratosis of the palmar and plantar surfaces together with a very destructive form of early-onset periodontitis. The periodontal destruction can be so rapid as to lead to complete loss (exfoliation) of all teeth by 3 to 4 years of age (Hattab et al 1995). The underlying mechanism responsible for the rapid periodontal breakdown is unclear, although some reports have implied that there may be inherent immunologic and neutrophil deficiencies (Van Dyke et al 1984).

Chromosomal Disorders

The best-recognized chromosome defect that has a periodontal component is trisomy 21 (Down Syndrome). Both early-onset periodontitis as well as advanced adult-type chronic inflammatory periodontitis have been noted in these individuals. A genetic compo-

nent to this condition is indicated by the fact that although individuals with either Down syndrome or non–Down syndrome retardation (eg, individuals with cerebral palsy complicated with retardation) have similar problems maintaining adequate oral hygiene, those with Down syndrome have a significantly greater amount of advanced periodontal destruction (Sznajder et al 1968; Cohen et al 1961; Cuttress 1971). Nevertheless, a number of other environmental factors such as whether the individual lives at home or in an institution, tongue abnormalities, tooth morphology, malocclusion, and chewing patterns may also impact on the periodontal disease in individuals with Down syndrome. The severity of the problem thus appears be a combination of both genetic and environmental influences.

Acquired Diseases of the Periodontium

This group of diseases includes gingivitis, periodontitis, drug-induced gingival overgrowth, and other diseases caused by agents of known and unknown etiology. Evolution of these diseases depends upon many factors including host, genetic, environmental, and microbial factors. The ultimate outcome of disease is intricately associated with disturbances to the balance between host defense mechanisms and microbial assault.

Gingivitis and Periodontitis

General concepts. Gingivitis and periodontitis are two of the most common chronic inflammatory diseases affecting humans as well as several, but not all, other animal species. These diseases are the result of an induction of host inflammatory responses to the accumulation of bacteria on tooth surfaces adjacent to the supra- and subgingival tissues.

Initially, gingivitis represents a generalized acute inflammatory response to the bacteria that colonize on the tooth surface adjacent to the gingiva. With time, gingivitis may become well-established, but remain confined to the superficial gingival connective tissues and manifest all of the classic features of a chronic inflammatory lesion. If the inflammatory response contained within the gingivitis lesion spreads to the deeper periodontal tissues, and alveolar bone is lost, the resultant lesion is called periodontitis. The precise mechanisms governing the progression of gingivitis to periodontitis are unclear. In some cases, gingivitis may represent the early stage in the evolution of periodontitis. However, in some individuals, gingivitis may exist as an independent clinical condition without progressing into periodontitis (Williams 1990). Indeed, the possibility exists that gingivitis and periodontitis are quite separate diseases.

Periodontitis is a family of related diseases that differ in their etiology, rate and pattern of progression, natural history, and response to therapy. Such variability can be attributed to differences in composition of the microbial flora, together with the presence of factors that might modify the host response to microbial assault, as well as factors that may predispose the individual to bacterial colonization at specific sites. Of these, it seems that the microfloral composition and the host modifying factors are the most important regarding manifestation of the various periodontal diseases.

While the host response and environmental factors that affect this response are important for disease manifestation, gingivitis and periodontitis cannot commence without the presence of bacteria. Nonetheless, it must be noted that although bacteria are necessary for disease initiation, they are not sufficient to cause disease progression unless there is an associated inflammatory response. The latter overrides its protective role and permits destruction to occur (Offenbacher 1996; Page et al 1997).

A large number of bacterial species colonize the teeth in the supra- and subgingival dental plaque. For gingivitis to develop, the type of bacteria present is relatively inconsequential since gingivitis is a nonspecific inflammatory response to dental plaque. However, approximately 20 microbes that inhabit the subgingival environment are considered to be significantly pathogenic to be associated with various forms of periodontitis. The most significant bacteria associated with periodontitis are *Actinobacillus actinomycetemcomitans, Porphyromonas gingivalis,* and *Bacteroides forsythus* (American Academy of Periodontology 1996). An important emerging concept with respect to the subgingival microflora is that it behaves as a biofilm that permits the occupants to survive as a community and resist common host defense mechanisms as well antibiotic exposure during therapy (Darveau et al 1997).

Gingivitis—pathology. Within days of supragingival plaque accumulation, bacterial components, especially lipopolysaccharides (LPS), interact through a serum protein with CD14–cell surface receptors of epithelial cells (keratinocytes). With their subsequent access to the gingival connective tissue, these substances may also interact with endothelial cells, fibroblasts, and leukocytes. Through these pathways, instructive messages reach the vasculature to initiate the earliest inflammatory responses, including margination and extravasation of polymorphonuclear leukocytes, together with vascular fluid exudation. Together, the fluid exudate and leukocytes flow toward the gingival sulcus to bathe the developing plaque. This early host response may be insufficient to contain the microbial challenge. With the emigration of polymorphonuclear leukocytes, the earliest stages of matrix destruction occur to make way for further cell migration and population of the gingival connective tissues.

If the bacterial plaque is permitted to accumulate, clinical evidence of gingivitis is seen. Early gingivitis becomes established some 4 to

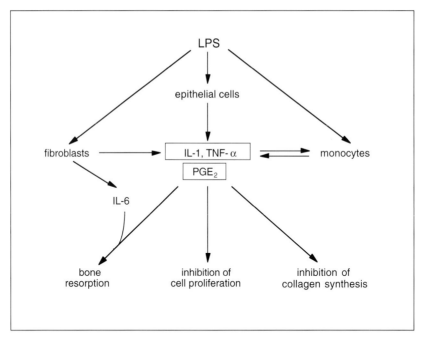

Fig 9-1 Possible mechanisms of cytokine induction that contributes to connective tissue alterations during inflammation. Bacterial substances, especially the LPS, stimulate keratinocytes and monocytes to produce IL-1, TNF-α, and PGE_2. Fibroblasts coming in contact with the LPS synthesize PGE_2 and IL-6. PGE_2 is a major mediator involved in tissue destruction; it inhibits fibroblast proliferation and collagen synthesis, and with IL-6, it causes bone resorption. Cytokines IL-1 and TNF-α activate the synthesis of MMP gene (see Fig 9-5).

7 days after plaque accumulation, and the inflammatory responses continue and begin to show signs of amplification with continued infiltration of macrophages and lymphocytes and further loss of collagen. At this stage, the inflammatory reaction may fulfill its protective role and the lesion may be contained. However, ongoing accumulation of plaque within the gingival sulcus contributes further to the overall magnitude of the inflammatory reactions occurring within the gingival connective tissues. By this stage, the gingival connective tissue is flooded with lymphocytes, macrophages, a plethora of cytokines, chemokines, lymphokines, enzymes, and other inflammatory products. The most significant molecules associated with disease are cytokines IL-1 and TNF-α, chemokines IL-8 and

MCP-1, and the lymphokine, IFN-γ. The cytokines, especially IL-1 and TNF-α, increase the production of PGE_2 by epithelial cells, monocytes and fibroblasts (Fig 9-1). All of these mediators, as well as the matrix metalloproteinases, are present in increased concentrations in the gingival crevicular fluid (Armitage 1996; Offenbacher 1996; Page et al 1997). Despite significant destruction of gingival connective tissue, no periodontal pocket has formed at this stage since there has been no loss of alveolar bone. Indeed, the lesion may still be contained by the host defense and remain localized within the gingival tissues. This stage is representative of chronic gingivitis, and its effects on the tissues are reversible following removal of the initiating factor, the dental plaque.

Periodontitis—pathology. Under certain conditions in a susceptible host, continuing accumulation of subgingival plaque will cause the situation to deteriorate even further. The defense mechanisms may be insufficient to contain the microbial challenge, and the gingivitis lesion may progress toward the deeper periodontal structures. Although several different types of periodontitis are recognized, the mechanisms of tissue destruction appear to be the same. Thus, the variability in disease manifestation most likely arises from the way in which the host defense mechanisms operate. In this regard, the speed, efficiency, and magnitude of the inflammatory response (all regulated by host modifying factors) appear to be the limiting features in disease manifestation.

The key players responsible for the clinical and biochemical features of periodontitis are bacterial substances and chemical mediators released by host cells. Among the multitude of factors present, several key elements seem to take an active role in leading to the bone destruction and pocket formation characteristic of periodontitis. The release of IL-1β by macrophages and resident fibroblasts, and the production of a significant amount of prostaglandin E_2 as a result of the inflammatory processes, are sufficient to induce osteoclast-driven resorption of the alveolar bone. With the loss of bone, the numerous proteases, in particular the matrix metalloproteinases, can destroy the collagenous components of the periodontal ligament and gingiva. These events then allow pocket formation through the apical migration of the junctional epithelium and, as its coronal portion separates it from the root surface, conversion of the junctional epithelium into pocket epithelium.

Thus, the development of periodontitis (regardless of its type) is a highly communicative and interactive process between pathogenic components in the dental plaque, the host tissues (including epithelium), the vasculature, the innate and humoral immune systems, and the connective tissue cells and their matrix

(Offenbacher 1996; Page et al 1997). In general, periodontitis manifests the classic clinical features of chronic inflammation with the infiltration of mononuclear cells, their conversion to macrophages, and antibody production by plasma cells. With a prolonged lesion, focal areas of fibrosis and granulation tissue develop. If left untreated, the biochemical changes described below will lead to alveolar bone loss, loss of connective tissue attachment to root surfaces, and eventually to tooth loss. These features are, for the most part, irreversible even if the initiating factors (ie, dental plaque) are removed.

Gingivitis and periodontitis—matrix changes. A hallmark of inflammatory periodontal diseases is the destruction of gingival connective tissue (Schluger et al 1990; Narayanan and Page 1983) (Fig 9-2). During the development of gingivitis, tissue destruction begins within the perivascular extracellular matrix where most of the collagen within the foci of inflammation is degraded. In gingivitis, the matrix destruction is mostly due to the activity of matrix metalloproteinases produced by polymorphonuclear leukocytes. In periodontitis however, matrix metalloproteinases produced by polymorphonuclear leukocytes, macrophages, keratinocytes, and fibroblasts contribute to matrix degradation. The gingivitis lesion may remain established for years, or even decades, and may recur with episodic phases of cyclic disease, during which the foci of inflammation manifest scarring and fibrosis. Such gingival fibrosis is seen in slowly progressive periodontitis in humans, baboons, and chimpanzees, but not in dogs (Page and Schroeder 1982).

Quantitative and qualitative changes occur in gingival collagen in patients with the above diseases. In gingiva, the collagen becomes more soluble, indicating new and active synthesis. Type I and III collagens are lost at foci of inflammation (Fig 9-3). The ratios of collagen types are altered; the amount of type V collagen increases, and its amount

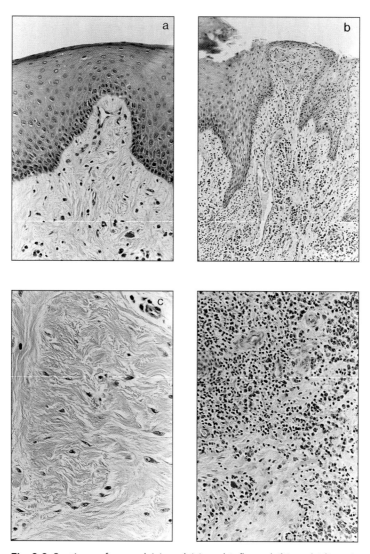

Fig 9-2 Sections of normal **(a)** and **(c)** and inflamed **(b)** and **(d)** periodontal tissues stained with hematoxylin and eosin. Note the dramatic loss of collagenous material from the sites of inflammatory cell infiltration. Original magnification: **a** and **b**, 100×; **c** and **d**, 200×.

may exceed that of type III, and a new collagen species, type I trimer, can be detected in inflamed gingiva. This collagen is a homotrimer of the $\alpha1[I]$ chain, which accumulates in the absence of functional $\alpha2[I]$ chains in certain collagen molecular diseases, embryonic tissues, and tumors. Noncollagenous gingival proteins are also destroyed along with the collagens. The destruction is carried out by matrix metalloproteinases, especially those released by polymorphonuclear leukocytes and macrophages. It is now recognized that pathologic breakdown of the matrix is due to an imbalance between the activated matrix metalloproteinases and their endogenous inhibitors (Reynolds and Meikle 1997; Ryan et al 1996; Birkedal-Hansen et al 1993).

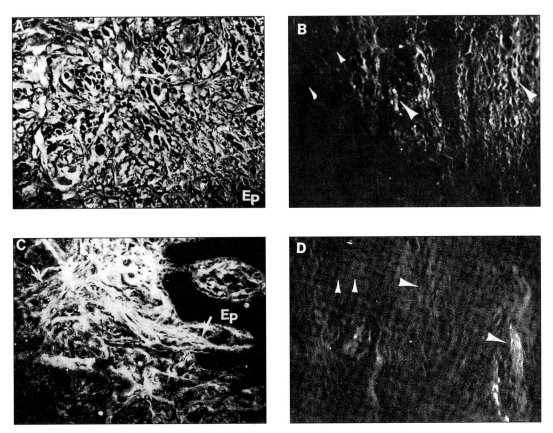

Fig 9-3 Sections of healthy and periodontitis-affected human gingival tissues in which collagens were visualized by immunostaining with type I (**a, b**) and III (**c, d**) collagens. (**a**) and (**c**) and are healthy, and (**b**) and (**d**) are inflamed areas. Original magnification 100×. (Reproduced with permission from Narayanan et al 1985.)

The gingival proteoglycans are also affected by inflammation, but the overall effect on these molecules is relatively smaller than on collagens. In inflamed gingival tissues, the amount of dermatan sulfate decreases while the concentration of chondroitin sulfate increases. Degradation of proteoglycan core proteins and hyaluronic acid are characteristic features of inflamed gingival connective tissues (Bartold and Page 1986). Proteoglycans are lost from sites of inflammatory foci, but they appear to increase in concentration around the periphery. Inflammatory cells also synthesize proteoglycans, especially proteoglycans containing chondroitin sulfate; therefore, the chondroitin sulfate content increases at these sites such that it predominates over the more common dermatan sulfate (Bartold et al 1989). The latter species is destroyed along with the collagens.

As the lesion of periodontitis develops, the junctional epithelium migrates apically and is responsible for the formation of the pocket epithelium. This process requires not only cell proliferation, but also migration of the cells over the connective tissue substratum that has been modified by the inflammatory process. Recent studies have identified variable expression of integrins and other adhesion molecules at the epithelial-connective tissue interface during the inflammatory process and subsequent migration of the junctional epithelium (Haapasalmi et al 1995). The integrin receptors, especially those on keratinocytes, play a significant role in the connective tissue alterations. For example $\alpha_5\beta_1$ and $\alpha_v\beta_6$ are not expressed in healthy epithelium, but they are induced by inflammation (Lajarva et al 1996).

The periodontal ligament manifests subtle topographical changes in the distribution of various glycosaminoglycans; the major change is an increase in the presence of chondroitin sulfate (Kirkham et al 1991; Kirkham et al 1992). Changes to the hard tissue matrices of bone and cementum differ significantly due to their different anatomical locations. Cementum may become altered due to its exposure to the oral or pocket environment in which there is a loss of collagenous attachment, and both its organic and inorganic content are changed (Selvig and Zander 1962; Stepnick et al 1975).

Attempts have been made to correlate connective tissue alterations to periodontal disease. The gingival crevicular fluid contains many breakdown products arising from inflammation, therefore studies have focused on measuring the levels in gingival crevicular fluid as well as in plasma proteins of collagen degradation products such as hydroxyproline and $\alpha1(I)$-N-propeptide (Fine and Mandel 1986). In addition, levels of cytokines such as IL-1 in gingival crevicular fluid have also been measured. However, differences between healthy and diseased tissues are subtle and do not appear to correlate well with the severity of disease. This is discussed in greater detail in the next chapter.

Gingival Overgrowth

The characteristic features of drug-induced gingival overgrowth and gingival fibromatosis are an increased gingival mass associated with fibroepithelial changes and an accumulation of connective tissue matrix (Fig 9-4). Gingival overgrowth is a common complication in some patients who take the antiepileptic drug diphenylhydantoin (phenytoin), immunosuppressants such as cyclosporine, calcium channel blockers such as nifedipine, and other drugs (Hassell and Hefti 1991).

The development of gingival inflammation is a common feature of medication-induced gingival overgrowth. However, while matrix elements are lost during gingivitis and periodontitis, they accumulate in gingival overgrowth. The lesions induced by these various drugs are indistinguishable. Ingestion of the drugs alone is insufficient for evolution of this lesion; it also requires a genetic component, bacterial plaque, and inflammation. In these lesions, the gingival margin and interdental papillae overgrow; the overgrowth may become so extensive that teeth are displaced and their crowns covered with overgrown gingival tissues. Clinically, these lesions have a cauliflowerlike appearance with enlarged epithelium and foci of infiltrating leukocytes. Although during early stages these lesions are highly cellular, in mature lesions the matrix-to-cell ratio is close to normal (Hassell and Hefti 1991; Hassell et al 1982).

The essential feature of all drug-induced gingival overgrowth is excessive accumulation of epithelial, as well as connective, tissue elements, especially collagen. Thus, it resembles other fibrotic lesions such as atherosclerosis and idiopathic pulmonary fibrosis. The localization of different collagen types in the various tissue components is similar to healthy tissues. For example, types I, III, V, and VI collagens and fibronectin are present and associated with the connective tissues in their characteristic structural forms, while type IV and VII collagens are associated with basement membrane structures (Romanos et al 1993). The amount of noncollagenous proteins also increases in phenytoin-induced gingival overgrowth. The noncollagenous matrix of the phenytoin lesion comprises approxi-

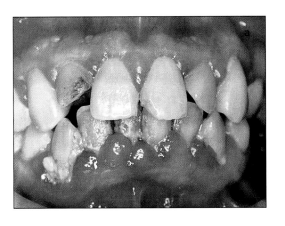
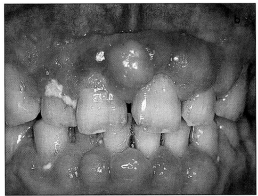
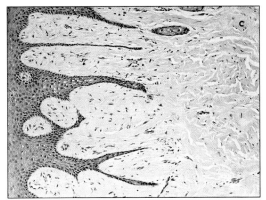
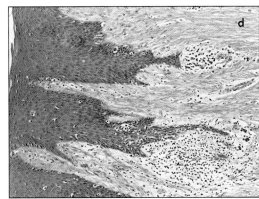

Fig 9-4 Medication-induced gingival overgrowth. Clinical appearance of **(a)** dilantin-induced gingival overgrowth and **(b)** cyclosporin-induced gingival overgrowth. Histologic appearance of tissue sections from **(c)** dilantin-induced gingival overgrowth and, **(d)** cyclosporine A–induced gingival overgrowth. Sections stained with hematoxylin and eosin. Original magnification 50×.

mately 20% of the dry weight, compared to approximately 7% in healthy tissues (Ballard and Butler 1974). They also have higher contents of hexosamine, uronic acid, glycosaminoglycans, and proteoglycans, and an increased number of glucocorticoid receptors (Suresh and Dhar 1991; Seymour et al 1996). Collagen content increases, and the type I/III ratio becomes different with some loss of type I and elevated levels of type III collagen (Narayanan and Hassell 1985).

Two complementary mechanisms appear to contribute to the accumulation of matrix proteins; these involve either a reduction of the levels or activities of matrix-degrading enzymes in these lesions, or the induction of matrix production. Induction of collagen production may occur by either the direct action of drugs on collagen synthesis machinery (Schincaglia et al 1992; Shikata et al 1993; Vernillo and Schwartz 1986), or indirectly, by decreasing the production of collagenase (Goultschin and Shoshan 1980; Vernillo and Schwartz 1987; Tipton et al 1991; McCulloch and Knowles 1993b). Increase in collagen can occur either by directly affecting the gene transcription rate, or indirectly through cytokines such as TGF-β and basic fibroblast growth factor (bFGF) (Li et al 1991; Saito et al 1996; Overall 1994; Shikata et al 1993;

Vernillo and Schwartz 1987; Vernillo et al 1986; Schincaglia et al 1992). In addition, changes in the levels of collagenase in these lesions may contibute to the excess amount of extracellular matrix (Hassell 1982; Goultschin and Shoshan 1980). For example, fibroblasts in gingiva manifest differential and heterogeneous responses to drugs in collagenase production (Tipton et al 1991), and phenytoin has been shown to reduce collagen degradation by gingival fibroblasts (Vernillo and Schwartz 1986).

Studies using cultured fibroblasts from these lesions have provided variable results when the effects of these drugs are examined by direct addition to cultures. However, cells derived from overgrown tissues, as well as those derived from other fibrotic organs, possess higher than normal rates of collagen synthesis, even in the absence of added drugs, and differ in ability to synthesize collagenase and tissue inhibitor of metalloproteinases (TIMP) as well as the ability to inhibit collagenase activity by TIMP (Tipton et al 1991; Tipton et al 1994). Such studies have given rise to the hypothesis that certain fibroblast subtypes with abnormal phenotypes are selected in these lesions (Narayanan and Page 1983).

Gingival fibromatosis is an idiopathic, progressive, and fibrous gingival enlargement that is inherited as an autosomal dominant disease. It may be focal or generalized and, unlike drug-induced gingival overgrowth, it does not have an inflammatory component.

Adaptive Changes of the Extracellular Matrix

Periodontal connective tissues also undergo age-related changes that affect their functions. The most significant changes occur in collagens, and decrease collagen solubility and increase the overall cross-linking. Interestingly, collagens of the gingiva and periodontal ligament retain their relatively high collagen-turnover rates with advancing age. Tissues of

all ages contain type I and III collagen fibers, however, the immunostaining capacity for type III, presumably due to reduced content, increases with age (Xu et al 1993). An anti-collagenase tissue inhibitor also appears to increase in this lesion (Morris et al 1993). In contrast to the fibroblasts, gingival epithelial cells do not manifest any age-related changes in proliferation rate or collagen synthesis, however, the proportion of noncollagenous proteins synthesized by these cells decreases to one half (Mariotti et al 1993).

Mechanisms of Periodontal Tissue Destruction

The biochemical composition of the periodontal connective tissues during health and disease is determined by the extents of degradation and synthesis of the matrix constituents (Reynolds and Meikle 1997). Degradation is a normal feature of the periodontal connective tissues and, as previously described, the gingival and periodontal ligament collagens have a high turnover rate relative to other tissues, even in adults. The degradation is a highly regulated process, however, it becomes excessive during inflammation, and may be impaired in hyperplasia. In this section we will review alterations in the regulatory mechanisms of matrix degradation in diseases of the periodontium.

The major change in the biochemical constituents of the connective tissue during gingivitis and periodontitis is the loss of collagens due to degradation. There are at least four different mechanisms by which the extracellular matrix can be degraded and modified during the establishment of periodontitis. These include the release of enzymes by host and bacterial cells, phagocytosis of matrix components, release of reactive oxygen species, and the release of a wide range of cytokines and other inflammatory mediators that affect enzyme release and fibroblast function.

Table 9-2. Matrix Metalloproteinases (MMPs) of Cells Residing in Periodontium

Cell Type	MMP Type	Inducers*
Fibroblast	Collagenase-1 (MMP-1) 72-kd gelatinase (MMP-2) SL-1 (MMP-3)	IL-1α, β; TNF-α PDGF
Keratinocytes	Collagenase-1 (MMP-1) 72-kd gelatinase (MMP-2) 92-kd gelatinase (MMP-9) SL-2 (MMP-10)	LPS, TGF-α
Monocytes, endothelial cells	Collagenase-1 (MMP-1) 72-kd gelatinase (MMP-2) 92-kd gelatinase (MMP-9) SL-1 (MMP-3)	...
PMN	Collagenase-2 (MMP-8) 92-kd gelatinase (MMP-9)	LPS

*In the context of periodontitis. These substances also suppress the transcription of TIMP genes. TGF-β and IFN-γ have an opposite effect. See Birkedal-Hansen 1993, Birkedal-Hansen et al 1993, and Reynolds and Miekle 1997 for detailed reviews.

IL-1β, interleukin 1β; TNF, tumor necrosis factor; PDGF, platelet-derived growth factor; LPS, lipopolysaccharide; TGF-α, transforming growth factor α; SL-1, stromelysin-1; SL-2, stromelysin-2; PMN, polymorphonuclear leukocytes.

Enzyme-Mediated Damage by Host Cells

Extracellular degradation of the matrix occurs via the release of numerous matrix metalloproteinases (MMP). These enzymes can efficiently degrade interstitial or basement membrane collagens, laminin, fibronectin, and the core proteins of proteoglycans. In the inflamed tissues, these enzymes are derived from polymorphonuclear leukocytes, macrophages, fibroblasts, keratinocytes, and endothelium. The secreted matrix metalloproteinases are subsequently activated by proteinases such as plasmin, which in turn are regulated by tissue protein factors such as plasminogen activators. The plasminogen activators are serine proteinases.

Matrix metalloproteinases. The types of matrix metalloproteinases, their substrates, and how their production and activities are regulated, have been discussed in Chapter 4. In the periodontium, many cell types express matrix metalloproteinases. These include fibroblasts, epithelial cells (keratinocytes), and endothelial cells, and inflammatory cells during inflammation (Birkedal-Hansen 1995). These cell types differ in the types of matrix metalloproteinases they produce (Table 9-2). Fibroblasts express several matrix metalloproteinases including collagenase-1 (MMP-1), but they do not produce collagenase-2 (MMP-8) or the 92-kd gelatinase (MMP-9). In contrast, polymorphonuclear leukocytes (PMN) secrete a specific type of collagenase (collagenase-2, MMP-8) and the 92-kd gelatinase (MMP-9) (Birkedal-Hansen 1993; Birkedal-Hansen et al 1993; Reynolds and Meikle 1997). The major matrix metalloproteinase types present in the gingival crevicular fluid of periodontitis patients are PMN-type collagenase (MMP-8) and 92-kd gelatinase (MMP-9), but not the 72-kd gelatinase (MMP-2) or stromelysin-1 (MMP-3) (Sorsa et al 1990; Golub et al 1976; Gangbar et al 1990; Uitto et al 1990; Ingman et al 1993; Villela et al 1987). These enzymes appear to be derived from polymorphonuclear leukocytes and they are believed to be primarily responsible for tissue destruction (Overall et al 1991; Sorsa et al 1990), whereas the enzymes

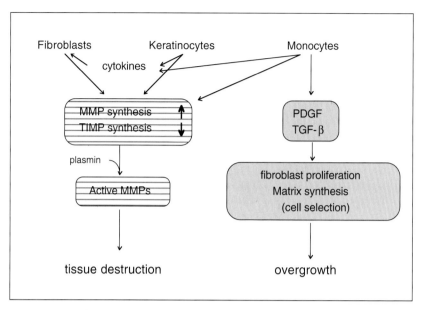

Fig 9-5 Possible mechanisms involved in connective tissue alterations in periodontitis and gingival overgrowth. In periodontitis, the major factors causing tissue destruction are the matrix metalloproteinases (MMP). In fibroblasts, the transcription of MMPs is activated by the cytokines IL-1β and TNF-α. In keratinocytes, LPS and TGF-β activate MMP synthesis. These substances also inhibit the synthesis of TIMPs. The MMPs become activated by plasmin and other serine proteinases and degrade matrix components. Oxygen-derived free radicals produced by inflammatory cells may also contribute to connective tissue destruction. In inflamed tissues, monocytes and platelets are triggered to produce growth factors such as PDGF and TGF-β continuously; these substances promote fibroblast proliferation and matrix synthesis associated with tissue overgrowth. Overgrowth may also be due selection of fibroblast subtypes with the disease phenotype.

synthesized by fibroblasts and epithelial cells are believed to be mostly involved in normal tissue remodeling (Sodek and Overall 1992; Lee et al 1995; Meikle et al 1994). LPS and TNF-α activate matrix metalloproteinase synthesis by keratinocytes. IL-1 enhances matrix metalloproteinase expression by fibroblasts, whereas LPS stimulate PGE_2 production by these cells (Fig 9-5, see Fig 9-1). The activities of PGE_2 include suppression of cell proliferation, inhibition of collagen synthesis, and, with IL-6, stimulation of bone resorption (Page et al 1997; Schwartz et al 1997).

Although distinct matrix metalloproteinase species are produced by the various periodon-

tal cell types, and the cells have a clear role during health and disease, the pattern of matrix metalloproteinase production by these cells is affected by several cytokines present in the inflamed periodontium. These include IL-1, TNF-α, cAMP, and PGE_2 (Tewari et al 1994; Gronowicz et al 1992; Overall et al 1991; Overall and Sodek 1990; Birkedal-Hansen 1993; Birkedal-Hansen et al 1993). Bacterial plaque products can also stimulate matrix metalloproteinase production by a variety of cells (Birkedal-Hansen 1993; Birkedal-Hansen et al 1993; Lyons et al 1993; Uitto and Raeste 1978). In general, the collagenase expression by cells of the periodontium may vary with different subpopulations (Tipton et al 1991; Birkedal-Hansen 1993; Birkedal-Hansen et al 1993; Overall et al 1991; Overall 1994). Many of the mediators that influence matrix metalloproteinase production and activity do so by not only directly increasing protein expression, but also indirectly by affecting TIMP production. For example, TGF-β, steroids, and interferon-γ induce the expression of TIMP-1 and TIMP-2.

Recently, tetracyclines and their analogues have been shown to inhibit the activity of some, but not all, matrix metalloproteinases associated with periodontal destruction (Ingman et al 1993; Golub et al 1991). This process is mediated via the ability of tetracycline to chelate divalent cations necessary for enzyme activity, thus making the enzyme structurally vulnerable to proteolytic degradation. Tetracycline, which also inhibits the expression 72-kd gelatinase (MMP-2; Uitto et al 1994), does not affect fibroblast collagenase, indicating that the matrix metalloproteinases in gingival crevicular fluid are derived from polymorphonuclear leukocytes (Ingman et al 1993; Golub et al 1995). Interestingly, while the collagenase of gingival crevicular fluid from patients with adult- and diabetes-associated periodontitis are susceptible to tetracyclines, those of localized juvenile periodontitis are more resistant (Ingman et al 1993).

Plasminogen activation system. Another matrix-degrading serine proteinase is plasmin, which is formed locally at sites of inflammation and repair by limited proteolysis of its inactive precursor, plasminogen. Plasminogen circulates in plasma and interstitial fluids (Deutsch and Mertz 1970), and its activation is by either urokinase-type plasminogen activator (u-PA) or tissue-type plasminogen activator (t-PA) (Saksela and Rifkin 1988). These catalytic reactions generally take place at the plasma membrane by u-PA, or on fibrin surfaces by t-PA. These activating enzymes are produced by a wide range of mesenchymal, epithelial, and endothelial cells in response to a variety of cytokines and growth factors. At sites of inflammation, the potential for up-regulation of the plasminogen activating system is high, and the resultant plasmin can degrade a wide range of substrates including matrix macromolecules other than collagens. The action of plasmin appears to be aimed toward degradation of components involved in temporization of the wound healing process (eg, fibrin and fibronectin), while the more permanent structures of the healed matrix (eg, collagens) seem to be relatively more resistant to the actions of plasmin. Nevertheless, plasmin can be associated with matrix degradation through its ability to activate matrix metalloproteinases. The activity of plasmin, and its activating proteinases, is regulated extracellularly through a number of proteinase inhibitors including α_2-macroglobulin, α_1-proteinase inhibitor, α_2-antiplasmin, plasminogen activator inhibitor-1 (PAI-1) and plasminogen activator inhibitor-2 (PAI-2).

The levels of plasminogen activators and plasmin have been reported to be elevated in chronically inflamed gingival tissues. u-PA, t-PA, PAI-1, and PAI-2 have been detected in gingival crevicular fluid, and their levels are reduced upon reduction of gingival inflammation (Kinnby et al 1991; Birkedal-Hansen 1993). The relative molar amounts of u-PA, t-PA, and PAI-2 in gingival crevicular fluid remain unaltered between diseased and healthy states, however it has been proposed that PAI-2 is an important inhibitor of tissue proteolysis in periodontal tissues (Kinnby et al 1994).

Tissue-Degrading Enzymes from Bacterial Plaque

A vast array of enzymes with the potential to degrade matrix components are secreted by many bacteria within the dental plaque. Microbial collagenases capable of hydrolyzing collagens to peptides are produced in culture by black-pigmented *Bacteroides*, *Porphyromonas gingivalis*, *Clostridium histolyticum*,

Treponema denticola, and *Bacteroides forsythus* (Kato et al 1992; Lawson and Meyer 1992; Mayrand and Holt 1988; Slots and Genco 1984). However, whether these enzymes are involved in the initial phases of tissue destruction is questionable (Overall et al 1987; Birkedal-Hansen 1993). Enzymes with trypsinlike activities have also been isolated from numerous oral bacteria including the putative periodontal pathogens *T denticola, B forsythus,* and *P gingivalis* (Inoue et al 1990; Smalley et al 1988; Mäkinen et al 1990; Söderling et al 1991). Neither these trypsinlike enzymes nor the bacterial collagenases have been detected in diseased periodontal tissues. Nevertheless, given their broad action, these enzymes would have the potential to degrade the noncollagenous and collagenous matrix proteins.

Although the most obvious mode of action of the bacterial proteinases would seem to be on substrates within the extracellular matrix, these enzymes may also contribute to the destructive phase of inflammatory periodontal disease in an indirect manner. For example, the bacterial enzymes may regulate matrix metalloproteinase activity by activating them proteolytically from inactive precursors, and by degrading matrix metalloproteinase inhibitors (Reynolds and Meikle 1997). Alternatively, bacterial enzymes could act as antigens, leading to the stimulation of cytokine production by host inflammatory cells.

Inflamed gingiva also contains numerous other hydrolytic enzymes capable of disrupting the extracellular matrix; these include β-glucuronidase, aryl sulfatase, hyaluronidase, heparinase, chondrosulfatase, and chondroitinase (Goggins et al 1968; Lamster et al 1987; Podhradsky et al 1982; Tam and Chan 1985; Tam et al 1982; Tipler and Embery 1985; Uitto et al 1986). The most likely substrates for such enzymes would be hyaluronan and the carbohydrate components of proteoglycans. However, direct evidence linking these enzymes to matrix destruction is not available. In light of biochemical analyses of inflamed

tissues that have demonstrated evidence of damage to proteoglycan core proteins while glycosaminoglycan chains were left relatively intact, the bacterial enzymes appear to have no primary role in the initial degradation of proteolgycans (Bartold 1987). More likely, these enzymes may be involved in the breakdown of glycosaminoglycan chains after initial proteolytic cleavage of proteoglycans.

Although depolymerization of hyaluronan has been noted in extracts of inflamed gingival tissues, the effect of enzymes such as hyaluronidase on hyaluronan is unclear because hyaluronan may be depolymerized by agents other than enzymes (eg, free radicals, see below).

As a final consideration of enzyme-mediated matrix destruction, it should be noted that at least three criteria must be fulfilled. In the first instance, the enzyme must be present in the tissues in an active or activated form such that it is neither complexed with an inhibitor nor present in a reactive configuration. Additionally, the enzyme must be in a suitable conformation to permit its catalytic site to be active. In this respect, not only is the presence or absence of precursor peptides instrumental in this function, but the surrounding matrix is also likely to play a significant role in the configuration of a molecule through the interplay of complex physicochemical interactions between the matrix and the enzyme. Finally, the substrate must be in a form that permits the enzyme access to cleavage sites. This point is critical in understanding the in vivo mechanisms of matrix destruction by enzymes. While collagenase may well degrade purified collagen in vitro, whether it can gain access to cleavage sites to degrade native collagens complexed with a number of other matrix components remains poorly studied.

Phagocytosis

During physiologic turnover of the periodontal connective tissues, phagocytosis of extracellular matrix components by fibroblasts and macrophages is believed to play a significant role in the degradative pathway for collagen (Deporter and Ten Cate 1973). The initial phagocytic process requires some form of proteolytic digestion prior to ingestion of collagens by the cell. Such proteolytic digestion may be via enzymes associated with either the cell surface or within the extracellular matrix immediately adjacent to the cell (lysosomal or matrix metalloproteinases). The precise mechanism by which collagen is phagocytosed is still unclear, however, phagocytosis has been noted to proceed even if such enzyme activity is blocked via blocking antibodies to collagenase or the addition of cysteine proteinase inhibitors (Everts et al 1985). Upon internalization, the vesicles within which the collagen peptides are entrapped (phagosomes) fuse with the lysosomes to form a phagolysosome and are degraded by lysosomal enzymes such as cathepsin L.

This intracellular mechanism of matrix turnover is believed to be involved in normal tissue remodeling, and whether it contributes to pathologic matrix destruction or other pathologies is not clear. For example, phagocytosis can be activated by concanavalin A, but not by IL-1 (Knowles et al 1991). The presence of cells defective in phagocytosis may contribute to tissue overgrowth (McCulloch and Knowles 1993a, b).

Free Radicals in Tissue Destruction

Free radicals are atoms, ions, or molecules capable of independent existence, which contain one or more unpaired electrons in their outer orbit. Of particular interest in tissue destruction are the oxygen-derived free radicals (ODFR) such as superoxide and hydroxyl radicals, which are integral products of normal cellular metabolism. In addition to the free radicals, other components of oxygen metabolism include hydrogen peroxide (H_2O_2) and hypochlorous acid (HOCl) (see Chapter 3). Reactive oxygen species are produced via a number of different pathways during normal cellular metabolism, and they are found in particularly high proportion in cells undergoing respiratory bursts at inflammatory sites. These are produced either by specific enzyme systems designed to produce free radicals, or as a consequence of electron transport chains or metabolic pathways. In some cases, auto-oxidation of small molecules may also generate radicals. Myeloperoxidase and NADPH oxidase are two enzymes that are particularly active in the respiratory burst of activated neutrophils and macrophages and lead to the formation of superoxide and hydroxyl radicals, as well as hypochlorite. The cascade of events associated with arachidonic acid metabolism has been found to generate free radicals.

Tissues may be exposed to a variety of free radicals during inflammatory reactions, particularly where polymorphonuclear leukocytes and macrophages are in abundance and respond with significant quantities of oxygen-derived free radicals, which may cause significant cellular and tissue damage. Of the reactive oxygen species produced, the superoxide radical has little direct toxicity on cells or tissues. However, this molecule may contribute to the pathogenesis of inflammation-mediated matrix disruption through its subsequent involvement in the production of hydroxyl radicals. The hydroxyl radical is very short-lived, but it can modify molecules within a few angstroms of its site of generation. On the other hand, hydrogen peroxide is more stable and it may cross lipid membranes to cause damage at sites quite distant from where it is produced. While there is little evidence to indicate that hypochlorous acid (HOCl; produced from Cl^-, H_2O_2, and myeloperoxidase) is involved in the cytotoxic actions of activated polymorphonuclear leukocytes, HOCl has significant effects on the tissues through activation of collagenases and gelatinase (Freeman and Crapo 1982; Henson and Johnston 1987). In general, the production of free radicals is self-perpetuating unless two radicals react with each other (with the subsequent formation of a stable pair of electrons in the outer shell of the product). Thus, even short-lived free radicals (such as the hydroxyl radical) can be generated in significant quantities through autocatalytic chain reactions.

The effects of free radicals on tissues and cells are many and varied, and include disruption to cellular proteins, nucleic acids, and membrane lipids, as well as causing the depolymerization of matrix components such as collagen, hyaluronan, and proteoglycans. These harmful effects are normally controlled by free radical scavengers such as glutathione, albumin, uronic acid, glucose, transferrin, lactoferrin, lipids, and immunoglobulins, and through specific enzyme systems, such as dismutase, that keep the levels of reactive oxygen at a low level, or by spontaneous dismutation.

Although they have not been investigated in great detail in the inflamed periodontium, free radicals may have the potential to play a role in matrix destruction in the inflamed periodontium. For example, oxygen-derived free radicals may depolymerize gingival proteoglycans and hyaluronan (Bartold et al 1984), activate neutrophil collagenase, and thus initiate matrix degradation (Sorsa et al 1989).

In recent years, nitric oxide has become recognized as a source of tissue-damaging free radicals. Originally identified in the exhaust fumes of motor vehicles, nitric oxide was recently shown to be produced by many cell types and is present in elevated amounts at sites of inflammation. To date, the effects of this radical are still unclear, but it does possess some cytotoxic and matrix-damaging properties similar to those of the hydroxyl free radical.

Effects of Soluble Mediators on Connective Tissue Cells

In soft periodontal connective tissues, fibroblasts are largely responsible for producing and maintaining the matrix constituents, whereas osteoblasts, and presumably cementoblasts, produce matrix in alveolar bone and cementum. A variety of factors present in the local environment dictate the activities of these cells, and the action of these molecules is described in Chapter 3.

The influence of many of these molecules has been studied on periodontal fibroblasts with respect to cell proliferation, and production of collagens and proteoglycans. Molecules examined include various isoforms of platelet-derived growth factor (PDGF), epidermal growth factor (EGF), prostaglandin E_2 (PGE$_2$), interferon-γ (IFN-γ), tumor necrosis factor α (TNF-α), and interleukin-1 (IL-1) (Narayanan and Bartold 1996). IL-1 is a major cytokine involved in matrix degradation in rheumatoid arthritis, periodontitis, and other inflammatory diseases, and in bone resorption. The mode of action of IL-1 appears to be through induction of genes for collagenase, gelatinases, and stromelysin-1 (Tewari et al 1994; Birkedal-Hansen 1993; Birkedal-Hansen et al 1993). Inflamed gingival tissues and gingival crevicular fluid contain IL-1α, IL-1β, TNF-α, IL-6, IL-8, and IFN-γ, and the presence of these cytokines is believed to contribute to higher levels of matrix-degrading enzymes in the gingival crevicular fluid (Alexander and Damoulis 1994).

The manner in which the fibroblasts respond to various agents depends upon several factors such as age of the cells, local environment, and the state of the cell cycle (Irwin et al 1994). For example, the matrix suppresses cell division and promotes differentiation, whereas in the absence of a matrix cells continue to divide (Schuppan et al 1994). The type and concentration of various substances present in the local environment determine the manner in which cells respond to, and regulate the progression of, healing and repair events. In particular, a recent study has noted that a specific genotype of the polymorphic IL-1 gene cluster leads to increased levels of IL-1 production and is a strong indicator for susceptibility to severe periodontitis in adults (Kornman et al 1997).

Synthesis of different matrix components, and how various cell types respond to specific cytokines, vary. For example, IL-1 enhances type VII collagen synthesis significantly, while type I is not affected (Mauviel et al 1994). This difference may also be manifested by different subpopulations of the same cell type because not all the resident cells in a tissue react in the same manner to the inflammatory mediators. Evidence indicates that fibroblast cultures obtained from same tissue explants consist of subtypes that differ in functional properties, such as growth rate and collagen synthesis, and that they respond differently to TGF-β, IFN-γ, PGE$_2$ and other substances (Bordin et al 1984; McCulloch and Bordin 1991; Fries et al 1994). Selective interactions between fibroblast subpopulations and inflammatory mediators have been shown to give rise to selection and enrichment of fibroblast subtypes, and presence of such subtypes is believed to be one factor contributing to disease phenotypes in inflammation and fibrosis (LeRoy et al 1990; Narayanan and Page 1983) (see Fig 9-5).

The activities of fibroblasts under healthy and pathologic conditions may be influenced by the factors derived from epithelium. Fibroses and overgrowths are often associated with enlarged epithelia, however, the interactions between epithelium and underlying connective tissue are poorly understood. Epithelium appears to be a significant source of PDGF in healthy and wounded dermis, and in gingiva (Ansel et al 1993; Green et al 1997).

Summary

The mechanisms by which matrix destruction of periodontal tissues can occur are many and varied. These processes may act in unison or individually, depending upon the initiating factors leading to their induction. In general, it is important to note that no single mechanism is likely to be responsible for matrix destruction. Rather, a combination of several different, but interrelated, processes is likely to be involved. This has significant ramifications for treatment, as any therapy aimed at reducing only one aspect of tissue degradation is unlikely to be of significant benefit since other mechanisms may gain prominence and lead to additional uncontrolled destruction.

References

Alexander MB, Damoulis PD. The role of cytokines in the pathogenesis of periodontal disease. Curr Opin Periodontol 1994:39.

Altman LC, Page RC, Vandesteen GE, Dixon LI, Bradford C. Abnormalities of leukocyte chemotaxis in patients with various forms of periodontitis. J Periodont Res 1985;20:553.

American Academy of Periodontology. 1996 World Workshop in Periodontics. Ann Periodontol 1996;1:926

Ansel JC, Tiesman JP, Olerud JE, et al. Human keratinocytes are a major source of cutaneous platelet-derived growth factor. J Clin Invest 1993;92:671.

Armitage GC. Periodontal diseases: diagnosis. World Workshop in Periodontics. Ann Periodontol 1996;1:37.

Ballard JB, Butler WT. Proteins of the periodontium. Biochemical studies on the collagen and noncollagenous proteins of human gingivae. J Oral Path 1974;3:176.

Barabas GM. The Ehlers-Danlos syndrome. Abnormalities of the enamel, dentine, cementum and the dental pulp: an histological examination of 13 teeth from 6 patients. Br Dent J 1969;126:509.

Bartold PM. Proteoglycans of the periodontium: structure, role and function. J Periodont Res 1987;22:431.

Bartold PM. Biochemical and immunohistochemical studies on overgrown gingival tissues associated with mannosidosis. Virchows Arch B 1992;62:391.

Bartold PM, Hayes DR, Vernon-Roberts B. The effect of mitogen and lymphokine stimulation on proteoglycan synthesis by lymphocytes. J Cell Physiol 1989;140:32.

Bartold PM, Page RC. The effect of chronic inflammation on gingival connective tissue proteoglycans and hyaluronic acid. J Oral Pathol 1986;15:367.

Bartold PM, Wiebkin OW, Thonard JC. The effect of oxygen-derived free radicals on gingival proteoglycans and hyaluronic acid. J Periodontal Res 1984;19:390.

Birkedal-Hansen H. Role of matrix metalloproteinases in human periodontal diseases. J Periodontol 1993;64:474.

Birdekal-Hansen H. Proteolytic remodeling of extracellular matrix. Curr Opin Cell Biol 1995;7:728.

Birkedal-Hansen H, Moore WGI, Bodden MK, et al. Matrix metalloproteinases: A Review. Crit Rev Oral Biol Med 1993;4:197.

Bordin S, Page RC, Narayanan AS. Heterogeneity of normal human diploid fibroblasts: Isolation and characterization of one phenotype. Science 1984;223:171.

Byers PH. Disorders of collagen biosynthesis and structure. In: Scriver CR, Beaudet AL, Sly WS, Valle D, eds. 7th ed. The Metabolic and Molecular Bases of Inherited Diseases. New York:McGraw-Hill; 1995:4029–4077.

Cawson RA. The oral changes in gargoylism. Proc R Soc Med 1962;55:1066.

Cohen MM, Winer RA, Schwartz S, Sklar G. Oral aspects of mongolism I. Periodontal disease in mongolism. Oral Surg Oral Med Oral Pathol 1961;14:92.

Crowley CA, Curnette JT, Rosin RE, et al. An inherited abnormality of neutrophil adhesion. Its genetic transmission and its association with a missing protein. New Engl J Med 1980;302:1163.

Cuttress TW. Periodontal disease and oral hygiene in trisomy 21. Arch Oral Biol 1971;16:1345.

Darveau RP, Tanner A, Page RC. The microbial challenge in periodontitis. Periodontology 2000. 1997;14:12.

Deasy MJ, Vogel RI, Macedo-Sobrinko B, Gertzman G, Simon B. Familial benign chronic neutropenia associated with periodontal disease. A case report. J Periodontol 1980;51:206.

Delgado WA, Calderon R. Acatalasia in two Peruvian siblings. Oral Surg Oral Med Oral Pathol 1979;8:358.

Deporter DA, Ten Cate AR. Fine structural localization of acid and alkaline phosphatase in collagen-containing vesicles of fibroblasts. J Anat 1973;114:457.

Deutsch DG, Mertz ET. Plasminogen: purification from plasma by affinity chromatography. Science 1970;127:1095.

Eaton JW, Ma M. Acatalasemia. In: Scriver CR, Beaudet AL, Sly WS, Valle D, eds. The Metabolic and Molecular Bases of Inherited Diseases, 7th ed. New York:McGraw-Hill 1995:2371.

Everts V, Beertsen W, Tigalchelaar-Gutter W. The digestion of phagocytosed collagen is inhibited by the proteinase inhibitors leupeptin and E-64. Coll Rel Res 1985;5:315.

Fine DH, Mandel ID. Indicators of periodontal disease activity. An evaluation. J Clin Periodontol 1986;13:533.

Freeman BA, Crapo JD. Biology of disease. Free radicals and tissue injury. Lab Invest 1982;47:412.

Fries KM, Bleiden T, Looney J, et al. Evidence of fibroblast heterogeneity and the role of fibroblast subpopulations in fibrosis. Clin Immunol Immunopathol 1994;72:283.

Gangbar S, Overall CM, McCulloch CAG, Sodek J. Identification of polymorphonuclear leukocyte collagenase and gelatinase activities in mouth rinse samples: correlation with periodontal disease activity in adult and juvenile periodontitis. J Periodont Res 1990;25:257.

Goggins JF, Fullmer HM, Steffeck AJ. Hyaluronidase activity of human gingiva. Arch Pathol 1968;85:272.

Golub LM, Ramamurthy NS, McNamara TF, Greenwald RA, Rifkin BR. Tetracyclines inhibit connective tissue breakdown: new therapeutic implications for an old family of drugs. Crit Rev Oral Biol Med 1991;2:297.

Golub LM, Siegel K, Ramamurthy NS, Mandel ID. Some characteristics of collagenase activity in gingival crevicular fluid and its relationship to gingival disease in humans. J Dent Res 1976;55:1049.

Golub LM, Sorsa T, Lee HM, et al. Doxycycline inhibits neutrophil (PMN)-type matrix metalloproteinases in human adult periodontitis gingiva. J Clin Periodontol 1995;22:100.

Goultschin J, Shoshan S. Inhibition of collagen breakdown by diphenylhydantoin. Biochim Biophys Acta 1980;631:188.

Green RJ, Usui ML, Hart CE, Ammons WF, Narayanan AS. Immunolocalization of platelet-derived growth factor A and B chains and PDGF-a and b receptors in human gingival wounds. J Periodont Res 1997;32:209.

Gronowicz G, Hadjimichael J, Richards D, Cerami A, Rossomando EF. Correlation between tumor necrosis factor-alpha (TNF-alpha)–induced cytoskeletal changes and human collagenase gene induction. J Periodont Res 1992;27:562.

Haapasalmi K, Mäkelä M, Oksala O, et al. Expression of epithelial adhesion proteins and integrins in chronic inflammation. Am J Pathol 1995;147:193.

Hamilton RE, Giansanti JS. Chediak Higashi syndrome: report of a case and review of the literature. Oral Surg Oral Med Oral Pathol 1974;37:754.

Hartsfield JK Jr, Kouseff BG. Phenotypic overlap of Ehlers-Danlos syndrome types IV and VIII. Am J Med Genet 1990;37:465.

Hassell TM. Evidence for production of an inactive collagenase by fibroblasts from phenytoin-enlarged human gingivae. J Oral Pathol 1982;11:310.

Hassell TM, Hefti AP. Drug induced gingival overgrowth: old problem, new problem. Crit Rev Oral Biol Med 1991;2:103.

Hassell TM, Roebuck S, Page RC, Wray SH. Quantitative histopathologic assessment of developing phenytoin-induced gingival overgrowth in the cat. J Clin Periodontol 1982;9:365.

Hattab FN, Rawashdeh MA, Yassin OM, Al-Momani AS, Al-Ubosi AA. Papillon-Lefevre syndrome: A review of the literature and report of 4 cases. J Periodontol 1995;66:413.

Henson PM, Johnston RB Jr. Tissue injury in inflammation. Oxidants, proteinases and cationic proteins. J Clin Invest 1987;79:669.

Ingman T, Sorsa T, Soumalainen K, et al. Tetracycline inhibition and the cellular source of collagenase in gingival crevicular fluid in different periodontal diseases. J Periodontol 1993;64:82.

Inoue J, Fukushima H, Onoe T, et al. Distribution of enzymatically pathogenic bacteria from periodontal pocket in advancing periodontitis. J Jap Assoc Periodontol 1990; 32:199.

Irwin CR, Schor SL, Fergusson MJW. Effects of cytokines on gingival fibroblasts *in vitro* are mediated by the extracellular matrix. J Periodont Res 1994;29:309.

Kato T, Takahashi N, Kuramitsu HK. Sequence analysis and characterization of the *Porphyromonas gingivalis* prtC gene, which expresses a novel collagenase activity. J Bacteriol 1992;174:3889.

Kinnby B, Lecander I, Martinsson G, Astedt B. Tissue plasminogen activator and placental plasminogen activator inhibitor in human gingival fluid. Fibrinolysis 1991;5:239.

Kinnby B, Matsson L, Lecander L. The plasminogen-activating system in gingival fluid from adults. Scand J Dent Res 1994;102:334.

Kirkham J, Robinson C, Smith AJ, Spence JA. The effect of periodontal disease on sulphated glycosaminoglycan distribution in the sheep periodontium. Arch Oral Biol 1992;37:1031.

Kirkham J, Robinson C, Spence JA. Effect of periodontal disease ("Broken Mouth") on the distribution of matrix macromolecules in the sheep periodontium. Arch Oral Biol 1991;36:257.

Kirstilia V, Sewon L, Laine J. Periodontal disease in three siblings with familial neutropenia. J Periodontol 1993; 64:566.

Knowles GC, McKeown M, Sodek J, McCulloch CA. Mechanism of collagen phagocytosis by human gingival fibroblasts: importance of collagen structure in cell recognition and internalization. J Cell Sci 1991;98:551.

Kornman KS, Crane A, Wang H-Y, et al. The interleukin-1 genotype as a severity factor in adult periodontal disease. J Clin Periodontol 1997;24:72.

Lamster IB, Harper DS, Fiorello LA, et al. Lysosomal and cytoplasmic enzyme activity, crevicular fluid volume, and clinical parameters characterizing gingival sites with shallow to intermediate probing depth. J Periodontol 1987; 58:614.

Larjava H, Haapsalmi T, Salo T, Wiebe C, Uitto V-J. Keratinocyte integrins in wound healing and chronic inflammation of the human periodontium. Oral Dis 1996;2:77.

Lawson DA, Meyer TF. Biochemical characterization of *Porphyromonas (Bacteroides) gingivalis* collagenase. Infect Immun 1992;60:1524.

Lee W, Aitken S, Sodek J, McCulloch CA. Evidence of a direct relationship between neutrophil collagenase activity and periodontal tissue destruction in vivo: role of active enzyme in human periodontitis. J Periodont Res 1995;30:23.

LeRoy EC, Trojanowska MI, Smith EA. Cytokines and human fibrosis. Eur Cytokine Netw 1990;1:215.

Li B, Sehajpal PK, Khama A, et al. Differential regulation of transforming growth factor β and interleukin 2 genes in human T cells; demonstration by usage of novel competitor DNA constructs in the quantitative polymerase chain reaction. J Exp Med 1991;174:1259.

Lyons JG, Birkedal-Hansen B, Pierson MC, Whitelock JM, Birkedal-Hansen H. Interleukin-1β and transforming growth factor/epidermal growth factor induce expression of Mr 95,000 type IV collagenase/gelatinase and interstitial fibroblast-type collagenase by rat mucosal keratinocytes. J Biol Chem 1993;268:19143.

Makinen KK, Chen C-Y, Makinen PL, Ohta K, Loesche WJ. The benzoylarginine peptidase from Treponema denticola (strain ASLM) a human oral spirochete: evidence for active carboxyl groups. Mol Microbiol 1990;4:1415.

Marazita ML, Lu H, Cooper ME, et al. Genetic segregation analysis of serum IgG2 levels. Am J Hum Genet 1996;58:1042.

Mariotti A, Hassell T, Kaminker P. The influence of age on collagen and non-collagen protein production by human gingival epithelial cells. Arch Oral Biol 1993; 38:635.

Mauviel A, Lapiere JC, Halcin C, Evans CH, Uitto J. Differential cytokines regulation of type I and VII collagen gene expression in cultured dermal fibroblasts. J Biol Chem 1994:269:25.

Mayrand D, Holt SC. Biology of asaccharolytic black-pigmented *Bacteroides* species. Microbiol Rev 1988;52:134.

McCulloch CA, Knowles G. Discrimination of two fibroblast progenitor populations in early explant cultures of hamster gingiva. Cell Tissue Res 1993a;264:87.

McCulloch CA, Knowles GC. Deficiencies in collagen phagocytosis by human fibroblasts in vitro: a mechanism for fibrosis? J Cell Physiol 1993b;155:461.

McCulloch CAG, Bordin S. Role of fibroblast subpopulations in periodontal physiology and pathology. J Periodont Res 1991;26:144.

Meikle MC, Hembry RM, Holley J, et al. Immunolocalization of matrix metalloproteinases and TIMP-1 (tissue inhibitor of metalloproteinases) in human gingival tissues from periodontitis patients. J Periodont Res 1994;29:118.

Morris ML, Harper E, McKenzie M. The presence of an inhibitor of human skin collagenase in the roots of healthy and periodontally diseased teeth. J Periodontol 1993; 64:363.

Nakao K, Yoneda K, Osaki T. Enhanced cytokine production and collagen synthesis of gingival fibroblasts from patients with denture fibromatosis. J Dent Res 1995;74: 1072.

Narayanan AS, Bartold PM. Biochemistry of periodontal connective tissues and their regeneration: A current perspective. Connect Tissue Res 1996;34:191.

Narayanan AS, Clagett JA, Page RC. Effect of inflammation on the distribution of collagen types I, III, IV, and V and type I trimer and fibronectin in human gingiva. J Dent Res 1985; 64:1111.

Narayanan AS, Hassell T. Characterization of collagens in phenytoin-enlarged human gingiva. Collagen Rel Res 1985;5:513.

Narayanan AS, Page RC. Connective tissues of the periodontium: A summary of current work. Collagen Rel Res 1983;3:33.

Offenbacher S. Periodontal diseases: Pathogenesis. Ann Periodontol (World Workshop in Periodontics) 1996;1:821.

Overall CM. Regulation of tissue inhibitor of matrix metalloproteinases expression. Ann NY Acad Sci 1994; 732:51.

Overall CM, Sodek J. Concanavalin A produces a matrix-degradative phenotype in human fibroblasts. Induction and endogenous activation of collagenase, 72-kDa gelatinase and Pump-1 is accompanied by the suppression of the tissue inhibitor of matrix metalloproteinases. J Biol Chem 1990;285:21141.

Overall CM, Wiebkin OW, Thonard JC. Demonstration of tissue collagenase activity *in vivo* and its relationship to inflammation severity in human gingiva. J Periodont Res 1987;22:81.

Overall CM, Wrana JL, Sodek J. Transcriptional and post-transcriptional regulation of 72-kDa gelatinase/type IV collagenase by transforming growth factor-beta 1 in human fibroblasts. Comparisons with collagenase and tissue inhibitor of matrix metalloproteinase gene expression. J Biol Chem 1991;266:14064.

Page RC, Baab DA. A new look at the etiology and pathogenesis of early onset periodontitis. Cementopathia revisited. J Periodontol 1985;56:748.

Page RC, Bowen T, Altman L, et al. Prepubertal periodontitis (I). Definition of a clinical disease entitiy. J Periodontol 1983;54:257.

Page RC, Offenbacher S, Schroeder HE, Seymour GJ, Kornman KS. Advances in the pathogenesis of periodontitis. Summary of developments, clinical implications and future direction. Periodontology 2000. 1997;14:216.

Page RC, Schroeder HE. Periodontitis in Man and Other Animals. A Comparative Review. Basel: Karger; 1982.

Plagmann HC, Kocher T, Kuhrau N, Caliebe A. Periodontal manifestation of hypophosphatasia. A family case report. J Clin Periodontol 1994;21:710.

Podhradsky J, J'any Z, Velgos S. Beta-glucuronidase activity in human gingiva in health and periodontal disease. Arch Oral Biol 1982;27:615.

Reynolds JJ, Meikle MC. Mechanisms of connective tissue matrix destruction in periodontitis. Periodontology 2000 1997;14:144.

Romanos GE, Strub JR, Bernimoulin JP. Immunohistochemical distribution of extracellular matrix proteins as a diagnostic parameter in healthy and diseased gingiva. J Periodont 1993;64:110.

Ryan ME, Ramamurthy S, Golub LM. Matrix metalloproteinases and their inhibition in periodontal treatment. Curr Opin Periodontol 1996;3:85.

Saito K, Mori S, Iwakura M, Sakamoto S. Immunohistochemical localization of transforming growth factor β basic fibroblast growth factor and heparan sulphate glycosaminoglycan in gingival hyperplasia induced by nifedipine and phenytoin. J Periodont Res 1996;31:545.

Saksela O, Rifkin DB. Cell-associated plasminogen activation: Regulation and physiological functions. Ann Rev Cell Biol 1988;4:93.

Schincaglia GAP, Forniti F, Cavallini R, et al. Cyclosporine-A increases type I procollagen production and mRNA level in human gingival fibroblasts in vitro. J Oral Pathol Med 1992;2:181.

Schluger S, Yuodelis RA, Page RC. Periodontal Disease. Philadelphia: Lea & Febiger; 1990.

Schuppan D, Somasundaram R, Dieterich W, Ehris T, Bauer M. The extracellular matrix in cellular proliferation and differentiation. Ann NY Acad Sci 1994;733:87.

Schwartz Z, Goultshin J, Dean DD, Boyan BD. Mechanisms of alveolar bone destruction in periodontitis. Periodontology 2000 1997;14:158.

Selvig KA, Zander H. Chemical analysis and microradiography of cementum and dentin from periodontally diseased human teeth. J Periodontol 1962;33:303.

Seymour RA, Thomason JM, Ellis JS. The pathogenesis of drug-induced gingival overgrowth. J Clin Periodontol 1996;23:165.

Shikata H, Utsumi H, Shimojima T, Oda Y, Okada Y. Increased expression of type VI collagen genes in drug-induced gingival enlargement. FEBS Lett 1993;334:65.

Slots J, Genco RJ. Black-pigmented *Bacteroides* species *Capnocytophaga* species and *Actinobacillus actinomycetemcomitans* in human periodontal disease: virulence factors in colonization, survival and tissue destruction. J Dent Res 1984;63:412.

Smalley JW, Birss AJ, Shuttleworth CA. The degradation of fibronectin and type I collagen by a trypsin-like enzyme and the extracellular vesicle fraction of *Bacteroides gingivalis*. Arch Oral Biol 1988;33:323.

Sodek J, Overall CM. Matrix metalloproteinases in periodontal tissue remodelling. Matrix 1992;1(suppl):352.

Söderling E. Mäkinen KK, Syed S, et al. Biochemical comparison of proteolytic enzymes present in rough- and smooth-surfaced capnocytophagas isolated from the subgingival plaque of periodontitis patients. J Periodont Res 1991;26:17.

Sorsa T, Saari H, Kontinen YT, et al. Non-proteolytic activation of latent human neutrophil collagenase and its role in matrix destruction in periodontal diseases. Int J Tissue Reac 1989;IX:153.

Sorsa T, Suomalainen K, Uitto VJ. The role of gingival crevicular fluid and salivary interstitial collagenases in human periodontal diseases. Arch Oral Biol 1990; 35(suppl):193S.

Stepnick RJ, Nakata TM, Zipkin I. The effects of age, fluoride exposure on fluoride, citrate and carbonate content of human cementum. J Periodontol 1975;46:45.

Stewart RE, Hollister DW, Rimoin DL. A new variant of the Ehlers-Danlos syndrome: an autosomal dominant disorder of fragile skin, abnormal scarring and generalized periodontitis. Birth Defects 1977;13:85.

Suresh R, Dhar SC. Increased glucocorticoid receptors in diphenylhydantoin induced human gingival overgrowth. Biochem Int 1991;24:669.

Sznajder N, Carraro JJ, Otero E, Carranza FA. Clinical periodontal findings in trisomy 21 (Mongolism). J Periodont Res 1968;3:1.

Tam Y-C, Chan EC. Purification and characterization of hyaluronidase from oral Peptostreptococcus species. Infect Immun 1985;47:508.

Tam Y-C, Harvey RF, Chas EC. Chondroitin sulfatase-producing oral bacteria associated with periodontal disease. J Can Dent Assoc 1982;48:115.

Temple TR, Kimball HR, Kakehashi S, Amen CR. Host factors in periodontal disease: periodontal manifestations of Chediak Higashi syndrome. J Periodont Res 1972; 10(suppl):26.

Tewari DS, Bian Y, Tewari M, et al. Mechanistic features associated with induction of metalloproteinases in human gingival fibroblasts by interleukin-1. Arch Oral Biol 1994;39:657.

Tipler LS, Embery G. Glycosaminoglycan-depolymerizing enzymes produced by an anaerobic bacteria isolated from the mouth. Arch Oral Biol 1985;30:303.

Tipton DA, Fry HR, Dabbous MK. Altered collagen metabolism in nifedipine-induced gingival overgrowth. J Periodont Res 1994;29:401.

Tipton DA, Stricklin GP, Dabbous Mk. Fibroblast heterogeneity in collagenolytic response to cyclosporine. J Cell Biochem 1991;46:152.

Uitto-VJ, Chan EC, Quee TC. Initial characterization of neutral proteinases from oral spirochetes. J Periodont Res 1986;21:95.

Uitto VJ, Firth JD, Nip L, Golub LM. Doxycycline and chemically modified tetracyclines inhibit gelatinase A (MMP-2) gene expression in human skin keratinocytes. Ann NY Acad Sci 1994;732:140.

Uitto VJ, Raeste AM. Activation of latent collagenase of human leukocytes and gingival fluid by bacterial plaque. J Dent Res 1978;57:844.

Uitto VJ, Suomalainen K, Sorsa AT. Salivary collagenase. Origin, characteristics and relationship to periodontal health. J Periodont Res 1990;25:135.

Van Dyke TE, Horoszwicz H, Cianciola LJ, Genco RJ. Neutrophil chemotaxis dysfunction in human periodontitis. Infect Immun 1980;27:124.

Van Dyke TE, Taubman MA, Ebersole JL, et al. The Papillon Lefevre syndrome: neutrophil dysfunction with severe periodontal disease. J Periodont Res 1984;20:503.

Vernillo AT, Schwartz NB. The effects of phenytoin o(5,5-diphenylhydantoin) on human gingival fibroblasts in culture. J Periodont Res 1987;22:307.

Vernillo AT, Schwartz NB. Stimulation of collagen and glycosaminoglycan production by phenytoin (5,5-diphenylhydantoin) in monolayer cultures of mesenchymal cells derived from embryonic chick sternae. Arch Oral Biol 1986;31:819.

Villela B, Cogen RB, Bartolucci AA, Birkedal-Hansen H. Collagenolytic activity in crevicular fluid from patients with chronic periodontitis, localized juvenile periodontitis and gingivitis, and from healthy control subjects. J Periodont Res 1987;22:381.

Waldrop TC, Hallmon WW, Mealey BL. Observations of root surfaces from patients with early-onset periodontitis and leukocyte adhesion deficiency. J Clin Periodontol 1995;22:168.

Whyte MP. Hypophosphatasia. In: Scriver CR, Beaudet AL, Sly WS, Valle D, eds. The Metabolic and Molecular Bases of Inherited Diseases. 7th ed. New York: McGraw-Hill;1995:4095.

Williams RC. Periodontal disease. New Engl J Med 1990; 322:373.

Wynne SE, Aldred MJ, Bartold PM. Hereditary gingival fibromatosis associated with hearing loss and supernumerary teeth. A new syndrome? J Periodontol 1995;66:75.

Xu LX, Ohsaki Y, Nagata K, Kurisu K. Immunohistochemical studies on the distributions and age-related changes of types I and III collagen in the oral mucosa of mice. J Dent Res 1993;72:1336.

Part IV

Clinical Aspects

Gingival Crevicular Fluid: Connective Tissue Elements as Diagnostic Markers

Introduction

Our understanding of the nature of periodontal disease has changed in the last two decades with evidence that periodontitis does not afflict all people and that it can be a site-specific problem that does not progress in a continuous manner. With this knowledge, and the fact that diagnostic techniques such as periodontal probing and radiographs give very limited information about current disease activity, there has been a surge in the interest in diagnostics. A diagnostic test that could differentiate between stable and progressive disease would ensure appropriate patient management and be of great clinical significance. At present there is no single reliable diagnostic indicator for active periodontal destruction (Beck 1995; Armitage 1996).

The events associated with the development of periodontitis can be divided into bacterial infection, genetic susceptibility, metabolic responses, and anatomical changes, each of which needs to be taken into account when diagnosing periodontal conditions. Given the multifactorial nature of the disease, it is un-

Table 10-1. Components of Gingival Crevicular Fluid

Cells	Bacteria
	Epithelial cells
	Leukocytes
Electrolytes	Calcium
	Sodium
	Fluoride
	Magnesium
	Phosphate
	Potassium
Microbial plaque products	Bacterial enzymes
	Cytotoxic substances
	Metabolic end products
	Lipopolysaccharide
Inflammatory cell products	Acute-phase proteins
	Cytokines
	Immunoglobulins
	Enzymes (matrix degrading)
	Lysosomal enzymes
	Prostaglandins
Host tissues	Complement
	Fibrin
	Fibronectin
	Collagens
	Osteocalcin
	Osteonectin
	Proteoglycans

likely that only one parameter will ever be used as a universal diagnostic aid. Nonetheless, markers of connective tissue disease activity may be of use when considering the metabolic responses of the disease process. Such connective tissue components may be divided into effectors of inflammation and products of inflammation (Embery and Waddington 1994).

Gingival crevicular fluid appears to be an ideal medium for monitoring the changes occurring during development of periodontal disease. It can be collected noninvasively, and its dynamics and composition are closely related to the environment of the periodontal tissues. As a result, many studies have focused on analyzing components of this inflammatory exudate in the hope of finding an indicator of active periodontal breakdown (Lamster and Grbic 1995; Armitage 1996). Specifically, plasma proteins, bacterial and mammalian enzymes, numerous inflammatory mediators, as well as products of matrix degradation have been among the myriad components studied in detail (Table 10-1). For the purposes of this chapter, only the elements associated with the extracellular matrix and its degradation will be considered in detail.

Diagnostic Tests for Periodontal Disease

Need for Diagnostic Tests

Prior to the 1980s, periodontitis was assumed to afflict all humans and to progress from gingivitis in a slow continuum until teeth were eventually lost (Marshall-Day et al 1955; Löe et al 1978). All pockets were thought to be active and thus needed treatment. Studies since then have demonstrated these assumptions to be untrue for some individuals. For example, disease activity may occur in episodes or bursts at a limited number of sites during a defined interval, with the clinical duration of activity occurring in short periods from days to months (Socransky et al 1984). On the other hand, there is evidence that indicates some sites in certain patients manifest periodontal breakdown that is slow but continuous in its progression (Jeffcoat and Reddy 1991). Importantly, there appears to be a small population of periodontal patients who do not respond to treatment and continue to lose attachment despite the best that our treatment procedures can provide. Our ability to identify these various types of patients and diseases is poor (Hirschfeld and Wasserman 1978).

To avoid overtreatment, and to treat progressive disease appropriately, there is a need to distinguish between stable and progressive disease sites and to assess when these sites are adequately treated. Traditional diagnostic instruments, such as the periodontal probe and radiographs, are inadequate in diagnosing disease activity as they indicate past tissue destruction and cannot distinguish prospectively between a progressive or a stable site (Haffajee et al 1983).

To develop a diagnostic test, one must first define the parameters to be analyzed. For periodontics, the principal feature to be established is the presence or absence of disease. However, other features such as disease severity, current disease status, and the possibility of future progression should also form part of the diagnostic process. A test that is easy to perform, particularly if it has a chairside application, and that is able to diagnose disease at a particular site will ensure periodontal treatment that is more effective and rational.

Since diagnosis involves many varied aspects, it becomes necessary to consider the initiator or driving force behind each event so that baselines may be developed. With respect to the periodontal diseases, at least three fundamental processes occur simultaneously: (1)

bacterial colonization, (2) host responses to the bacteria, and (3) metabolic events arising from the host response. Each of these parameters will have a bearing on past disease activity, current disease activity, and the likelihood of future breakdown. In addition to this, it must be remembered that the ultimate outcome of the disease process is further complicated by numerous modifying and predisposing factors that must be recognized for successful periodontal therapy, and that may compromise universal utilization of periodontal diagnostic tests.

Requirements of a Diagnostic Test

A diagnostic test that will be valuable clinically must add to the information already gained by traditional methods of diagnosis. As such, a useful diagnostic test should be able to detect subclinical disease and thereby lower the detection threshold as compared to current clinical measures (Offenbacher et al 1993). The information gained should be relevant to diagnosis, treatment, or predictive tests. In addition, the test should be able to be accurately repeated in a number of different clinical situations and levels of disease severity (Offenbacher et al 1993).

The value of diagnostic tests should relate to their clinical utility. At least four different uses have been suggested for periodontal diagnostic tests (McCulloch 1994):

1. To detect disease presence and evaluate severity.
2. To predict the subsequent clinical course and prognosis.
3. To estimate responsiveness to treatment before therapy.
4. To assess actual response to treatment after completion.

Numerous authors have stressed the need for a diagnostic test to not only distinguish between gingivitis and periodontitis, but to also distinguish between disease-active and disease-inactive sites (Curtis et al 1989; Fine 1992; McCulloch 1994). However, this distinction is difficult because periods of active periodontal destruction are usually accompanied by an acute phase of inflammation in which gingivitis and progressive periodontitis may produce similar byproducts from the acute inflammatory response that then appear in the gingival crevicular fluid.

Markers of gingival inflammation cannot be assumed to be markers of destructive periodontitis. Therefore, the search for a component in gingival crevicular fluid that is specifically related to active phases of periodontitis has become a goal of diagnostic testing. Products arising from bone destruction that are specific to the molecular composition of bone and not found in soft tissue may have considerable potential as markers of tissue destruction.

For a diagnostic test to be useful it should be both specific and sensitive. That is, it should be able to distinguish between those individuals (or sites around teeth) with periodontal disease and those who are disease free (Beck 1995). Sensitivity is the probability that the disease is present when test results are positive. Specificity is the probability that the disease is absent when test results are negative (Armitage 1992). Usually a test does not have both good sensitivity and good specificity; often, the more sensitive the test, the lower the specificity (Beck 1995). It has been proposed that a test erring on the side of false positives but with higher sensitivity is the choice in diagnosing periodontal disease, as the consequences of a false positive for periodontal disease diagnosis are milder than the consequences of a false negative (Beck 1995). Since 100% sensitivity and 100% specificity are impossible to obtain, threshold values of the ratio between sensitivity and specificity should be set for a diagnostic test based on treatment philosophies, cost, and manpower (Listgarten 1986). Another term used to describe a diagnostic test is the predictive value of a test. This refers to the probability of disease being present given the result of the test (Beck 1995). Thus, a positive predictive value would refer to active disease returning a positive result.

To determine these aspects of a diagnostic test, the marker in question must be assessed in longitudinal trials to correlate changes in attachment level to changes in the marker. This will provide sensitivity and specificity data, and allow determination of cutoff values for a screening test (Offenbacher 1993).

Rationale for the Use of Gingival Crevicular Fluid as a Diagnostic Test

Saliva, serum, and gingival crevicular fluid have all been studied as vehicles for assessing periodontal disease activity (Curtis et al 1989; Mandel 1991; Taubman et al 1992). Saliva, however, has a number of drawbacks as it is made up of components derived from multiple sources including salivary glands, serum, gingival crevicular fluid, sloughed epithelial cells, bacteria, and foreign substances introduced into the oral cavity (Lamster and Grbic 1995). Gingival crevicular fluid offers an advantage over serum in that it is easily and noninvasively collected (Fig 10-1), and contains products of the host, the plaque, and their interactions (Curtis et al 1989).

Prior to the appearance of gingival crevicular fluid in the gingival crevice, the exudate from the gingival microcirculation traverses the inflamed periodontal tissues and is thought to collect molecules of potential interest en route that may reflect the underlying disease or health status of the tissues (Page 1992). Gingival crevicular fluid will thus contain, in varying amounts, components derived from plasma, from locally produced host factors, and from microbial sources. The concentrations of these will depend on a wide range of variables such as the composition of the plaque, the rate of turnover of the connective tissue, the permeability of the epithelium, and the degree of inflammation (Curtis et al

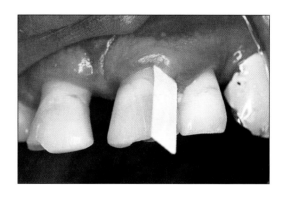

Fig 10-1 Sampling and collection of human gingival crevicular fluid onto filter-paper strips. The strips are placed at the gingival crevice and left in place for specified periods to allow the crevicular fluid to impregnate the filter paper. Note that the strip is placed atraumatically so as not to induce any bleeding, which might interfere with the fluid composition.

1989). As gingival crevicular fluid is derived from the periodontal tissues, analysis of its constituents may provide an early indicator of changes in the tissue. Thus, crevicular fluid contains many of the reaction products associated with periodontal inflammation, and as such, provides a rich source of potential markers (Page 1992). While many approaches and components have been identified as potentially useful, few have been adequately evaluated in carefully designed longitudinal studies. Indeed, some have suffered from (or are in danger of) being prematurely introduced into the market without appropriate long-term studies to determine their usefulness.

Unfortunately, a serious drawback of most of these potential markers studied in gingival crevicular fluid is that they reflect processes occurring in the gingival connective tissues and tell us little about attachment loss or bone loss. Thus, it can be difficult to make any clear distinction between gingivitis and periodontitis. However, due to the site specificity of some matrix components (see Chapter 8), the possibility exists for their detection and measurement in crevicular fluid and correlate their presence with site-specific and tissue-specific periodontal destruction. In assessing the usefulness of any component in the gingival crevicular fluid for assisting periodontal diagnosis, the limitations of gingival

crevicular fluid as a diagnostic medium and the requirements of a diagnostic test need to be recognized.

Limitations of Gingival Crevicular Fluid as a Diagnostic Medium

One of the major limitations in the interpretation of information obtained from a diagnostic test is the lack of a gold standard against which the test can be evaluated (Listgarten 1986; Beck 1995). Often, the standard itself may be less than ideal. Thus, any comparisons to an inadequate standard can lead to false impressions and inaccurate conclusions.

Another limitation of gingival crevicular fluid as a diagnostic test is the unknown dynamics of the complex gingival environment. Our knowledge is limited regarding what happens to the fluid as it traverses the tissues, with respect to the binding, metabolism, and redistribution of fluid components. The gingival sulcus contains a large number of different molecules with interactions that are not fully understood. Thus, determining the levels of one specific enzyme or tissue product may be meaningless without knowing how it is affected by various bacteria, their products, and other host enzymes (McCullough 1994).

Crevicular Fluid and Matrix Destruction

More than 40 components have been identified in the gingival crevicular fluid and have been classified by Cimasoni (1983) into cellular elements, electrolytes, organic compounds, bacterial products, metabolic products, enzymes, and enzyme inhibitors (see Table 10-1). In particular, attention has focused on biochemical mediators of inflammation, tissue-degrading enzymes, and tissue breakdown products in the gingival crevicular fluid as markers of the inflammatory response and possible indicators of some aspects of periodontal disease activity (Lamster et al 1985).

Biochemical Mediators and Products of Inflammation

From the earliest phases of gingival inflammation involving the recruitment of inflammatory cells into the gingival connective tissues, there is a significant release of numerous cytokines, lymphokines, chemokines, and other inflammatory mediators, together with large amounts of antibodies. Many of these components have been investigated for their potential to correlate with phases of active periodontal destruction.

Antibodies to periodontal bacteria. Antibodies to periodontopathic bacteria are found in both serum and gingival crevicular fluid of patients with a history of periodontal infection (Ebersole et al 1984). The fact that antibodies are found in gingival crevicular fluid implies that these antibodies are produced locally in response to the bacteria inhabiting the periodontal pocket. However, this issue is complex since the gingival crevicular fluid is itself a serum exudate, and the likelihood that antibodies in this exudate arise from the serum cannot be discounted. Studies investigating levels of antibodies in gingival crevicular fluid reactive with periodontal pathogens have, in general, shown inconclusive results due to large site-to-site variations leading to insignificant differences (Page 1992). However, one study, which investigated immunoglobulin G (IgG) subclasses in gingival crevicular fluid, noted that the subclasses IgG_1 and IgG_4 were elevated at periodontitis sites (Reinhardt et al 1989). In particular, elevated levels of IgG_4 were found at sites of periodontal disease activity and demonstrated a positive correlation with bleeding on probing and disease progression (Reinhardt et al 1989; Wilton et al 1993). Gingival crevicular fluid IgG levels to specific periodontal pathogens such as *Porphyromonas gingivalis* have also been found to correlate with probing pocket depth, and these levels decrease significantly following subgingival débridement (Sengupta et al 1988; Johnson et al 1993). To date, these studies have provided some interesting insights into the host responses to periodontal infections, but are inconclusive as to their clinical utility as a diagnostic aid for determining disease activity.

Cytokines. Cytokines, specifically interleukin (IL)-1α, IL-1β, IL-6, IL-8, and tumor necrosis factor (TNF)-α, have been found in gingival crevicular fluid and studied in relation to their role in the progression of periodontal destruction (Masada et al 1990; Rossomando et al 1990; Reinhardt et al 1993a; Payne et al 1993; Tsai et al 1995). Of these, IL-1 has been studied in greatest detail. This cytokine, which is released by activated macrophages, polymorphonuclear leukocytes, lymphocytes, and fibroblasts, is involved in proinflammatory processes, matrix destruction, and wound healing (see Chapter 3). Due to its strong relationship with bone resorption, this cytokine has received considerable attention as a potential marker for active periodontal tissue destruction. Both the IL-1α and IL-1β forms have been detected in gingival crevicular fluid; IL-1β concentrations increase significantly during episodes of periodontal inflammation

(Masada et al 1990; Reinhardt et al 1993b). Cross-sectional studies have indicated that the levels of IL-1β are increased at periodontitis sites compared to gingivitis and healthy sites (Preiss and Meyle 1994; Kinane et al 1992). To date, there have been too few longitudinal studies investigating the relationship between IL-1 levels in gingival crevicular fluid to make any conclusive statement regarding its usefulness as a diagnostic marker for periodontal disease activity (Armitage 1996).

Complement. Activated forms of the complement system have also been found in the gingival crevicular fluid (Niekrash and Patters 1986) and are important in defense against foreign substances. An increase in C3 cleavage has been noted to correlate positively with plaque accumulation and subsequent development of gingivitis (Patters et al 1989). Whether there is a similar correlation with the development of periodontitis is not clear.

Prostaglandins. Prostaglandins, which are derived from arachidonic acid metabolism, are found in abundance at sites of inflammation (see Chapter 3). These potent molecules are associated with tissue destruction, changes in fibroblast metabolism, and bone resorption (Keuhl and Egan 1980). Recently, the levels of prostaglandin E_2 (PGE_2) in gingival crevicular fluid have been reported to correlate positively with periodontal inflammation and impending tissue destruction (Offenbacher et al 1986; Offenbacher et al 1991). In addition, PGE_2 levels have been noted to be elevated in the gingival crevicular fluid from patients with juvenile periodontitis compared to patients with adult-type periodontitis and gingivitis (Offenbacher et al 1984). Although only one longitudinal study investigating PGE_2 levels in crevicular fluid and its correlation with periodontal disease activity has been reported, this marker is considered to have considerable potential as a diagnostic marker of active disease (Page 1992). Unfortunately, the currently available tests required to detect

PGE_2 in gingival crevicular fluid are, in general, complex and not easy to perform as chairside diagnostic tests.

$α_2$-Macroglobulin and $α_1$-antitrypsin. The proteinase inhibitors $α_2$-macroglobulin and $α_1$-antitrypsin are acute-phase proteins found at all sites where there is active acute inflammation occurring with concomitant tissue destruction. Under conditions of experimental gingivitis, both of these proteins have been found in elevated amounts in gingival crevicular fluid (Adonogianaki et al 1992). However, at sites of active periodontal inflammation that show significant bone loss, the levels of $α_2$-macroglobulin appear to decrease (Skaleric et al 1986). Whether this finding reflects the formation of macromolecular complexes that are not readily detected in gingival crevicular fluid remains to be established. To date, measurement of these proteinases in gingival crevicular fluid has been unable to distinguish between gingivitis and periodontitis.

C-reactive protein. C-reactive protein is another acute-phase protein derived from serum; it is found in most inflammatory exudates. This protein coats bacteria and aids complement binding. While it is an important component of the inflammatory exudate, and is found in increased levels at sites of inflammation, this protein does not show any differences in concentration in gingival crevicular fluid between sites of gingivitis or periodontitis (Sibraa et al 1991).

Lysozyme. Lysozyme, which is found in the azurophil granules of polymorphonuclear leukocytes, is released at sites of acute inflammation. This enzyme acts as a bactericidal agent by cleaving the peptidoglycan component of bacterial cell walls. Levels of this enzyme in gingival crevicular fluid do not distinguish between adult periodontitis and gingivitis lesions (Modeer and Twetman 1979). However, elevated levels have been noted in samples taken from patients with lo-

229

calized juvenile periodontitis compared to samples from patients with gingivitis or adult periodontitis (Friedman et al 1983). To date, too few studies have been carried out on this component to make any firm conclusions regarding its potential as a biochemical marker of disease activity.

Lactoferrin. Lactoferrin is also found within polymorphonuclear leukocytes; it has antibacterial properties due to its high affinity for iron, which is required for bacterial growth. In contrast to lysozyme, lactoferrin levels do not differ significantly between different disease conditions (Friedman et al 1983). However, since the concentration of lactoferrin in normal crevicular fluid is some two- to tenfold greater than that of lysozyme and because lactoferrin levels are not influenced by disease whereas lysozyme levels are, changes in the ratio of lysozyme to lactoferrin may be of diagnostic value in distinguishing gingivitis and periodontitis sites (Friedman et al 1983). However, more studies are needed before this can be confirmed.

Transferrin. Transferrin is an antibacterial serum protein found at inflammatory sites; it acts in a manner similar to lactoferrin by binding iron required for bacterial growth. In experimental gingivitis studies, the level of transferrin in gingival crevicular fluid has been noted to increase with the development of gingivitis (Adonogianaki et al 1994). However, when oral hygiene is resumed, the levels of transferrin in the crevicular fluid do not return to baseline levels. Similarly elevated levels of transferrin have been noted in crevicular fluid sampled from periodontitis sites. These early studies imply that the presence of this protein does not distinguish between gingivitis and periodontitis sites.

Myeloperoxidase. Myeloperoxidase is a component of granules within polymorphonuclear leukocytes; it is released at sites of inflammation. Although it has not been extensively studied in gingival crevicular fluid, this enzyme has been noted to be elevated at periodontitis sites compared to control sites, and its concentration decreases following treatment (Smith et al 1986; Cao and Smith 1989).

Acid phosphatase. Acid phosphatase is an intracellular enzyme commonly used to determine lysosomal activity. However, its presence in gingival crevicular fluid does not correlate well with the presence of disease (Binder et al 1987). This poor correlation is presumably due to its broad distribution in inflammatory cells as well as in desquamated epithelial cells, bone cells, and bacteria.

Host-Derived Enzymes

It has been suggested that levels of proteolytic and hydrolytic enzymes in crevicular fluid could be of potential value as diagnostic markers (Bowers and Zahradnik 1989; Lamster 1991). A number of enzymes may be released by host cells, including collagenase, elastase, and a wide battery of lysosomal enzymes including the cathepsins, acid phosphatase, alkaline phosphatase, β-glucuronidase, lactate dehydrogenase, and arylsulfatase (Lamster 1991). It is important to note that the activity of many of these enzymes is modulated by specific enzymes and proteins either locally produced or circulating in the plasma. Therefore, the mere presence of an enzyme should not be mistaken to indicate biologic activity in situ. Indeed, many enzymes are released in an inactive form or may be complexed with other tissue proteins and rendered inactive. A common misconception in identifying enzymes in crevicular fluid is that their presence implies, or equates with, tissue destruction. This clearly cannot be the case unless the presence of active enzyme is demonstrated. Nonetheless, the presence of an enzyme (either active or inactive) may be the harbinger of impending tissue destruction, and as such, may still correlate with disease status and be of diagnostic use.

Collagenase. The presence of collagenases in gingival crevicular fluid has been of particular interest as collagens constitute one of the major extracellular matrix proteins in the periodontium, and because significant destruction of collagens occurs during periodontal destruction (see Chapter 9). Collagenases may be derived from host cells, including polymorphonuclear leukocytes, macrophages, fibroblasts, keratinocytes, and osteoclasts, as well as from bacteria. Since it appears that the collagenase secreted by polymorphonuclear leukocytes is the most important in the degradation of periodontal collagens, this collagenase has received prominent attention (Overall and Sodek 1987; Overall et al 1991; Birkedal-Hansen 1993). Several studies have indicated that collagenase levels are increased in gingival crevicular fluid at both gingivitis and periodontitis sites (Larivée et al 1986; Sorsa et al 1990). In addition, levels of collagenase in crevicular fluid have been noted to correlate specific forms of periodontitis, including adult-type periodontitis and localized juvenile periodontitis (Villela et al 1987a, 1987b). However, the usefulness of this enzyme as a diagnostic marker is questionable, because differentiation between gingivitis and periodontitis has been difficult (Overall et al 1991). In general, the levels of this enzyme in gingival crevicular fluid show marked fluctuations with regard to site, disease status, and treatment. These differences may be related to the many sources of collagenase and thus make it an unreliable marker of disease activity.

Elastase. Neutrophil elastase is a serine endopeptidase that can degrade both collagenous and noncollagenous extracellular matrix proteins; it is released at sites of inflammation. The levels of this enzyme in gingival crevicular fluid have been noted to increase with the development of gingivitis, as well at sites of established periodontitis (Meyle et al 1992; Gustafsson et al 1992). In addition, the levels of neutrophil elastase have been found to decrease following treatment of affected periodontal sites (Meyle et al 1992). Longitudinal studies have indicated that gingival crevicular fluid levels of neutrophil elastase have some predictive value for identifying sites at risk of further breakdown (Armitage et al 1994). While further studies are needed, this enzyme shows some promise as a diagnostic marker for active periodontal disease.

Cathepsins. The cathepsins are a group of lysosomal cysteine proteinases that are released in high levels at inflammatory sites; they can degrade numerous components of the extracellular matrix. In gingival crevicular fluid, cathepsins B, D, G, H, and L have been identified (Ishikawa et al 1972; Kunimatsu et al 1990; Kunimatsu et al 1995). To date, little evidence exists to support a role for these enzymes in the diagnosis of periodontal disease, although they may have some utility for determining tissue responses to treatment (Eley et al 1991; Cox and Eley 1992, Eley and Cox 1996).

Alkaline phosphatase. Alkaline phosphatase is a lysosomal enzyme found in osteoblasts, fibroblasts, neutrophils, and bacteria; it is found in serum and in gingival crevicular fluid. Since the levels of alkaline phosphatase are normally higher in gingival crevicular fluid than in serum, it is possible that the alkaline phosphatase noted in gingival crevicular fluid arises from local production by cells in the gingival environment. Increased levels of alkaline phosphatase have been noted in experimental gingivitis studies and at periodontitis sites (Ishikawa and Cimasoni 1970; Binder et al 1987). The level of alkaline phosphatase at periodontitis sites showed a strong positive correlation with a predictive value of 73% of active sites being detected (true positive) and 36% of inactive sites being included (false positive).

Arylsulfatase and β-glucuronidase. Of all the lysosomal enzymes, arylsulfatase and β-glucuronidase have been studied in considerable detail because of their relationship to polymorphonuclear leukocyte function, as well as their ability to degrade some components of the extracellular matrix (Lamster et al 1988; Lamster et al 1993). The enzyme β-glucuronidase degrades disaccharide and tetrasaccharide components of proteoglycans and glycoproteins, while arylsulfatase catalyzes the release of O-sulfate ester groups from sulfated glycosaminoglycans and other sulfated glycoproteins. The action of these enzymes is secondary to initial enzymatic cleavage of proteoglycans, and it may not be of major importance in the initiation of matrix destruction. A positive correlation between the presence of these two enzymes in crevicular fluid and periodontal disease has been noted (Bang et al 1970; Oshrain et al 1984). More recently, both cross-sectional and longitudinal studies have shown that the levels of both β-glucuronidase and arylsulfatase increase with increasing levels of periodontal destruction, and that these levels return to near baseline following treatment (Lamster et al 1987; Lamster and Grbic 1995). In addition, β-glucuronidase levels may be positively associated with the presence of numerous periodontopathic bacteria in the subgingival flora (Harper et al 1989). To date, these two enzymes show some promise for further development as diagnostic aids for detecting active periodontal diseases.

Aspartate aminotransferase. Aspartate aminotransferase is a cytoplasmic enzyme released upon cell death. Since cell death is an integral part of periodontal destruction, levels of this enzyme have been studied as a possible marker of disease activity (Persson et al 1990). Good correlation between the level of aspartate aminotransferase in gingival crevicular fluid and disease activity, as well as disease progression, has been demonstrated (Persson et al 1991; Magnusson et al 1996). However,

it should be noted that few longitudinal studies have been carried out to determine the usefulness of this marker as a diagnostic aid. Thus, it may suffer from problems similar to other test systems currently available, namely a lack of specificity for disease prediction.

Extracellular Matrix Components in Gingival Crevicular Fluid

The tissues of the periodontium exist in a delicate balance between health and disease as well as between repair and regeneration. During periods of active periodontal disease, tissue destruction will exceed synthesis. However, synthetic mechanisms will also be enhanced as the repair events seek to overcome injury to the tissue. Thus, both catabolic and anabolic products from the extracellular matrix may be present in the gingival crevicular fluid; these are potentially important markers of disease and tissue turnover (Embery et al 1991).

Collagen. Collagen represents the most abundant structural protein in the periodontium. Type 1 collagen predominates in gingival connective tissue, periodontal ligament, and alveolar bone; there are lesser amounts of type III and V collagen (see Chapter 8). Early studies on the turnover of periodontal collagens focused on measuring the hydroxyproline levels in gingival tissue extracts and crevicular fluid in an attempt to monitor periodontal breakdown (Hara and Takahashi 1975). The hydroxyproline content of gingival crevicular fluid and serum has been noted to decrease significantly following periodontal surgery (Hara and Takahashi 1975). In a ligature-induced periodontitis model, the levels of hydroxyproline in gingival crevicular were highest in samples taken 4 days after ligature removal (Svanberg 1987a, 1987b). However in this study, no indication was given regarding the extent of tissue destruction at this time point. Furthermore, the source of these collagenous components (ie, hard or soft tissues) is unknown. Indeed, due to the relative nonspecificity of such assays (ie, all collagens contain hydroxyproline), no correlation between the presence of hydroxyproline and its site or source of breakdown can be made.

Other structural components of gingival collagens have been monitored in gingival crevicular fluid to evaluate collagen degradation and turnover. The detection of type I collagen carboxyterminal propeptide, N-propeptide alpha I type I collagen, and type II collagen aminoterminal propeptide have all been used to study collagen synthesis and turnover (Talonpoika and Hämäläinen1992; Talonpoika and Hämäläinen 1993a). Other studies have described the pyridinoline–cross-linked type I collagen carboxy terminal telopeptide in gingival crevicular fluid as a measure of collagen degradation (Talonpoika and Hämäläinen 1994). However, as for hydroxyproline assays, the detection of such telopeptides is still relatively nonspecific since measurement of type I collagen C-terminal telopeptide is unable to distinguish the source, which may be gingiva, periodontal ligament, or alveolar bone.

Recently, interest has focused on the development of methods to identify pyridinium cross-links in collagens that might be specific for bone. Pyridinium cross-links result from a series of reactions occurring during the maturation of collagen and lead to the formation of pyridinoline (also referred to as hydroxylysyl pyridinoline) and deoxypyridinoline (lysyl pyridinoline). The pattern of collagen cross-linking appears to be tissue specific. For example, pyridinoline is found mainly in cartilage, but also in bone, tendon, and blood vessels, whereas deoxypyridinoline is found exclusively in bone and dentin. Neither pyridinoline nor deoxypyridinoline are found in skin (Delmas 1993). Therefore, deoxypyridinoline has been targeted as a specific marker for mature bone. Because these cross-links result from posttranslational modifications of collagen, and thus cannot be reutilized during collagen synthesis, they represent a true indicator of bone resorption. Preliminary studies have identified pyridinium cross-links in crevicular fluid; these may correlate with sites undergoing active bone resorption (Meng et al 1991; Giannobile et al 1995). If these observations are confirmed, then the possibility of using the presence of pyridinium cross-links in crevicular fluid as a marker of active bone destruction is very attractive.

Proteoglycans and glycosaminoglycans. The measurement of proteoglycans, and their glycosaminoglycan components, in crevicular fluid shows some potential for monitoring active periodontal destruction (Embery et al 1982; Last et al 1985; Giannobile et al 1993). The sulcular fluid appears to be rich in metabolic or degradative products of the proteoglycans found in the various periodontal tissues. Some site specificity for various glycosaminoglycans in the periodontium has been noted; the gingival connective tissue is rich in dermatan sulfate, while the alveolar bone is rich in chondroitin sulfate (see Chapter 8).

The application of histochemical dyes to exudate collected onto filter-paper strips to indicate the presence of glycosaminoglycans in sulcular fluid was first reported by Sueda et al in 1966. Chemical analysis identified uronic acid in sulcular fluid, and thus confirmed the presence of glycosaminoglycans (Hara and Löe 1969). More recently, these studies have been extended to include identification of the types of glycosaminoglycans present in crevicular fluid. Hyaluronan is a ubiquitous component of sulcular fluid, regardless of the site sampled (inflamed or noninflamed). Chondroitin sulfate is the principal sulfated glycosaminoglycan identifiable in crevicular fluid; small amounts of heparan sulfate and dermatan sulfate are also present (Last et al 1985; Shibutani et al 1993). The high concentration of chondroitin sulfate in crevicular fluid sampled from sites of active bone resorption has been interpreted to indicate that this component originates from the matrix of the alveolar bone (Last et al 1985; Samuels et al 1993; Smedberg et al 1993). However, the precise origin of this glycosaminoglycan has not been determined. An alternative source could be the relatively high cellular composition of inflamed tissues, from which cell-surface chondroitin sulfate may be sequestered. Nonetheless, the observation that high levels of chondroitin sulfate are noted in samples taken from noninflamed sites undergoing orthodontic tooth movement does imply a close association between the appearance of chondroitin sulfate in crevicular fluid and bone resorption (Last et al 1988; Samuels et al 1993). While the usefulness of monitoring glycosaminoglycans in crevicular fluid awaits the appropriate longitudinal studies, the potential for chondroitin sulfate to be a useful marker of active bone resorption is good and warrants further detailed investigation.

Osteonectin. Osteonectin is a noncollagenous protein of mineralized tissue; it is thought to play a role in the mineralization process, thus its presence may indicate active bone turnover (see Chapter 5). This protein has been detected in gingival crevicular fluid in a cross-sectional study of patients with periodontal disease; the amount of protein increased with increasing pocket depth (Bowers et al 1989). However, osteonectin can be liberated from many different cell types as a heat-shock protein. While the role of heat-shock proteins is not fully understood, studies have shown that heat, a major clinical sign of inflammation, induces their synthesis (Polla 1988). Thus, osteonectin in gingival crevicular fluid may also relate to inflammation in general, and therefore it may discriminate poorly between gingivitis and periodontitis.

Osteocalcin. Osteocalcin, another bone matrix protein, is synthesised by osteoblasts. Osteocalcin has been identified in gingival crevicular fluid and studied in relation to clinical parameters (Kunimatsu et al 1993). No significant levels of osteocalcin were detected in the crevicular fluid of a small group of patients with gingivitis while patients with untreated periodontitis showed levels of osteocalcin in their crevicular fluid of 200 to 500 times higher than serum levels. The authors concluded that osteocalcin levels may be considered to reflect the severity of periodontal breakdown.

Fibronectin. Fibronectin, a normal component of serum and connective tissue, has been related to periodontal disease activity. Both host responses and bacterial enzymes are capable of degrading fibronectin. The resultant fibronectin fragments have different biologic properties compared to the intact molecule (Vartio 1983) and may be involved in the pathogenesis and healing of periodontal lesions. The levels of fibronectin in gingival crevicular fluid have been studied; more intact molecules are present in healthy sites than at sites of periodontitis (Talonpoika et al 1989; Cho 1984; Talonpoika et al 1993b). However, whether the appearance of fibronectin in gingival crevicular fluid reflects tissue remodeling or serum exudation is unclear.

Peri-Implant Sulcular Fluid

The relevance of the components of crevicular fluid around dental implants is now recognized as diagnostically significant. Indeed, because the anatomy of the soft tissue to implant interface is reasonably similar to teeth with respect to epithelial attachment and the presence of a peri-implant sulcus, there is no reason to expect that peri-implant sulcular fluid could not provide useful information regarding the integration, or otherwise, of osseointegrated dental implants. Since the flow and volume of peri-implant sulcular fluid appears to be similar to those of gingival crevicular fluid, peri-implant sulcular fluid has been suggested as a suitable medium for monitoring osseointegration and changes associated with peri-implantitis (Apse et al 1989).

Peri-implant sulcular fluid around two-stage implants has been studied following second-stage surgery to expose the integrated implant through to occlusal loading (Beck et al 1991; Last et al 1995). In particular, the levels of chondroitin-4-sulfate were found to be high immediately following exposure and also following occlusal loading of the implant. These studies provide evidence for the use of chondroitin-4-sulfate in gingival crevicular fluid as a potential marker of bone breakdown, since any contribution to the composition of the fluid by the periodontal ligament can be discounted. As these studies did not find dermatan sulfate, a major component of gingival connective tissue, the authors concluded that breakdown products from the soft tissues can be discounted as contributing to the composition of the peri-implant sulcular fluid.

In addition to the above studies, other connective tissue elements studied in peri-implant sulcular fluid include proteolytic and lysosomal enzymes, such as cathepsins, elastase, dipeptidyl peptidase, myeloperoxidase, β-glucuronidase, and trypsin—all correlate positively with peri-implant inflammation and bone resorption (Eley et al 1991; Boutros et al 1996). However, as for the gingival sulcular fluid, detailed longitudinal studies are required before peri-implant sulcular fluid analyses can become an accepted diagnostic aid.

Summary

Although good clinical judgments can be made using existing conventional periodontal diagnostic procedures, the decisions made are very subjective and can be quite unreliable. There is no doubt that clinical experience may often be the only diagnostic procedure relied upon in periodontics. Therefore, it is clear there is need for a more informed decision making process to be developed based upon sound diagnostic criteria. Diagnostic tests that provide more accurate assessment of periodontal disease activity than currently available methods should have a significant impact on disease management. As a result, it can be anticipated there will be continuing efforts in the development of diagnostic test systems. Gingival crevicular fluid is an easily and noninvasively collected medium for assessing changes in the periodontal tissues. Numerous components in the gingival crevicular fluid have been studied for their potential as markers of periodontal breakdown, however, many of these fall short of the ideal requirements of a diagnostic test. As periodontitis is characterized by loss of periodontal attachment with concomitant loss of alveolar bone, a marker specific to the bone matrix may be a reliable indicator of disease activity.

Care should be taken in evaluating these systems before committing oneself to the additional time, cost, and follow-up needed to implement such tests. It should be borne in mind that it is very unlikely that one test will provide both the needed sensitivity and the needed specificity. Rather, tests based on bacterial etiology, genetic susceptibility, host response, and metabolic events associated with the development, progression, and resolution of periodontal disease will be used in conjunction with traditional measures of anatomical changes to provide an accurate picture of past disease activity, current disease status, likelihood of future breakdown, and response to treatment.

References

Adonogianaki E, Moughal NA, Mooney J, Stirrups D, Kinane DF. Acute-phase proteins in gingival crevicular fluid during experimentally induced gingivitis. J Periodont Res 1994;29:196.

Adonogianaki E, Mooney J, Kinane DF. The ability of gingival crevicular fluid acute phase proteins to distinguish healthy, gingivitis and periodontitis sites. J Clin Periodontol 1992;19:98.

Apse P, Ellen RP, Overall CM, Zarb GA. Microbiota and crevicular fluid collagenase activity in the osseointegrated dental implant sulcul. A comparison of sites in edentulous and partially edentulous patients. J Periodont Res 1989; 24:96.

Armitage GC. Diagnostic tests for periodontal diseases. Curr Opin Dent 1992;2:53.

Armitage GC. Periodontal diseases: Diagnosis. Ann Periodontol 1996;1:37.

Armitage GC, Jeffcoat MK, Chadwick DE, et al. Longitudinal evaluation of elastase as a marker for the progression of periodontitis. J Periodontol 1994;65:120.

Bang J, Cimasoni G, Held AJ. Beta-glucuronidase correlated with inflammation in the exudate from human gingiva. Arch Oral Biol 1970;15:445.

Beck CB, Embery G, Langley MS, Waddington RJ. Levels of glycosaminoglycans in peri-implant sulcus fluid as a means of monitoring bone response to endosseous dental implants. Clin Oral Impl Res 1991;2:179.

Beck JD. Issues in assessment of diagnostic tests and risk for periodontal disease. Periodontol 2000 1995;7:100.

Binder TA, Goodson JM, Socransky SS. Gingival fluid levels of acid and alkaline phosphatase. J Periodont Res 1987;22:14.

Birkedal-Hansen H. Role of matrix metalloproteinases in human periodontal disease. J Periodontol 1993;64:474.

Boutros SM, Michalowicz BS, Smith QT, Aeppli DM. Crevicular fluid enzymes from endosseous dental implants and natural teeth. Int J Oral Maxillofac Implants 1996;11;322.

Bowers JE, Zahradnik RT. Evaluation of a chairside gingival protease test for use in periodontal diagnosis. J Clin Dent 1989;1:106.

Bowers M, Fisher LW, Termine JD, Somerman MJ. Connective tissue-associated proteins in crevicular fluid: Potential markers for periodontal disease. J Periodontol 1989;60:448.

Cao CF, Smith QT. Crevicular fluid myeloperoxidase at healthy, gingivitis, and periodontitis sites. J Clin Periodontol 1989;16:17.

Cho MI, Garant PT, Lee YL. Immunohistological localization of collagen (I and III) and fibronectin in inflamed and noninflamed gingival connective tissue and sulcular fluid of beagle dogs. J Periodont Res 1984;19:638.

Cimasoni, G. Crevicular fluid updated. Monogr Oral Sci Vol. 12. Basel: Karger;1983.

Cox SW, Eley BM. Cathepsin B/L-, elastase-, tryptase-, trypsin- and dipeptidyl peptidase IV-like activities in gingival crevicular fluid. A comparison of levels before and after basic periodontal treatment of chronic periodontitis patients. J Clin Periodontol 1992;19:333.

Curtis MA, Gillet IR, Griffiths GS, et al. Detection of high risk groups and individuals for periodontal diseases: Laboratory markers from analysis of gingival crevicular fluid. J Clin Periodontol 1989;16:1.

Delmas PD. Biochemical markers of bone turnover for the clinical investigation of osteoporosis. Osteoporosis Int 1993;1(suppl):S81.

Ebersole JL, Taubman MA, Smith DJ, Goodson JM. Gingival crevicular fluid antibodies to oral microorganisms. I. Method of collection and analysis of antibody. J Periodont Res 1984;19:124.

Eley BM, Cox SW. The relationship between gingival crevicular fluid cathepsin B activity and periodontal attachment loss in chronic periodontitis patients: a 2-year longitudinal study. J Periodont Res 1996;31:381.

Eley BM, Cox SW, Watson RM. Protease activities in peri-implant sulcus fluid from patients with permucosal osseointegrated dental implants. Correlation with clinical parameters. Clin Oral Impl Res 1991;2:62.

Embery G, Oliver WM, Stanbury JB, Purvis JA. The electrophoretic detection of acidic glycosaminoglycans in human gingival sulcus fluid. Arch Oral Biol 1982;27:177.

Embery G, Waddington R. Gingival crevicular fluid: biomarkers of periodontal tissue activity. Adv Dent Res 1994;8:329.

Embery G, Waddington RJ, Last KS. The connective tissues of the periodontium and their breakdown products in gingival crevicular fluid as markers of periodontal disease susceptibility and activity. In: Johnson NW, ed. Risk Markers for Oral Diseases, vol. 3. Cambridge: Cambridge University Press; 1991:338.

Fine DH. Incorporating new technologies in periodontal diagnosis into training programs and patient care: A critical assessment and a plan for the future. J Periodontol 1992;63:383.

Friedman SA, Mandel ID, Herrera MS. Lysozyme and lactoferrin quantitations in the crevicular fluid. J Periodontol 1983;54:347.

Giannobile WV, Lynch SE, Denmark RG, Paquette DW, Fiorellini JP, Williams RC. Crevicular fluid osteocalcin and pyridinoline cross-linked carboxyterminal telopeptide of type I collagen (ICTP) as markers of rapid bone turnover in periodontitis. A pilot study in beagle dogs. J Clin Periodontol 1995;22:903.

Giannobile WV, Riviere GR, Gorski JP, Tira DE, Cobb CM. Glycosaminoglycans and periodontal disease: Analysis of GCF by Safranin O. J Periodontol 1993;64:186.

Gustafsson A, Åsman B, Bergström K, Söder P-Ö. Granulocyte elastase in gingival crevicular fluid. A possible discriminator between gingivitis and periodontitis. J Clin Periodontol 1992;19:535.

Haffajee AD, Socransky SS, Goodson JM. Clinical parameters as predictors of destructive periodontal disease activity. J Clin Periodontol 1983;10:257.

Hara K, Löe H. Carbohydrate components of the gingival exudate. J Periodont Res 1969;4:202.

Hara K, Takahashi T. Hydroxyproline content in gingival exudate before and after periodontal surgery. J Periodont Res 1975;10:270.

Harper DS, Lamster IB, Celenti R. Relationship of subgingival plaque flora to lysosomal and cytoplasmic enzyme activity in gingival crevicular fluid. J Clin Periodontol 1989;16:164.

Hirshfeld L, Wasserman B. A long term study of tooth loss in 600 treated patients. J Periodontol 1978;49:225.

Ishikawa I, Cimasoni G. Alkaline phosphatase in human gingival fluid and its relation to periodontitis. Arch Oral Biol 1970;15:1401.

Ishikawa I, Cimasonin G, Ahmad-Zadeh C. Possible role of lysosomal enzymes on cathepsin D in human gingival fluid. Arch Oral Biol 1972;17:111.

Jeffcoat MK, Reddy MS. Progression of probing attachment loss in adult periodontitis. J Periodontol 1991; 62:185.

Johnson V, Johnson BD, Sims TJ, et al. Effects of treatment on antibody titre to *Porphyromonas gingivalis* in gingival crevicular fluid of patients with rapidly progressive periodontitis. J Periodontol 1993;64:559.

Keuhl FA, Egan RW. Prostaglandins, arachidonic acid and inflammation. Science 1980;210:978.

Kinane DF, Winstanley FP, Adonogianaki E, Moughal NA. Bioassay of interleukin 1 (IL-1) in human gingival crevicular fluid during experimental gingivitis. Arch Oral Biol 1992;37:153.

Kunimatsu K, Mine N, Muraoka Y, et al. Identification and possible function of cathepsin G in gingival crevicular fluid from chronic adult periodontitis patients and from experimental gingivitis subjects. J Periodont Res 1995; 30:51.

Kunimatsu K, Yamamoto K, Ichimaru E, Kato Y, Kato I. Cathepsins B, H and L activities in gingival crevicular fluid from chronic adult periodontitis patients and experimental gingivitis subjects. J Periodont Res 1990;25:69.

Kunimatsu K, Mataki S, Tanaka H, et al. A cross sectional study on osteocalcin levels in gingival crevicular fluid from periodontal patients. J Periodontol 1993;64:865.

Lamster IB. Host derived enzyme activities in gingival crevicular fluid as markers of periodontal disease susceptibility and activity: historical perspective, biological significance and clinical implications. In: Johnson NW, ed. Risk Markers for Oral Diseases, vol. 3. Cambridge: Cambridge University Press; 1991:277.

Lamster IB, Celenti RS, Jans HH, Fine JB, Grbic JT. Current status of tests for periodontal disease. Adv Dent Res 1993;7:182.

Lamster IB, Grbic JT. Diagnosis of periodontal disease based on analysis of the host response. Periodontol 2000 1995;7:83.

Lamster IB, Harper DS, Fiorello KA, Oshrain RL, Celenti RS, Gordon JM. Lysosomal and cytoplasmic enzyme activity, crevicular fluid volume and clinical parameters characterizing gingival sites with shallow to intermediate probing depths. J Periodontol 1987;58:614.

Lamster IB, Hartley LJ, Vogel RI. Development of a biochemical profile for gingival crevicular fluid. Methodological considerations and evaluation of collagen-degrading and ground substance degrading enzyme activity during experimental gingivitis. J Periodontol 1985;56:13.

Lamster IB, Oshrain RL, Harper DS, Celenti RS, Hovliaris CA, Gordon JM. Enzyme activity in crevicular fluid for detection and prediction of clinical attachment loss in patients with chronic adult periodontitis. J Periodontol 1988;59:516.

Larivée J, Sodek J, Ferrier JM. Collagenase and collagenase inhibitor activities in crevicular fluid of patients receiving treatment for localized juvenile periodontitis. J Periodont Res 1986;21:702.

Last KS, Cawood JI, Howell RA, Embery G. Monitoring of Tubingen endosseous dental implants by glycosaminoglycans analysis of gingival crevicular fluid. Int J Oral Maxillofac Implants 1991;6:42.

Last KS, Donkin C, Embery G. Glycosaminoglycans in human gingival crevicular fluid during orthodontic movement. Arch Oral Biol 1988;33:907.

Last KS, Smith S, Pender N. Monitoring of IMZ titanium endosseous dental implants by glycosaminoglycan analysis of peri-implant sulcul fluid. Int J Oral Maxillofac Impl 1995;10:58.

Last KS, Stanbury JB, Embery G. Glycosaminoglycans in human gingival crevicular fluid as indicators of active periodontal disease. Arch Oral Biol 1985;32:275.

Listgarten MA. A perspective on periodontal diagnosis. J Clin Periodontol 1986:13:175.

Löe H, Anerud A, Boysen H, Smith M. The natural history of periodontal disease in man. The rate of periodontal destruction before forty years of age. J Periodontol 1978;4:607.

Magnusson I, Persson RG, Page RC, et al. A multi-center clinical trial of a new chairside test in distinguishing between diseased and healthy periodontal sites. II. Association between site type and test outcome before and after therapy. J Periodontol 1996;67:589.

Mandel ID. Markers of periodontal disease susceptibility and activity derived from saliva. In: Johnson NW, ed. Risk Markers for Oral Diseases, vol. 3. Cambridge: Cambridge University Press;1991:228.

Marshall-Day CD, Stephens RG, Quigley LF. Periodontal disease: Prevalence and incidence. J Periodontol 1955; 26:185.

Masada MP, Persson R, Kenney JS, Lee SW, Page RC, Allison AC. Measurement of interleukin-1α and -1β in gingival crevicular fluid: implications for the pathogenesis of periodontal disease. J Periodont Res 1990;25:156.

McCulloch CAG. Host enzymes in gingival crevicular fluid as diagnostic indicators of periodontitis. J Clin Periodont 1994;21:497.

Meng HX, James IT, Skingle L, Johnson NW, Thompson PW. Collagen cross links in human gingival crevicular fluid. J Dent Res 1991;70:714. Abstract.

Meyle J, Zell St, Brecx M, Heller W. Influence of oral hygiene on elastase concentration of gingival crevicular fluid. J Periodont Res 1992;27:226.

Modeer T, Twetman S. Lysozyme activity in saliva from children with various degrees of gingivitis. Swed Dent J 1979;3:63.

Niekrash CE, Patters MR. Assessment of complement cleavage in gingival fluid in humans with and without periodontal disease. J Periodont Res 1986;21:233.

Offenbacher S, Collins JG, Arnold RR. New clinical diagnostic strategies based on pathogenesis of disease. J Periodont Res 1993;28:523.

Offenbacher S, Odle BM, Gray RC, Van Dyke TE. Crevicular fluid prostaglandin E levels as a measure of the periodontal disease status of adult and juvenile periodontitis patients. J Periodont Res 1984;19:1.

Offenbacher S, Odle BM, VanDyke TE. The use of crevicular fluid prostaglandin E$_2$ levels as a predictor of periodontal attachment loss. J Periodont Res 1986;21:101.

Offenbacher S, Soskolne WA, Collins JG. Prostaglandins and other eicosanoids in gingival crevicular fluid as markers of periodontal disease activity. In: Johnson NW, ed. Risk Markers for Oral Diseases, vol. 3. Cambridge: Cambridge University Press; 1991:313.

Oshrain RL, Lamster IB, Hartley LJ, Gordon JM. Arylsulphatase activity in human gingival crevicular fluid. Arch Oral Biol 1984;29:399.

Overall CM, Sodek J. Initial characterization of a neutral metalloproteinase, active on native 3/4-collagen fragments, synthesized by ROS17/2.8 osteoblastic cells, periodontal fibroblasts and identified in crevicular fluid. J Dent Res 1987;66:1271.

Overall CM, Sodek J, McCulloch CAG, Birek P. Evidence for polymorphonuclear leukocyte collagenase and 92-kilodalton gelatinase in gingival crevicular fluid. Infect Immun 1991;59:4687.

Page RC. Host response tests for diagnosing periodontal diseases. J Periodontol 1992;63:356.

Patters MR, Niekrash CE, Lang NP. Assessment of complement cleavage in gingival fluid during experimental gingivitis in man. J Clin Periodontol 1989;16:33.

Payne JB, Reinhardt RA, Masada MP, DuBois LM, Allison AC. Gingival crevicular fluid IL-8: Correlation with local IL-1β levels and patient estrogen status. J Periodont Res 1993;28:451.

Persson GR, DeRouen TA, Page RC. Relationship between levels of aspartate aminotransferase in gingival crevicular fluid and gingival inflammation. J Periodont Res 1990;25:17-24.

Persson GR, Imrey PB, Cohen RL, Crawford JM, Alves MEAF, McSwiggin TA. A longitudinal study of aspartate aminotransferase in human gingival crevicular fluid. J Periodont Res 1991;26:65.

Polla BS. A role for heat shock proteins in inflammation. Immunol Today 1988;9:134.

Preiss DS, Meyle J. Interleukin-1β concentration of gingival crevicular fluid. J Periodontol 1994;65:423.

Reinhardt RA, Masada MP, Johnson GK, DuBois LM, Seymour GJ, Allison AC. IL-1 in gingival crevicular fluid following closed root planing and papillary flap debridement. J Clin Periodontol 1993b;20:514.

Reinhardt RA, Masada MO, Kaldahl WB, et al. Gingival fluid IL-1 and IL-6 levels in refractory periodontitis. J Clin Periodontol 1993a;20:225.

Reinhardt RA, McDonald TL, Bolton RW, DuBois LM, Kaldahl WB. IgG subclasses in gingival crevicular fluid from active versus stable periodontitis sites. J Periodontol 1989;60:44.

Rossomando EF, Kennedy JE, Hadjimichael J. Tumor necrosis factor alpha in gingival crevicular fluid as a possible indicator of periodontal disease in humans. Arch Oral Biol 1990;35:431.

Samuels RHA, Pender N, Last KS. The effects of orthodontic tooth movement on the glycosaminoglycan components of gingival crevicular fluid. J Clin Periodontol 1993;20:371.

Sengupta S, Lamster IB, Khocht A, Duffy TA, Gordon JM. The effect of treatment on IgG, IgA, IgM and α-2-macroglobulin in gingival crevicular fluid from patients with chronic adult periodontitis. Arch Oral Biol 1988;33:425.

Shibutani T, Nishino W, Shiraki M, Iwayama Y. ELISA detection of glycosaminoglycans in gingival crevicular fluid. J Periodont Res 1993;28:17.

Sibraa PD, Reinhardt RA, Dyer JK, DuBois LM. Acute phase protein detection and quantification in gingival crevicular fluid by direct and indirect immunoblot. J Clin Periodontol 1991;18:101.

Skaleric U, Zajsek P, Cvetko E, Lah T, Babnik J. Alpha 2-macroglobulin in gingival fluid: correlation with alveolar bone loss in periodontal disease. J Clin Periodontol 1986;13:833.

Smedberg J-I, Beck CB, Embery G. Glycosaminoglycans in peri-implant sulcus fluid from implants supporting fixed or removable prostheses. Clin Oral Impl Res 1993;4:137.

Smith QT, Hinrichs JE, Melnyk RS, Gingival crevicular fluid myeloperoxidase at periodontitis sites. J Periodont Res 1986;21:45.

Socransky SS, Haffajee A, Goodson M, Lindhe J. New concepts of destructive periodontal disease. J Clin Periodontol 1984;11:21.

Sorsa T, Suomalainen K, Uitto V-J. The role of gingival crevicular fluid and salivary interstitial collagenases in human periodontal disease. Arch Oral Biol 1990;35:193S.

Sueda T, Cimasoni G, Held AJ. Histochemical study of human gingival fluid. Paradontologie 1966;20:141.

Svanberg GK. Hydroxyproline determination in serum and gingival crevicular fluid. J Periodont Res 1987a;2:133.

Svanberg GK. Hydroxyproline titers in gingival crevicular fluid. J Periodont Res 1987b;22:212.

Talonpoika J, Paunio K, Söderling E. Molecular forms and concentrations of fibronectin and fibrin in human gingival crevicular fluid before and after periodontal treatment. Scand J Dent Res 1993b;101:375.

Talonpoika JT, Hämäläinen MM. Collagen III aminoterminal propeptide in gingival crevicular fluid before and after periodontal treatment. Scand J Dent Res 1992; 100:107.

Talonpoika JT, Hämäläinen MM. Type I carboxyterminal telopeptide in human gingival crevicular fluid in different clinical conditions and after periodontal treatment. J Clin Periodontol 1994;21:320.

Talonpoika JT, Hämäläinen MM. Collagen I carboxyterminal propeptide in gingival crevicular fluid before and after periodontal treatment. Scan J Dent Res 1993a; 101:154.

Talonpoika J, Heino J, Larjava H, Häkkinen L, Paunio K. Gingival crevicular fluid fibronectin degradation in periodontal health and disease. Scand J Dent Res 1989;97:415.

Taubman MA, Haffajee AD, Socransky SS, Smith OJ, Ebersole JL. Longitudinal monitoring of humoral antibody in subjects with destructive periodontal diseases. J Periodont Res 1992;27:511.

Tsai C-C, Ho Y-P, Chen C-C. Levels of interleukin-1β and interleukin-8 in gingival crevicular fluids in adult periodontitis. J Periodontol 1995;66:852.

Vartio T. Fibronectin: multiple interactions assigned to structural domains. Med Biol 1983;61:283.

Villela B, Cogen RB, Bartolucci AA, Birkedal-Hansen H. Collagenolytic activity in crevicular fluid from patients with chronic adult periodontitis, localized juvenile periodontitis and gingivitis and from healthy control subjects. J Periodont Res 1987a;22:381.

Villela B, Cogen RB, Bartolucci AA, Birkedal-Hansen H. Crevicular fluid collagenase activity in healthy, gingivitis, chronic adult periodontitis and localized juvenile periodontitis patients. J Periodont Res 1987b;22:209.

Wilton JMA, Bampton JLM, Hurst TJ, Caves J, Powell JR. Interleukin-1β and IgG subclass concentration in gingival crevicular fluid from patients with adult periodontitis. Arch Oral Biol 1993;38:55.

Periodontal Regeneration

Introduction

Periodontal disease is an all-encompassing term relating to inflammatory disorders of the periodontium. These range from the relatively benign form known as gingivitis, to the more aggressive forms of early-onset periodontitis and rapidly progressive periodontitis. All forms of inflammatory periodontal diseases are associated with bacterial deposits on the root surfaces (Offenbacher 1996; Page et al 1997). One of the most significant outcomes of periodontal inflammation is connective tissue damage. The tissue damage caused by gingivitis is reversible, provided all causative agents are removed, as the gingival tissue has a remarkable capacity to regenerate to its original form and function (Melcher 1976) (Fig 11-1). However, with long-term plaque deposition the disease may become established. Depending upon host, genetic, environmental, and other factors, there may be subsequent loss of connective tissue attachment to the root surface, bone resorption, and formation of a periodontal pocket (see Chapter 9). In contrast to gingivitis, with the establishment of periodontitis many of the architectural

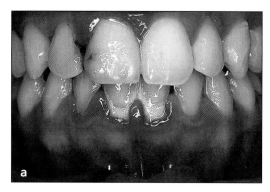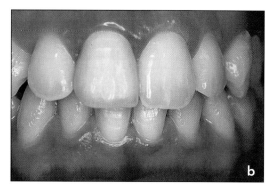

Fig 11-1 Clinical picture showing resolution of gingivitis. **(a)** Appearance of gingival tissues prior to treatment. **(b)** Appearance of tissues after treatment consisting of oral hygiene instruction together with plaque and calculus removal. Note complete restoration of the architecture of the gingival tissues.

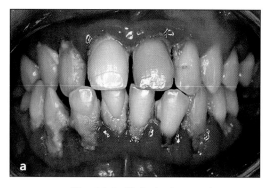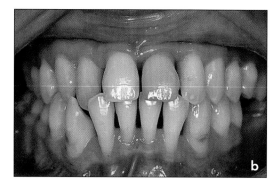

Fig 11-2 Clinical picture showing resolution of periodontitis with associated anatomical deficiencies. **(a)** Appearance of periodontal tissues prior to treatment. **(b)** Appearance of periodontal tissues after treatment consisting of oral hygiene instruction together with plaque and calculus removal. Note incomplete restoration of architecture of the gingival tissues.

changes to the hard and soft connective tissues are irreversible—even if the causative inflammation is controlled (Fig 11-2).

The goal of periodontal therapy is to restore periodontal tissues affected by disease to their original architectural form and function. This requires regeneration of the gingival connective tissues destroyed by inflammation, formation of cementum, restoration of lost bone, and reestablishment of connective tissue fibers into previously diseased root surfaces. However, predictable and complete re-

generation of the diseased periodontium has been difficult to achieve. Nonetheless, studies over the past 15 years have demonstrated that regeneration is biologically possible and clinically feasible. The objective of this chapter is to discuss the basic principles involved in periodontal regeneration, and how evolving concepts of wound healing apply to periodontal healing. In recent years, some of these principles have been experimentally tested in periodontal therapy with varying degrees of success; we review some of these procedures.

Definitions and Objectives

To determine the outcomes of therapy precisely, the terms involved are defined as follows (American Academy of Periodontology 1992):

Periodontal repair is the restoration of new tissue that does not replicate the structure and function of lost tissue, and is analogous to scar tissue formation.

Periodontal reattachment is the reunion of connective tissue to the root surface (separated by incision or injury) on which viable periodontal ligament is still present.

Periodontal new attachment is the reunion of connective tissues with a pathologically exposed root surface that is deprived of its periodontal ligament and may or may not include new cementum.

Periodontal regeneration is defined histologically as regeneration of the tooth's supporting tissues, including alveolar bone, periodontal ligament, and cementum over a diseased root surface.

Bone fill is the clinical restoration of bone tissue in treated periodontal defects.

Ankylosis is the fusion of the tooth and alveolar bone.

Resorption is the degradation of native mineralized tissue, alveolar bone, and root in the periodontium.

Processes Involved in Periodontal Regeneration

The basic processes involved in periodontal healing are largely the same as those described in Chapter 3 for other systems, however, there are some significant differences. Inflammation is a major requirement, and a blood clot is needed at the site to be healed to provide a provisional matrix that is subsequently organized into a granulation tissue. Formation of granulation tissue and fibroblast proliferation

are features of chronic periodontitis associated with healing and repair. The granulation tissue is subsequently remodeled into scar tissue or regenerated tissue. Periodontal regeneration is unique because it involves soft (gingival and periodontal ligament) and mineralized (bone and cementum) connective tissues. The healing of all periodontal components needs to be coordinated and integrated in order for regeneration to occur. Many molecules and cell types presumably participate in this process. The cellular events required are migration of cells by chemotaxis, their adhesion, proliferation, differentiation, and production of matrix components (Fig 11-3). One of the crucial cellular events is recruitment of cells as the cell-type selection determines whether healing occurs by repair or regeneration. The mechanisms involved in cell selection are unknown, although they are likely to involve selective chemotaxis, adhesion, and specific cell-molecule interactions.

Embryology in Relation to Periodontal Regeneration

In order to appreciate the cellular and molecular events necessary for periodontal regeneration to occur, an appreciation of the developmental processes and an understanding of the healing potential of the mature periodontium are necessary. In this section, only the developmental processes that might provide an insight into regenerative mechanisms are discussed. For a more detailed description of the development of the periodontium, the reader is referred to Chapter 7.

During the development of the periodontal tissues, the cells of the dental follicle are separated from the newly formed root dentin by the cells of Hertwig's epithelial root sheath, which secrete a fine layer of enamel-like proteins onto the dentin surface, known as the hyaline layer (Lindskog 1982; Slavkin et al 1988). After some as yet unclear biologic events, the Hertwig's epithelial root sheath

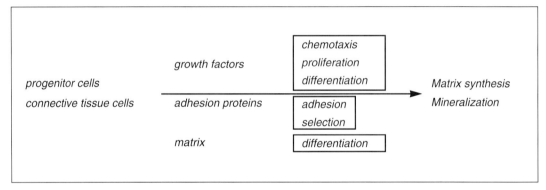

Fig 11-3 Interaction of molecules with periodontal cells and outcomes. Polypeptide growth factors are chemotactic to these cells and they promote their proliferation and differentiation. Adhesion molecules promote their adhesion, and these molecules may promote the establishment of certain specific cell types depending upon their ability to promote the adhesion of certain cell types. Matrix is necessary for the differentiation of these cells. Such interactions, which are as yet unclear, participate in the recruitment of progenitor cells, which differentiate into functional connective tissue cells such as cementoblasts. The final outcome, regeneration or repair, depends upon the differentiated functions of these cells.

fragments and permits direct contact between the cells of the dental follicle and the newly formed hyaline layer. This leads to the first appearance of cementoblasts, which have presumably differentiated from the cells of the dental follicle, and thus cementogenesis proceeds. With continued root development in an apical direction and the coordinated formation of periodontal ligament fibers and alveolar bone, the attachment apparatus consisting of the periodontal ligament fibers, cementum, and alveolar bone, becomes complete.

The concept that cementum deposition may be associated with deposition of a matrix first secreted by epithelial cells is not new (Ten Cate 1996, 1997). However, it does have important ramifications for regeneration around mature teeth. While the exact biochemical nature of this material is not known, it has been proposed to contain a number of enamel proteins (Schonfeld and Slavkin 1977), presumably including amelogenin, and may act as a reservoir of biologic factors in stimulating the migration, adhesion, and

differentiation of cells (Ten Cate 1996; Hammarström et al 1996; Harrison and Roda 1995). It follows from this hypothesis that acellular cementum can only be formed during tooth formation, since the epithelial cells (except for those in the rests of Malassez) responsible for the formation of the hyaline layer are no longer present in the adult periodontium. Thus, reformation of acellular cementum during adult life becomes unlikely. This tissue is particularly well-suited for connective tissue attachment, while simultaneously it is the tissue most frequently exposed to gingival inflammation and root planing. This creates the dilemma regarding the ideal clinical treatment of the root surface during periodontal therapy.

In an extension of traditional concepts of embryonal origins, Ten Cate and associates have suggested that the tissues of the periodontium arise from the ectomesenchymal cells surrounding the dental papilla (Ten Cate 1975; Freeman and Ten Cate 1971). Furthermore, they indicated that the fibroblasts of the periodontal ligament near the cementum are derivatives of the ectomesenchymal cells of the investing layer, while fibroblasts near the alveolar bone seam are derived from perivascular mesenchyme. These tissues, therefore, have a high specificity of both origin and function. In support of such interpretations, experimental data indicate that the mitotic activity and collagen turnover rates within the periodontal ligament at the tooth surface are different from those found in the ligament near the alveolar bone, particularly when the periodontal attachment unit is challenged by factors affecting the equilibrium of the periodontal structures, such as trauma from occlusal imbalances (Beertsen 1975).

Molecules Involved in Periodontal Regeneration

A variety of molecules participate in the regulation of processes involved in periodontal regeneration. These substances, many of which were discussed in Chapters 2 and 3, can be divided into three types based on their action: (1) growth factors and other inflammatory mediators, including cytokines, lymphokines, and chemokines; (2) adhesion molecules, such as fibronectin and laminin; and (3) matrix components such as collagens, proteoglycans, and hyaluronan. The first group of molecules regulate the migration and proliferation of cells during inflammation and wound repair. These substances are usually pleiotropic in their action, and their effects depend upon many factors, especially the nature of the extracellular matrix (see Chapter 2). Adhesion molecules localize cells at required sites and may be specific to certain cell types or nonspecific in their interactions. Specific promotion of attachment is likely to be a factor that determines whether recruitment of the needed cell types occurs, and absence of the correct molecule or cell can be expected to affect the course of healing. Matrix components such as collagens and proteoglycans are neces-

sary for the structural and physiologic integrity of the new tissue, and these are also needed for other functions, particularly for cell differentiation. All three groups of molecules may participate in healing by regulating cellular activities alone and together (see Chapter 2). The origins of these molecules may be from the circulation, or produced locally by cells residing in the tissue matrix. Thus, growth factors such as IGF-I and adhesion molecules such as vitronectin are derived from the blood plasma, while PDGF, fibronectin TGF-β, IL-1, and IFN-γ are secreted by fibroblasts and inflammatory cells. Many growth factors, including IGF-I, FGF-1, and FGF-2, are also bound within the extracellular matrix, and these, together with degradation products of the matrix, are released during inflammation.

Cell Populations and Periodontal Regeneration

Apart from inflammatory cells, periodontal regeneration involves several cell types: fibroblasts for soft connective tissues, cementoblasts for cementogenesis, osteoblasts for bone, endothelial cells for angiogenesis, and epithelial cells for the epithelium (Pitaru et al 1994). During the regenerative process, these cells must interact with a variety of soluble mediators mentioned above, such that the course of regeneration is dictated by cell-molecule, cell-matrix, and cell-cell interactions. Very little is known about these interactions or about the signaling events that mediate them. The periodontal connective tissues contain heterogeneous populations of cells with diverse properties and functions (McCulloch and Bordin 1991; Phipps et al 1997). The noninflammatory cell populations of the periodontium can be classified into four main groups: synthetic cells, resorptive cells, progenitor cells, and miscellaneous cells. The synthetic cells include (1) osteoblasts lining the surface of bone; (2) cementoblasts lining the

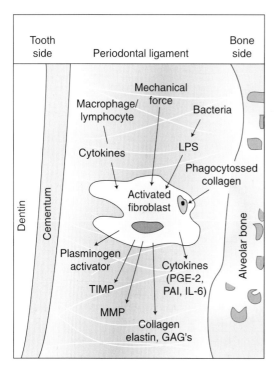

Tooth side	Periodontal ligament	Bone side

Fig 11-4 Schematic representation of the location of periodontal ligament cell progenitors and their migration pathways. Progenitor cells are located in the paravascular regions of the periodontal ligament located close to the alveolar bone, and line the vascular channels in the contiguous alveolar bone. Migration of the cells is along collagen fibers and in an apicocoronal direction during tooth eruption. (Reproduced with permission from Lekic and McCulloch, 1996.)

From the point of view of regeneration, progenitor cells are of particular interest since these are the cells that may be considered to be the parent cells for the three synthetic cells. Due to cell death or terminal differentiation into specific cells (eg, osteoblasts or cementoblasts), the synthetic cell population needs to be renewed constantly in order to maintain normal physiologic homeostasis. The biologic requirements of these progenitor cells include the capacity to undergo continuous division to maintain their progeny, and the ability to give rise to cells that have the capacity to form one or more of the periodontal tissues (cementum, bone, or periodontal ligament).

Several studies have demonstrated that the progenitor cells for periodontal tissues are located close to the blood vessels in periodontal ligament (Gould et al 1980; Iglhaut et al 1987; McCulloch and Melcher 1983). It has been demonstrated that the progenitor cells divide slowly, but continually, in paravascular zones, and that daughter cells migrate away from the paravascular zones toward the root surface, alveolar bone, or into the body of the periodontal ligament (McCulloch and Melcher 1983; McCulloch et al 1987). Because there are numerous vascular channels in the alveolar bone connecting the periodontal ligament compartment with the bone stromal compartment, the progenitor or stem cells may actually originate from the bone stromal compartment (Fig 11-4). This possibility is supported by the in vitro observation that cells cultured from bone have the capacity to form cementum-like material (Melcher et al 1986). When periodontal tissues are wounded under experimental conditions, the progenitor cells located in the paravascular zones undergo rapid cell division and presumably supply the wounded site with cell populations that synthesize new extracellular matrix (Gould et al 1980; Iglhaut et al 1987).

Current evidence indicates that fibroblasts and osteoblasts are responsible for the restoration of soft connective tissue and bone, respectively (Fig 11-5). As mentioned in Chap-

cementum surface; (3) fibroblasts located within the gingiva, periodontal ligament, and periosteum of alveolar bone; (4) blood vessel endothelial cells; and (5) the highly replicative epithelial cells. Of these, the epithelial cells have the greatest replication rate and potential to promote repair relative to other connective tissue cell types. Connective tissue cells show considerable variability among different groups and within the same cell type in replication potential and other properties (Aukhill 1991; McCulloch and Bordin 1991; Phipps et al 1997).

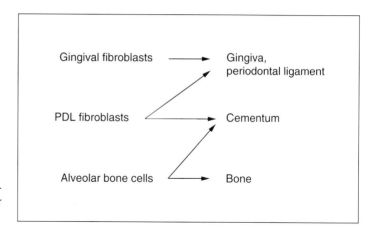

Fig 11-5 Major periodontal connective tissue cell types and their product tissues.

ter 8, periodontal ligament cells consist of two fibroblast types, one existing as soft tissue fibroblasts and the other manifesting high alkaline phosphatase levels as do osteoblasts. The cells with high alkaline phosphatase levels can form bone- and cementum-like structures in vitro, and it appears likely these cells are capable of becoming cementoblasts that synthesize extrinsic (Sharpey's) fibers of the cementum (Cho et al 1995; Schroeder 1992).

The so-called miscellaneous cells in the periodontal ligament include all the remaining cell types. Most notable among these are the remnants of Hertwig's epithelial root sheath seen during root development. These epithelial remnants appear as clusters or small islands of cells, and are also referred to as cell rests of Malassez. The clinical significance of these cells in tissue regeneration has not been determined.

Formation of New Cementum

Regenerative cementogenesis on previously diseased root surfaces is unpredictable, even under the most conducive conditions available today. The most common outcome is the formation of new tissue that resembles cementum or bone, is cellular, and contains collagen fibers; however, the fibers are not functionally attached to previously diseased root surfaces. New matrix does not interdigitate with the root surface or become stabilized by mineralization.

As described earlier in this chapter, the cells that form cementum during odontogenesis are derived from the dental follicle and are exposed to differentiation signals in an appropriate time sequence for cementogenesis to take place along a coronoapical gradient. In order for periodontal regeneration to occur, this process must be repeated. However, the necessary signals, types of cells, and their interactions are not yet fully elucidated.

Available evidence indicates that systemic and local factors are likely to participate in the regeneration process, including new cementum formation. The role of local factors is especially relevant in cementum, which, like other calcified structures, stores a variety of growth factors and adhesion molecules, yet does not readily regenerate (MacNeil and Somerman 1993; Narayanan and Bartold 1996). These molecules are expected to regulate cementum formation (and regeneration) in several ways. In particular, these molecules are likely to be the motivating force to recruit cells to the dentinal (root) surface, select or induce the cementoblast phenotype, permit their attachment to the dentin surface, and encourage their proliferation. Thus, through a sequence of selective and inductive processes coordinated by local factors, the recruited cells will be induced to differentiate into cementoblasts and their genes regulated to express proteins consistent with their differentiated phenotype.

Healing Following Conventional Periodontal Therapy

Following mechanical or surgical periodontal therapy, healing may occur in one of six ways:

1. Control of inflammation (repair).
2. Long junctional epithelium (repair).
3. Connective tissue attachment to the root surface (reattachment or new attachment).
4. New bone separated from the root surface by long functional epithelium (repair).
5. New bone with root resorption or ankylosis or both (repair).
6. New functional attachment apparatus with formation of cementum, periodontal ligament, and alveolar bone (regeneration).

In light of the above, it can be seen that periodontal wound healing is more complicated than simple soft tissue healing because of the requirement for the involvement of at least four different tissues, each of which is structurally and biologically unique.

Periodontal Healing Following Scaling and Root Planing

The histologic and clinical responses to scaling and planing of the tooth root have been well documented over the years (Stahl et al 1972; Lindhe et al 1982). The local measures of thorough root surface débridement cause obvious changes to the histologic picture of the periodontally diseased pocket. The differences between responses occurring following ultrasonic instrumentation and conventional hand instrumentation are slight; both result in the removal of cementum from the tooth

surface and the removal of the epithelial lining of the pocket, and whether or not intentional, the root surfaces so produced are similar (Torfason et al 1979).

Within 1 week following subgingival débridement, a marked reduction in the inflammatory infiltrate is the most striking histologic observation (Tagge et al 1975). Subsequently, apical migration of the junctional epithelium occurs along the root surface, extending to the level of instrumentation. This epithelium is adherent to the tooth surface. The routine histologic observation of a long junctional epithelium abutting the root surface following scaling and root planing was considered to be a nonideal situation, and one that predisposed the tissues to future breakdown and pocket formation (Levine and Stahl 1972). This concept has since been demonstrated not to be valid (Magnusson et al 1983). Nonetheless, the formation of a long junctional epithelial attachment to the root surface does not fulfill the criteria for regeneration of a lost attachment, and at best may be considered a form of tissue repair.

Periodontal Healing Following Surgery

The manipulation of the gingival and periodontal tissues for therapeutic reasons results in a definite sequence of healing events. As well as the elimination of etiologic factors such as subgingival plaque and calculus deposits, goals for these procedures may include the reduction in pocket depth, removal of infected or granulomatous tissues, or access to the root surface. These goals may be achieved via excision of the tissues, or by the attempted replacement and attachment of the tissues to the root surface achieved by the formation of a long junctional epithelium, or by connective tissue attachment to the root surface.

Healing following gingivectomy occurs first by the production of a clot over the wound surface. This is followed by granulation tissue formation and the migration of epithelial cells from the wound margins to cover the exposed tissues (Henning 1968). This is healing via secondary intention. Within two weeks, gingivectomy wounds form a completely new junctional epithelium that is derived from daughter cells located in the basal layer of the adjacent oral epithelium (Listgarten 1972).

The healing dynamics following flap surgery differ from gingivectomy wounds in that wound coverage is obtained postsurgically, and hence healing may occur more rapidly (Wikesjö et al 1992). The events are very similar to healing of any incisional wound (see Figure 3-5). Clot formation is initially noted between the flap and the underlying tissues. This is subsequently infiltrated with granulation tissue, and epithelial cells traverse the distance between the flap margin and the tooth. There is a small amount of resorption of the alveolar bone; the amount depends upon the surgical procedure. After primary healing, there is remodeling of the area, such that some of the resorbed bone may be replaced. Following this type of surgery, there is minimal connective tissue attachment to the root surface; junctional epithelium migrates to the most-apical area exposed during the procedure. The formation of a long junctional epithelium is a common feature of healing following most periodontal surgical procedures.

As a result of the above observations, it was considered that the junctional epithelium would remain unchanged in its position on the root surface following surgical treatment. However, it has been noted that in rats, coronal migration of the most apical extension of the junctional epithelium occurs over time, with its replacement by a connective tissue attachment to the root (Listgarten et al 1982). This observation has challenged the concept that the periodontium remains static following healing.

Thus, following both surgical and nonsurgical periodontal therapy, it has been well established that the epithelium from the wound margin has a strong ability to migrate apically along the root surface (Stahl and Froum 1977; Caton et al 1980). The resultant long junctional epithelium that is either attached to, or very closely adapted to, the root surface can be established as early as 7 to 10 days after instrumentation. Ultrastructural studies have shown that the newly established long junctional epithelium resembles normal junctional epithelium (Listgarten 1972). This epithelium is derived from the gingival epithelial tissues in cases where the original junctional epithelium has been completely removed, or from a combination of this epithelium and residual junctional epithelium in other situations.

Although healing by formation of a long junctional epithelium can be associated with acceptable clinical results, re-establishment of connective tissue attachment onto the root surface is preferable for the following reasons:

1. A connective tissue attachment on the root surface generally favors more regeneration of bone.
2. A connective tissue attachment consists of reservoirs of cells with the potential to form new bone, cementum, and periodontal ligament.
3. A connective tissue attachment can also mean a normal junctional epithelium, suggesting a shallower pocket depth and thus easier maintenance.

Traditionally, the failure to obtain a new connective tissue attachment after conventional (surgical or nonsurgical) periodontal therapy has been attributed to the rapid migration of the oral epithelium and the reformation of subgingival plaque on the root surface. This rapid apical migration of the junctional epithelium can prevent other cell types (gingival or periodontal ligament fibroblasts) from making contact with the root surface. These observations led investigators to speculate that regeneration of a connective tissue attachment to the root surface could be possible if the oral epithelium could be excluded from the site of its apical migration (Melcher 1976).

The above observations and speculations led to an important series of experiments designed to address the regenerative capacity of the periodontal tissues (Karring et al 1980; Nyman et al 1980; Nyman et al 1982a). These studies indicated that if teeth were partially deprived of their periodontal tissues by root planing, and then reimplanted with the prepared root surface facing either alveolar bone or gingival connective tissue (with complete exclusion of the epithelium), then healing adjacent to the root surface denuded of its periodontal ligament was characterized by external root resorption in the case of the side contacting the gingival tissues, and by ankylosis on the side contacting bone. Of particular note was the observation that, regardless of the tissue interface (gingiva or bone), those root surfaces that had intact periodontal ligament on the root surface at the time of implantation demonstrated a reformed and functionally oriented attachment apparatus. These findings led to the hypothesis that cells in the gingival connective tissues, bone, and epithelium did not possess the capacity to form new connective tissue attachments onto root surfaces denuded of their periodontal ligament. As such, it was proposed that only the cells residing in the periodontal ligament possessed such regenerative capacity, and that in order for regeneration to occur, the epithelial cells had to be excluded from the regenerating site.

This concept was subsequently tested in an elegant series of experiments in which root surfaces were exposed via surgical fenestration of the alveolar bone, and the periodontal ligament at this site was then denuded (Nyman et al 1982a). The cells from the periodontal ligament were preferentially allowed to repopulate this wound site by the draping of a millipore filter as a barrier membrane over the surgical site prior to replacement of the mucoperiosteal flap. The rationale for the barrier membrane was to provide a physical barrier to exclude both gingival connective tissue and gingival epithelium from the healing wound site. The results demonstrated the formation

of new cementum together with inserting collagen fibers and new bone. While these results were not consistent along the entire apico-coronal dimension of the root surface, in that some areas in the coronal portion showed connective tissue adhesion to the root surface only (no cementum or bone formation), this was the first demonstration that periodontal ligament cells possessed the ability to re-form connective tissue attachment to a denuded root surface, and that periodontal regeneration was biologically possible around fully formed teeth.

Regenerative Procedures

Over the years, many techniques have been used in attempts to increase the amount of connective tissue reattachment to tooth roots following periodontal treatment. The following is a discussion of the major developments over the last 20 years.

Root Surface Conditioning

The root surface must serve as a suitable site for cell attachment and fiber development during regeneration. Diseased root surfaces are contaminated by bacterial products, and are characterized by loss of collagen and alterations in surface composition and mineral density. They do not support the attachment or growth of fibroblasts, but promote epithelial migration along the root surface. For these reasons, attempts have been made to modify the diseased root surfaces to make them conducive to the attachment of connective tissue cells.

Citric acid. In animals, the ability of mesenchymal cells to differentiate into osteoblasts following their exposure to demineralized dentin matrix has been well documented (Yeomans and Urist 1967; Urist 1971). Believing that demineralized root surfaces held an induction potential for bone and cementum formation, Register (1973) carried out the first studies involving acid treatment of root surfaces in situ in a series of animals, and noted accelerated healing and new cementum formation on acid-treated tooth surfaces as compared to untreated surfaces.

In addition to the possible inductive effect of root surface demineralization on bone and cementum formation, it was postulated that such root surface treatment resulted in removal of the smear layer formed following root planing of the root surface and exposure of the ends of collagen fibrils present within the dentin, which subsequently allowed improved attachment of newly formed collagen fibrils from the adjacent connective tissue (Daryabegi et al 1980; Polson et al 1984). In addition, it was proposed that the effects of root surface conditioning with citric acid could be due to the impedance of epithelial migration across the tooth surface (Larjava et al 1988).

Despite these encouraging results, subsequent studies in humans indicated that citric acid treatment of root surfaces did not accelerate cementogenesis, nor did it appear to augment the connective tissue reattachment to the diseased root surfaces. Thus, it was concluded that the treatment of root surfaces with citric acid was not a reliable clinical procedure (Stahl and Froum 1977; Frank et al 1983; Marks and Mehta 1986; Fuentes et al 1993).

Tetracycline. Tetracycline has been proposed as a useful root surface conditioning agent. It is an acidic compound with several pharmacologic actions. It is a bacteriostatic antibiotic with collagenase inhibitory properties (Golub et al 1984). The effect of tetracycline on the root surface has been described as similar to that obtained using citric acid (Wikesjö et al 1986; Lafferty et al 1993). The poor clinical results achieved with citric acid have been attributed, in part, to bacterial contamination of the root surface. Therefore, due to the im-

mediate antibiotic effect of tetracycline, its substantive properties (Baker et al 1983), and its retarding effect on plaque formation (Bjorvatn 1986), together with its etching properties, tetracycline has been proposed as a root surface conditioning agent of some promise.

Early studies using tetracycline as a root surface conditioning agent, on the basis of the above assumptions, produced promising results both in vitro and in vivo (Claffey et al 1987; Terranova et al 1986). However, other studies have shown variable results following root surface conditioning with tetracycline, ranging from some minor improvement in clinical parameters to no improvement at all (Alger et al 1990; Parashis and Mitsis 1993).

To date, reports on the clinical and histologic effects of tetracycline in humans are too few to draw any meaningful conclusions regarding the use of tetracycline as a root surface conditioning agent of any significant clinical consequence.

Fibronectin. Fibronectin is a glycoprotein component of the extracellular matrix. Its main function is the promotion of cell adhesion, although it may have a significant chemoattractant property for fibroblasts and other mesenchymal cells (see Chapter 5). It has been established that both fibronectin and laminin are involved in the attachment of gingival fibroblasts to root surfaces (Terranova and Martin 1982). Thus, there has been considerable interest in utilizing fibronectin as a clinical agent to promote fibroblast attachment to root surfaces and establishing new attachment (Holden and Smith 1983; Fernyhough and Page 1983). An early in vitro study demonstrated enhanced fibroblast attachment to freshly cleaned root surfaces following topical application of fibronectin (Aleo et al 1975). This accelerated attachment was later suggested to have been the result of opsonization of root-bound endotoxin (Porvaznick et al 1982), or related to the function of fibronectin in the initial stages of cell attachment (Weiss and Reddi 1980).

Fibronectin has also been proposed to play a significant role in the formation of new attachment to acid-treated root surfaces, whereby enhanced fibroblast attachment to the collagen exposed by demineralization was mediated by naturally occurring fibronectin (Boyko et al 1980). In an extension of this concept, it has been proposed that significant reattachment to reimplanted teeth treated with citric acid was due to a thin linkage of fibrin with exposed collagen, mediated via fibronectin (Polson and Proye 1983). The combination of acid demineralization of root surfaces and application of fibronectin may enhance cellular proliferation of the gingival tissues, and promote wound healing following periodontal surgery (Caffesse et al 1985).

While fibronectin binds to demineralized tooth and bone and promotes cell attachment in vitro (Terranova and Martin 1982), the situation may be quite different in vivo since the sites available for this binding are rapidly saturated with fibronectin derived from normal serum (Pearson et al 1988). Thus, although benefits have been noted with the application of fibronectin to root surfaces, no increased benefit is derived at concentrations above serum levels (Smith et al 1987). Hence the application of exogenous fibronectin to root surfaces would appear to be of limited benefit.

Other conditioners. Other materials have been used in attempts to improve reattachment procedures. Two detergents (cetylpyridinium chloride and sodium *N*-lauroyl sarcosine) have been found to aid in root surface decontamination and can lead to significant amounts of new attachment (Blomlöff et al 1987). However, the application time of these detergents (30 minutes) probably precludes them from becoming clinically useful. Using sodium deoxycholate (a bile salt) and plasma factor Cohn IV in monkeys resulted in a significant increase in attachment (compared to the controls) (Wirthlin and Hancock 1982). Chlorhexidine has also been used, but it was found to significantly inhibit fibroblast at-

tachment when applied to root surfaces (Alleyn et al 1991).

Graft Materials Used for Periodontal Regeneration

Regeneration of bone defects associated with periodontal disease and restoration of architectural form of the alveolar arch due to tooth loss remain significant problems in dentistry. Ingrowth of soft connective tissue into such defects often occurs; this prevents the formation of new bone tissue, causing aberrations and functional disturbances. In efforts to stimulate osteogenesis, various grafting procedures and materials have been developed (Mellonig 1992). However, the search for an ideal graft material continues to be a challenge.

Several philosophies have developed regarding the importance of repairing bony defects caused by chronic periodontal diseases. The rationale behind the use of bone grafts in angular bony defects is that the presence of bone tissue close to a scaled and root-planed surface would stimulate the formation of a connective tissue attachment. However, such concepts have been questioned because, on biologic grounds, the use of bone transplants for the management of periodontal defects is highly questionable (Karring et al 1984).

Boyne (1973) stated that an ideal graft material should: (1) exist in an unlimited supply, without the need for violation of a distant donor site; (2) provide immediate osteogenesis for rapid consolidation; (3) illicit no adverse host responses, such as immune reactions; (4) facilitate revascularization, which assists early healing and resistance to infection; (5) stimulate osteoinduction of recipient site cells; (6) be adaptable to a variety of physical requirements; (7) cause no impediment to growth or orthodontic tooth movement; (8) provide support and stability where discontinuity or mobility exists; (9) provide a framework for osteoconduction; and (10) be completely replaced by host bone of the same or superior quality and quantity as quickly as possible. In light of our current understanding of the contribution of specific components of the periodontium, an ideal graft material for periodontal defects should also induce or enhance cementogenesis and the formation of a new attachment apparatus (new bone, cementum, and periodontal ligament). To date there is no such material.

Many osseous grafting materials have been used towards the goal of obtaining periodontal regeneration.

Autografts. An autograft is a graft transferred from one site to another within the same individual.

Cortical bone. Chips or shavings of cortical bone have been used with some success in periodontal defects (Nabers 1984; Langer et al 1986). However, because of their large size, these types of grafts have a tendency to sequestrate. Attempts to improve the success of cortical bone grafts by reducing the size of grafted osseous particles have included mixing the bone with blood and pulverizing it into a coagulum, and using pulverized cortical or cancellous bone alone (Froum et al 1976; Jacobs and Rosenberg 1984).

Cancellous bone, marrow, and bone blend. Cancellous bone and marrow obtained from either intraoral or extraoral donor sites, or a combination (bone blend), can also be used in autografts. The potential advantage of using these is the inclusion of marrow osteogenic stem cells within the scaffold provided by the bone. Iliac crest grafts have been shown to be more effective than intraoral bone grafts, presumably due to the greater number of viable stem cells present (Hiatt and Schallhorn 1973). One of the inherent problems of using hematopoietic cells is that they contain the monoblastic precursors to osteoclasts and therefore might lead to root resorption if the graft is juxtaposed to tooth root surfaces. Furthermore, ankylosis may be a complication of using fresh marrow in filling a periodontal defect (Ellegard et al 1973).

Allografts. Allografts are grafts transferred between genetically dissimilar members of the same species. Three types of bone allografts may be used clinically: (1) viable cancellous bone and marrow, (2) freeze-dried bone, (3) demineralized freeze-dried bone. Due to the obvious problems with donor-recipient cross-matching, and the potential for disease transmission, viable cancellous bone and marrow allografts are not considered a suitable option for periodontal therapy.

Freeze-dried bone has been used in either undemineralized or decalcified form. Undemineralized freeze-dried bone allografts (FDBA) were introduced into periodontal therapy by Mellonig et al (1976). The freeze-drying process removes approximately 95% of the water from the bone, kills all the cells, but maintains the original morphology and chemical structure of the bone graft. Although freeze-dried bone has been reported to improve approximately 60% of periodontal defects with up to 50% bone fill (Mellonig et al 1976; Sepe et al 1978), this still represents a less-than-ideal healing response. The osteogenic potential of freeze-dried cadaver bone is low; it probably acts as a scaffold for new bone growth, when it works at all. Freeze-dried bone allografts and fresh bone autografts in combination have been associated with somewhat greater success in filling periodontal defects, probably because of the bone growth inherent in the live bone cells from the autograft (Sanders et al 1983).

The enhanced osteoinductive potential of demineralized cortical bone has been demonstrated (Urist 1965). This process is thought to expose the bone morphogenetic proteins, located in the bone matrix, which enhance new bone formation by stimulating host cells into differentiating into osteoblasts (Urist and Strates 1970; Urist and Iwata 1973). Following these studies, it was proposed that demineralized freeze-dried bone might be a useful allograft material to induce new bone.

Following the introduction of demineralized freeze-dried bone allografts into periodontics (Libin et al 1975), numerous studies have been carried out to evaluate the clinical efficacy of this graft material. In general, these studies have compared grafts with nongrafted controls and shown significant increases in probing depth and gains in clinical attachment levels (Bowers et al 1989a; Bowers et al 1989b; Pearson et al 1981; Quintero et al 1982; Mellonig 1984; Rummelhart et al 1989). Unfortunately, very few of these studies presented any histologic data to confirm either the osteogenic potential of the graft materials or their periodontal regenerative capacity. Of the few studies that have looked at the histologic response to demineralized freeze-dried bone allografts, most have shown a remarkably poor osteogenic response in relation to the claimed clinical results (Libin et al 1975; Becker et al 1994; Brugnami et al 1996; Xiao et al 1996).

Heterografts. Heterografts (or xenografts) are grafts taken from a donor of another species. Heterografts have been found to be generally ineffective due to the induction of an immune response at the graft site due to the molecular divergence between the tissues of different species, and hence are generally not used.

Alloplastic materials. Alloplastic or synthetic grafts are artificial materials used as inert foreign-body implants to induce osteogenesis in bony defects. The literature contains references to an enormous range of alloplastic grafting materials. However, the commonly used materials for periodontal reconstruction are the calcium phosphate ceramics: namely the relatively nonresorbable hydroxyapatites, and the resorbable tricalcium phosphates. The use of these materials has been reviewed (Shetty and Han 1991). These materials are devoid of any osteogenic potential, but do permit osseous deposition by providing a lattice structure for osteoblasts. However, some studies have shown that these materials do not stimulate bone formation, and merely act as fillers, becoming encapsulated by fibrous tissue (Stahl and Froum 1986).

Regardless of their mode of action, the ultimate goal in the use of alloplastic materials is to fill the periodontal defect so that bone can adhere to the exterior surface of the implant material, infiltrate the interstices through pores, or biodegrade in advance of osteogenesis. Whether these are rational biologic and clinical goals is questionable in light of their inability to induce new cementum formation or new connective tissue attachment to the root surface.

Summary of grafting materials. The use of various grafting materials may produce radiographic evidence of bone fill and clinical evidence of improvement in probing depths and clinical attachment levels. However, several studies have shown that even though there is some bone growth around the graft particles, there is substantial fibrous encapsulation of the graft (Fig 11-6). In addition, there is an interposed layer of epithelial cells present on the root of the tooth, and consequently, no connective tissue reattachment (Yukna 1976; Listgarten and Rosenberg 1979; Caton et al 1980). Consequently, the relevance of these materials to the regeneration of the periodontium can be questioned.

Guided Tissue Regeneration

Principles. By the early 1980s, a number of important observations had been made in relation to periodontal regeneration. These have been summarized by Cárd et al (1987) and are presented here in slightly modified form:

1. Regeneration is biologically possible, but can be verified only by histologic analysis.
2. Epithelial migration and formation of a long junctional epithelium is a fundamental healing process occurring after either surgical or nonsurgical periodontal therapy.
3. Formation of a long junctional epithelium prevents root resorption by gingival connective tissue, but also impedes new con-

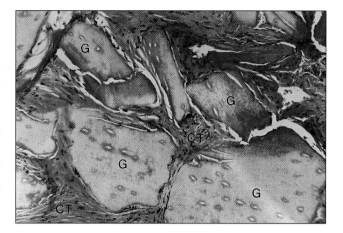

Fig 11-6 Human histologic response to demineralized freeze-dried bone allografts 9 months after implantation. Note that the graft particles (G) are embedded within a fibrous connective tissue matrix. No evidence of new bone formation is evident. Hematoxylin and eosin (original magnification 40×).

nective tissue attachment onto the root surface.

4. Periodontal ligament cells colonize root surfaces more quickly than do bone-derived cells, thus preventing ankylosis.

5. New attachment can be obtained onto a root surface that has been exposed to the oral environment.

6. Gingival connective tissue cells and bone cells do not appear to have the ability to form new connective tissue attachment onto a root surface.

7. Cells derived from the periodontal ligament appear to have the potential to form new connective tissue attachment onto a root surface.

8. In order for regeneration to occur, selective repopulation of the wound site must occur with cells possessing the potential to form new cementum, periodontal ligament, and alveolar bone.

From the above observations, a clinical procedure based on the principles of guided tissue regeneration was developed (Nyman et al 1982b). This method relies on draping a barrier membrane from the root surface over the periodontal defect and onto adjacent alveolar bone prior to replacement of a full-thickness mucoperiosteal flap (Fig 11-7). In doing so, a space is provided into which cells from the periodontal ligament may migrate, and an effective barrier prevents both gingival connective tissue and epithelium from occupying this space during the healing (regenerative) phase. Apart from exclusion of gingival epithelium and connective tissue from the healing site, the wound stability, the adhesion of the blood clot to the tooth surface, and the provision of adequate space by the barrier membrane also contribute to the successful outcome of guided tissue regeneration therapy (Scantlebury 1993).

While the literature is replete with studies extolling the virtues of guided tissue regeneration, there are few studies of a long-term nature that have followed the effectiveness of these treatments (Minabe 1991; Machtei et al 1996). In general, the long-term studies indicate that the procedure is predictable and stable for the management of class II furcations as well as two- and three-wall infrabony defects (Machtei et al 1995). However, the management of class III furcations and one-wall infrabony defects with guided tissue regeneration is not very predictable (Gottlow et al 1992; Becker and Becker 1993).

From the published studies to date, it has become apparent that gains in both probing and attachment levels can be expected following guided tissue regeneration procedures, although there is significant variability de-

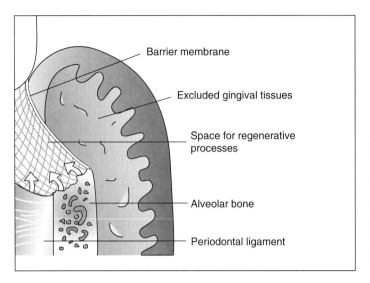

Barrier membrane

Excluded gingival tissues

Space for regenerative processes

Alveolar bone

Periodontal ligament

Fig 11-7 Schematic representation of guided tissue regeneration. The barrier membrane is draped over the periodontal defect so as to allow sufficient space for cells from the periodontal ligament to repopulate this space. The gingival tissues are physically excluded from access to the wound space by the membrane.

pending on numerous clinical parameters (Demolon et al 1993; Tonetti et al 1993; Mellonig et al 1994; Machtei et al 1994). Some of the major limiting factors include defect size and location, type of furcation defect, degree of membrane exposure during the healing period, and degree of microbial contamination.

At the time of membrane removal (for nonresorbable membranes), the regenerating tissues forming underneath the membrane have a soft, gelatinous consistency (Becker et al 1988). With time, this tissue may mature into bone—although this appears to be a rather variable response. Indeed, current data indicate that the predominant healing process is via new connective tissue attachment to the root surface, with minor contributions of new cementum and bone formation (Becker et al 1988; Lekovic et al 1989; Proestakis et al 1992; Flores-de-Jacoby et al 1994; Selvig et al 1992). Therefore, by definition, regeneration has not occurred.

Types of barrier membranes

Nonresorbable membranes. Prior to commercialization of guided tissue regeneration membranes, the original experiments in this field used Millipore filters (type GS: Millipore A, Mosheim, France: pore size of 0.22 μm)

(Nyman et al 1982b). Since these early experiments, the material most rigorously developed has been Gore-Tex Periodontal Material (W.L. Gore & Associates, Flagstaff, AZ). These membranes are made from expanded polytetrafluoroethylene (ePTFE) cut into specific configurations for various periodontal defects. This material is nontoxic; no adverse effects have been noted to date (Caffesse and Quinones 1993; Scantlebury 1993). These membranes are composed of an open microstructure collar and an occlusive apron (Fig 11-8). The collar is designed to impede epithelial down-growth, while the occlusive apron is designed to prohibit both gingival epithelium and connective tissue from gaining access to the healing periodontal defect.

As a result of considerable investigations into the use of this material, five essential design criteria have been proposed for guided tissue regeneration membranes (Scantlebury 1993).

1. Tissue integration—have an open microstructure to encourage tissue integration and limit epithelial migration, while creating a stable site for wound healing.
2. Cell occlusivity—membranes should separate all cell types so that the desired cells can repopulate the defect area.

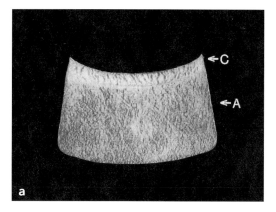
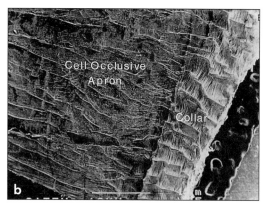

Fig 11-8 (a) Macroscopic view of a "single tooth wide" Gore-Tex periodontal membrane made from expanded polytetrafluorethylene (original magnification 2×). **(b)** Scanning electron microscopic appearance of a Gore-Tex periodontal membrane (original magnification 25×). Note the open microstructure collar (C) and the cell occlusive apron (A) portions of the membrane.

3. Clinical manageability—membranes should be easy to cut and shape to fit particular periodontal defects.
4. Spacemaking—membranes should resist collapse from the pressure of overlying tissues so that they can maintain adequate space during the healing period.
5. Biocompatibility—membranes should be nontoxic, nonantigenic, and induce minimal inflammatory response from the host.

Since ePTFE is not resorbable, it is used in a two-stage procedure (Fig 11-9). The first stage involves elevation of a full-thickness mucoperiosteal flap, thorough débridement of the site to be treated, trimming of the selected membrane to fit the site, and replacement of the flap. The membrane is then left in situ for 4 to 6 weeks, during which a very high level of oral hygiene is required for an acceptable clinical outcome. In the second stage, the membrane is removed under surgical conditions, taking care not to disturb the regenerating tissues located under the membrane. After removal of the membrane, the flap is repositioned to cover all of the newly formed tissue.

Resorbable membranes. Materials other than the synthetic ePTFE membranes have been used with varying degrees of success in guided tissue regeneration procedures. Materials such as collagen, polylactic acid, polyglycolic acid, and copolymers have been used (Magnusson et al 1988; Gottlow 1993). Autograft and allograft materials have also been used (Lekovic et al 1991; Yamaoka et al 1996).

As for the nonresorbable membranes, specific design criteria have been proposed for resorbable membranes. These include the five criteria listed above, as well as two additional criteria (Gottlow 1993):

1. Membrane stability—membrane must remain in situ to allow progenitor cells adequate time to repopulate the defect site without interference from gingival connective tissue or epithelium.
2. Membrane resorption—membrane should be degraded, replaced, or incorporated into the healing flap after cell selection is complete.

Similar results regarding tissue regeneration have been achieved with resorbable membranes compared to nonresorbable membranes (Gottlow 1993). Although resorbable membranes negate the need for second-stage surgery, problems are encountered with regards to their stability in situ. Thus,

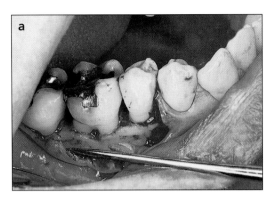
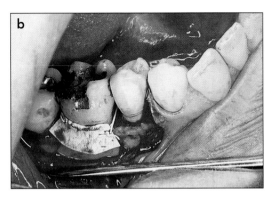
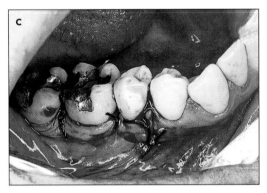
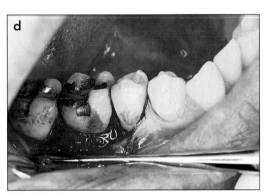

Fig 11-9 Clinical procedure for placement of a nonresorbable membrane and its subsequent removal. **(a)** Class II furcation defect on lower first molar exposed via a full thickness mucoperiosteal flap. **(b)** Gore-Tex membrane sutured into position. **(c)** Replacement of tissue flap. **(d)** Appearance of the defect 6 weeks after placement of the membrane. Note complete fill of the furcation defect with a red gelatinous tissue—at this stage this material has not formed bone.

resorbable membranes must remain intact long enough to allow the regenerative process to mature prior to bioresorption of the membrane. By virtue of their resorbable nature, together with the multitude of biologic agents proposed as degradable membrane, care must be taken to ensure that these types of membrane are suitable for clinical use from both an ethical and efficacy standpoint (Fig 11-10).

Combinations of guided tissue regeneration and regenerative agents. One challenge of regenerative therapies has been to achieve alveolar bone replacement in furcation, dehiscence, and horizontal defects coronal to the existing bony crest level. Guided tissue regenerative techniques alone have failed to achieve this.

More recently, a combination of grafting treatments and barrier membranes was used in attempts to augment the technique of guided tissue regeneration. These were often combined with root demineralization techniques. The combinations include resorbable or nonresorbable barrier membranes with bone grafts or synthetic grafts placed under them, and coronally positioned flaps. Several studies have reported some improvement in the healing of furcation defects when a combination of guided tissue regeneration membranes and demineralized freeze-dried bone allografts or dura mater membrane were used (Anderegg et al 1991; Schallhorn and McClain 1988; Zaner et al 1989). These assessments were, however, based solely on clinical criteria and no histo-

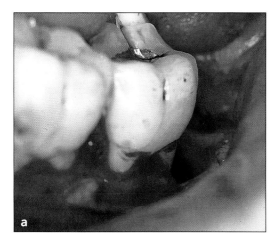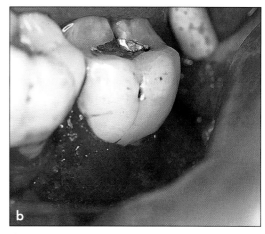

Fig 11-10 Clinical picture of the placement of a resorbable membrane. **(a)** Appearance of a periodontal defect on the distal surface of a lower second molar. **(b)** Appearance of a resorbable Resolut (Gore-Tex) membrane in place. Since these materials resorb, no reentry retrieval surgery is required.

logic data were available. More recently, the effects of guided tissue regeneration, with and without demineralized freeze-dried bone allografts, in the treatment of furcation defects in dogs with naturally occurring periodontal disease have been evaluated (Caffesse et al 1993). In this histologic study, adjunctive bone grafting did not appear to enhance regeneration. In a human study comparing demineralized freeze-dried bone allografts with and without ePTFE membranes in periodontal defects, using allografts as controls, it was concluded that utilization of ePTFE membranes, in addition to demineralized freeze-dried bone allografts, did not lead to additional radiographic gains in the defect area (Guillemin et al 1993). Thus, the overall conclusion of these studies is that the results are variable and benefits, if any, are only marginal.

Guided bone regeneration. The principle of guided tissue regeneration is applicable for tissues other than the periodontal ligament connective tissue cells. During the healing of an osseous defect, soft connective tissue ingrowth into the defect is the normal means of healing. Thus, because of the soft tissue ingrowth, the surrounding cells with osteogenic

potential are unable to populate the wound site and osteogenesis cannot proceed in any significant manner. With these concepts in mind, it has been demonstrated that by placing a barrier membrane over an osseous defect to exclude ingrowth of the soft connective tissues, bone can be encouraged to grow in the defect site (Buser et al 1990). Such a response occurs if adequate space is maintained by the membrane for clot formation and subsequent population by cells with osteogenic potential. Guided bone regeneration in periodontics has been developed over the past few years, particularly in the field of implantology, and has become a very predictable procedure (Dahlin 1994). Despite its clinical success, the precise molecular and cellular mechanisms operating to permit predictable new bone growth are poorly understood. Nonetheless, several criteria have been cited as important for new bone formation through the principles of guided bone regeneration (Dahlin 1994).

1. A viable source of bone cells must be available from the surrounding bone.
2. New bone formation requires an adequate blood supply.

3. The wound must remain mechanically stable during healing.
4. Adequate space must be created and maintained between the membrane and the bone surface.
5. Soft tissue cells must be excluded from the space created by the barrier membrane.

In addition to the above criteria, another important feature for success in guided bone regeneration is the need to obtain primary closure of the soft tissues over the barrier membrane. In doing so, the wound site is completely protected from the oral environment and regeneration can proceed unimpeded by the complicating factors of plaque, saliva, and mechanical instability. This feature is in clear contrast to the situation created when using guided periodontal regeneration procedures, and most likely is a very important factor in the exceptional clinical predictability of the guided bone regeneration procedure.

Growth Factors in Periodontal Regeneration

Various wound healing events and cellular activities associated with healing are regulated by polypeptides (see Chapters 2, and 3). Therefore it is logical to utilize the potentials of growth factors to promote periodontal regeneration (Tables 11-1 and 11-2) (Caffesse and Quinones 1993; Terranova 1993; Gian-

Table 11-1. Growth Factor Families and Their Members

Platelet-derived growth factors	PDGF-AA
	PDGF-BB
	PDGF-AB
	Vascular endothelial cell growth factor
Epidermal growth factors	Epidermal growth factor
	Transforming growth factor-α
	Amphiregulin
Fibroblast growth factors	Acidic fibroblast growth factor (FGF-1)
	Basic fibroblast growth factor (FGF-2)
Insulinlike growth factors	Insulinlike growth factor-I
	Insulinlike growth factor-II
Transforming growth factors	Transforming growth factor-β
	Bone morphogenetic proteins 2 and 8

Table 11-2. Growth Factors of Potential Use in Periodontal Regeneration

Properties	Growth factor					
	FGFs	PDGF	IGF	TGF-β	EGF	BMPs
Competence factor	X	X				
Progression factor			X			
Fibroblast mitogen	X	X	X		X	
Neovascularization	X	X		X	X	
Stimulate epithelial cells	X				X	
Stimulate osteoblasts	X	X	X	X		
Stimulate matrix synthesis	X	X	X	X		
Clinical trials underway	X	X	X			X

nobile 1996). With this rationale, several growth factors have been utilized to treat natural and experimentally induced periodontal defects in animal models. Despite their lack of specificity (Chao 1992), many growth factors have been examined, alone and in combination, and the results of these studies have been critically evaluated (Graves and Cochran 1994; Garrett 1996).

The first studies to show an effect of growth factors in relation to periodontal regeneration used a combination of platelet-derived growth factor (PDGF)-BB and insulin-like growth factor (IGF)-1 (Lynch et al 1989; Lynch et al 1991). After surgical access and débridement of the root surface, the roots were treated with a combination of PDGF-BB and IGF-I in an aqueous gel, or with the gel alone (control). Significant amounts of cementum and bone deposition at the treated surgical sites in test teeth were noted, as compared to the controls (Fig 11-11). These important studies paved the way for a great deal of activity and interest in the use of growth factors for periodontal regeneration. Later, a study in monkeys using a ligature-induced model of periodontitis assessed the effects of PDGF-AA/IGF-I or PDGF-BB/IGF-I, or a control gel. Both homodimers of PDGF appeared to stimulate a significant amount of new attachment onto the débrided root surfaces compared to the controls (Rutherford et al 1992). In a subsequent study, Rutherford et al (1993) demonstrated that a combination of PDGF and dexamethasone could also promote periodontal regeneration in monkeys. On the basis of still further encouraging results using PDGF-BB and IGF-1 in dogs (Giannobile et al 1994; Cho et al 1995), it would seem that these agents would be suitable for use in human clinical trials. A recent report concerning a phase I/II clinical trial to evaluate a combination of recombinant human platelet–derived growth factor-BB and recombinant insulin-like growth factor-1 in patients with periodontitis has indicated that this form of ther-

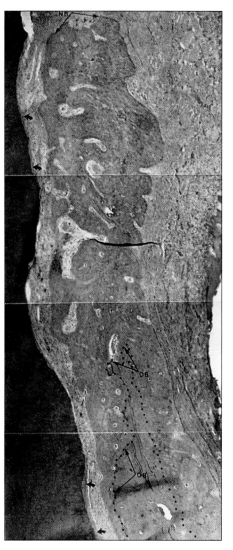

Fig 11-11 Histologic picture of the effects of treating a root surface with a combination of PDGF-BB and IGF-1. New bone (NB) is present coronal to the original alveolar crest (OB). New cementum (arrows) has been deposited on the root surface adjacent to the new bone. A physiologic periodontal ligament space appears to have been regenerated. Original magnification ×40. (Reproduced with permission from Lynch 1994.)

apy has considerable promise (Howell et al 1997). However, more studies are needed, as it is still not clear which factors are needed for regeneration, and which variables affect regeneration (Graves and Cochran 1994).

To date, the only other growth factors studied in any detail in humans with regards to periodontal regeneration are the bone morphogenetic proteins (BMPs). An early study did not demonstrate a stimulatory effect for osteogenin (BMP-3) in the healing of periodontal defects (Bowers et al 1991). More recently, BMP-2 has been found to significantly increase alveolar bone healing in furcation defects in baboons (Ripamonti et al 1994). In addition, BMP-2 has been found to significantly increase bone and cementum formation in periodontal defects in dogs, when used in a carrier gel or underneath barrier membranes (Sigurdsson et al 1995; Sigurdsson et al 1996).

Summary

Numerous techniques have been tried and tested to regenerate tissues lost to periodontal disease. Success is largely dependent upon an understanding of the biology of the regenerative process. The relevance of the recreation of a connective tissue attachment has been questioned, due to the fact that a long junctional epithelial attachment to the tooth was shown to be no more susceptible to further breakdown in a diseased site than in a nondiseased site. Despite this, regenerative procedures have been developed and found to be successful at the histologic level. However, the techniques currently under use that show the greatest promise (ie, guided tissue regeneration and growth factors) are still clinically unpredictable due to their highly technique-sensitive nature. The next phase in regenerative technologies will undoubtedly involve a deeper understanding of the molecular signaling (both intra- and extracellular) and cellular differentiation processes involved in the regenerative processes.

References

Aleo J, De Renzis FA, Farber PA. *In vitro* attachment of human gingival fibroblasts to root surfaces. J Periodontol 1975;46:639.

Alger FA, Solt CE, Vuddhakanok S, Miles K. The histologic evaluation of new attachment in periodontally diseased human roots treated with tetracycline-hydrochloride and fibronectin. J Periodontol 1990;61:447.

Alleyn CD, O'Neal RB, Strong SL, et al. The effect of chlorhexidine treatment of root surfaces on the attachment of human gingival fibroblasts in vitro. J Periodontol 1991; 62:434.

American Academy of Periodontology. Glossary of Periodontic Terms. 3rd ed. 1992.

Anderegg CR, Martin SJ, Gray JL, Mellonig JT, Gher ME. Clinical evaluation of the use of decalcified freeze-dried bone allograft with guided tissue regeneration in the treatment of molar furcation invasions. J Periodontol 1991; 62:264.

Aukhill I. Biology of tooth-cell adhesion. Dent Clin North Am 1991;35:459.

Baker PJ, Evans RT, Coburn R, Genco RJ. Tetracycline and its derivatives strongly bind to and release from the tooth surface in active form. J Periodontol 1983;54:580.

Becker W, Becker B. Treatment of 3-wall intrabony defects by flap debridement and expanded polytetrafluoroethylene barrier membranes. Long term evaluation of 32 treated patients. J Periodontol 1993;64:1138.

Becker W, Becker B, Berg L, Prichard J, Caffesse R, Rosenberg E. New attachment after treatment with root isolation procedures: Report for treated class III and class II furcations and vertical osseous defects. Int J Periodont Rest Dent 1988;3:9.

Becker W, Becker B, Caffesse R. A comparison of demineralized freeze-dried bone and autologous bone to induce bone formation in human extraction sockets. J Periodontol 1994;65:1128.

Beertsen W. Migration of fibroblasts in the periodontal ligament of the mouse incisor as revealed by autoradiography. Arch Oral Biol 1975;20:659.

Bjorvatn K. Scanning electron microscope study of pellicle and plaque formation on tetracycline impregnated dentin. Scand J Dent Res 1986;94:89.

Blomlöff L, Lindskog S, Appelgren R, Jonsson B, Weintraub A, Hammarström L. New attachment in monkeys with experimental periodontitis with and without removal of the cementum. J Clin Periodontol 1987;14:136.

Bowers G, Felton F, Middleton C, et al. Histologic comparison of regeneration in human intrabony defects when osteogenin is combined with freeze-dried bone allograft with purified bovine collagen. J Periodontol 1991;62:690.

Bowers GM, Chadroff B, Carnevale R, et al. Histologic evaluation of new attachment apparatus formation in humans, part III. J Periodontol 1989b;60:683.

Bowers GM, Chadroff B, Carnevale R, Mellonig JT, Corio R. Histologic evaluation of new attachment apparatus formation in humans, part II. J Periodontol 1989a;60:675.

Boyko GA, Brunette DN, Melcher AH. Cell attachment to demineralized root surfaces *in vitro*. J Periodont Res 1980;15:297.

Boyne PJ. Induction of bone repair by various bone grafting materials. Hard tissue growth, repair and regeneration. Ciba Found Symp 1973;11:121.

Brugnami F, Then PR, Moroi H, Leone CW. Histologic evaluation of human extraction sockets treated with demineralized freeze dried bone allograft (DFDBA) and cell occlusive membrane. J Periodontol 1996;67:821.

Buser D, Bragger U, Lang NP, Nyman S. Regeneration and enhancement of jaw bone using guided tissue regeneration. Clin Oral Impl Res 1990;1:1990.

Caffesse RG, Holden MJ, Kon S, Nasjleti CE. The effect of citric acid and fibronectin on healing following surgical treatment of naturally occurring periodontal disease in beagle dogs. J Clin Periodontol 1985;12:578.

Caffesse RG, Nasjleti CE, Plotzke AE, Anderson GB, Morrison EC. Guided tissue regeneration and bone grafts in the treatment of furcation defects. J Periodontol 1993;64:1145-1153.

Caffesse RG, Quinones CR. Polypeptide growth factors and attachment proteins in periodontal wound healing and regeneration. Periodontol 2000 1993;1:69.

Card SJ, Caffesse RG, Smith WA. A historical perspective of current new attachment procedures. J West Soc Periodontol 1987;35:93.

Caton J, Nyman S, Zander H. Histometric evaluation of periodontal surgery. II. Connective tissue attachment levels after four regenerative procedures. J Clin Periodontol 1980;7:224.

Chao MV. Growth factor signaling: Where is the specificity. Cell 1992;68:995.

Cho MI, Lin W-LL, Genco RJ. Platelet-derived growth factor modulated guided tissue regenerative therapy. J Periodontol 1995;66:522.

Claffey N, Bogle G, Bjorvatn K, Selvig KA, Egelberg J. Topical application of tetracycline in regenerative surgery in beagles. Acta Odontol Scand 1987;45:141.

Dahlin C. Scientific background of guided bone regeneration. In: Buser D, Dahlin C, Schenk RK, eds. Guided Bone Regereration in Implant Dentistry. Chicago: Quintessence; 1994:13.

Daryabegi P, Pameijer CH, Ruber MP, Richetti PA. Root surface–soft tissue interface. J Periodontol 1980;51:77.

Demolon IA, Persson GR, Moncla BJ, Johnson RB, Ammons WF. Effects of antibiotic treatment on clinical conditions and bacterial growth with guided tissue regeneration. J Periodontol 1993;64,609.

Ellegard B, Karring T, Listgarten MA, Löe H. New attachment after treatment of interradicular lesions. J Periodontol 1973;44:209.

Fernyhough W, Page RC. Attachment, growth and synthesis by human gingival fibroblasts on demineralized or fibronectin-treated normal and diseased tooth roots. J Periodontol 1983;54:133.

Flores-de-Jacoby L, Zimmermann A, Tslaikis L. Experiences with guided tissue regeneration on the treatment of advanced periodontal disease. A clinical re-entry study, part 1. Vertical, horizontal and combined vertical and horizontal periodontal defects. J Clin Periodontol 1994;21:113.

Frank RM, Fiore-Donno G, Cimasoni G. Cementogenesis and soft tissue attachment after citric acid treatment in a human. An electron microscopic study. J Periodontol 1983;54:389.

Freeman E, Ten Cate AR. Development of the periodontium. An electron microscopic study. J Periodontol 1971;42:387.

Froum SJ, Oritiz RT, Witkins R, Thaler R, Scopp IW, Stahl SS. Autografts III. Comparison of osseous coagulum-bone blend implants with open curettage. J Periodontol 1976;47:287.

Fuentes P, Garrett S, Nails R, Egelberg J. Treatment of periodontal furcation defects. Coronally positioned flaps with or without citric acid root conditioning in Class II defects. J Clin Periodontol 1993;20:425.

Garrett S. Periodontal regeneration around natural teeth. Ann Periodontol 1996;1:621.

Giannobile WV, Finkelman RD, Lynch SE. Comparison of canine and non-human primate animal models for periodontal regenerative therapy: Results following a single administration of PDGF/IGF-1. J Periodontol 1994;65:1158.

Giannobile WV. Periodontal tissue engineering by growth factors. Bone 1996;19:23S.

Golub LM, Ramamurthy TF, McNamara TF, et al. Tetracyclines inhibit tissue collagenase activity. A new mechanism in the treatment of periodontal disease. J Periodont Res 1984;19:651.

Gottlow J. Guided tissue regeneration using bioresorbable and non-resorbable devices: initial healing and long term results. J Periodontol 1993;64:1157.

Gottlow J, Nyman S, Karring T. Maintenance of new attachment gained through guided tissue regeneration. J Clin Periodontol 1992;19:315.

Gould TRL, Melcher AH, Brunette DM. Migration and division of progenitor cell populations in periodontal ligament after wounding. J Periodont Res 1980;15:20.

Graves DT, Cochran DL. Periodontal regeneration with polypeptide growth factors. Curr Opin Periodontol 1994: 178–186.

Guillemin MR, Mellonig JT, Brunsvold MA, Steffensen B. Healing in periodontal defects treated by decalcified freeze-dried bone allografts in combination with ePTFE membranes. Assessment by computerized densitometric analysis. J Clin Periodontol 1993;20:520.

Hammarström L, Atali I, Fong CD. Origins of cementum. Oral Diseases 1996;2:63.

Harrison JW, Roda RS. Intermediate cementum. Development, structure, composition and potential function. Oral Surg Oral Med Oral Pathol 1995;79:624.

Henning FR. Healing of gingivectomy wounds in the rat: Re-establishment of the epithelial seal. J Periodontol 1968;39:265.

Hiatt WH, Schallhorn RC. Intraoral transplants of cancellous bone and marrow in periodontal lesions. J Periodontol 1973;44:194.

Holden MJ, Smith BA. Citric acid and fibronectin in periodontal therapy. J West Soc Periodontol 1983;31:45.

Iglhaut J, Suggs C, Borjesson B, Aukhil I. Apical migration of oral epithelium in experimental dehiscence wounds. J Clin Periodontol 1987;14:508.

Jacobs JE, Rosenberg ES. Management of an intrabony defect using osseous coagulum from a lingual torus. Compend Contin Ed Dent 1984;5:57.

Karring T, Nyman S, Lindhe J. Healing following implantation of periodontitis affected roots into bone tissue. J Clin Periodontol 1980;7:96.

Karring T, Nyman S, Lindhe J, Sirirat M. Potentials for root resorption during periodontal wound healing. J Clin Periodontol 1984;11:41.

Lafferty TA, Gher ME, Jonathan GL. Comparative SEM study on the effect of acid etching with tetracycline HCl or citric acid on instrumented periodontally-involved human root surfaces. J Periodontol 1993;64:689.

Langer B, Wegengerg B, Langer L. Ther use of frozen autogenous bone in grafting procedures. Int J Periodont Rest Dent 1986;6:68.

Larjava H, Salonen J, Hakkinen L, Narhi T. Effect of citric acid on the migration of epithelium on root surfaces *in vitro*. J Periodontol 1988;59:95.

Lekic P, McCulloch CAG. Periodontal ligament cell populations: The central role of fibroblasts in creating a unique tissue. Anat Rec 1996;245:327.

Lekovic V, Kenney EB, Carranza FA, Martignoni M. The use of autogenous periosteal grafts as barriers for the treatment of class II furcation involvements in lower molars. J Periodontol 1991;62:775.

Lekovic V, Kenney EB, Kovacevic K, Carranza FA. Evaluation of guided tissue regeneration in class II furcation defects. A clinical re-entry study. J Periodontol 1989;60:694.

Levine HL, Stahl SS. Repair following periodontal flap surgery with retention of gingival fibers. J Periodontol 1972;43:99.

Libin BM, Ward H, Fishman L. Decalcified, lyophilized bone allografts for use in human periodontal defects. J Periodontol 1975;46:51-56.

Lindhe J, Westfelt E, Nyman S, Socransky SS, Heijl L, Bratthall G. Healing following surgical/non-surgical treatment of periodontal disease. A clinical study. J Clin Periodontol 1982;9:115.

Lindskog S. Formation of intermediate cementum I. Early mineralization of aprismatic enamel and intermediate cementum in monkey. J Craniofac Genet Dev Biol 1982; 2:147.

Listgarten MA. Ultrastructure of the dento-gingival junction following gingivectomy. J Periodont Res 1972;7:151.

Listgarten MA, Rosenberg MM. Histologic study of repair following new attachment procedures in human periodontal lesions. J Periodontol 1979;50:333.

Listgarten MA, Rosenberg S, Lerner S. Progressive replacement of epithelial attachment by a connective tissue junction after experimental periodontal surgery in rats. J Periodontol 1982;53:659.

Lynch SE. The role of growth factors in periodontal repair and regeneration. In: Polson AM, ed. Periodontal Regeneration. Current Status and Directions. Chicago: Quintessence; 1994:179.

Lynch SE, de Castilla GR, Williams RC, et al. The effects of short-term application of a combination of platelet-derived and insulin-like growth factors in periodontal wound healing. J Periodontol 1991;62:458.

Lynch SE, Williams RC, Polson AM, et al. A combination of platelet-derived and insulin-like growth factors enhances periodontal regeneration. J Periodont Res 1989;16:545.

Machtei EE, Cho MI, Dunford R, Norderyd J, Zambon JJ, Genco RJ. Clinical, microbiological and histological factors which influence the success of regenerative periodontal therapy. J Periodontol 1994;65,154.

Machtei EE, Grossi SG, Dunford R, Zambon JJ, Genco RJ. Long term stability of class II furcation defects treated with barrier membranes. J Periodontol 1996;67:523.

Machtei EE, Schallhorn RG. Successful regeneration of mandibular class II furcation defects: An evidence-based treatment approach. Int J Periodont Rest Dent 1995;15: 146.

MacNeil RL, Somerman MJ. Factors regulating development and regeneration of cementum. J Periodont Res 1993;28:550.

Magnusson I, Batich C, Collins BR. New attachment formation following controlled tissue regeneration using biodegradable membranes. J Periodontol 1988;59:105.

Magnusson I, Runstead L, Nyman S, Lindhe J. A long junctional epithelium — A *locus minoris resistentiae* in plaque infection? J Clin Periodontol 1983;10:333.

Marks SC, Mehta NR. Lack of effect of citric acid treatment of root surfaces on the formation of new connective tissue. J Clin Periodontol 1986;13:109.

McCulloch CAG, Bordin S. Role of fibroblast subpopulations in periodontal physiology and pathology. J Periodont Res 1991;26:144.

McCulloch CAG, Melcher AH. Cell migration in the periodontal ligament of mice. J Periodont Res 1983;18:339.

McCulloch CAG, Nemeth E, Lowenberg B, Melcher AH. Paravascular cells in endosteal spaces of alveolar bone contribute to periodontal ligament cell populations. Anat Rec 1987; 219:233.

Melcher AH. On the repair potential of periodontal tissues. J Periodontol 1976;47:256.

Melcher AH, Cheong T, Cox J, Nemeth E, Shiga A. Synthesis of cementum-like tissue *in vitro* by cells cultured from bone. A light and electron microscope study. J Periodont Res 1986;21:592.

Mellonig JT. Decalcified freeze-dried bone allograft as an implant material in human periodontal defects. Int J Periodont Rest Dent 1984;4:41.

Mellonig JT. Autogenous and allogenic bone grafts in periodontal therapy. Crit Rev Oral Biol Med 1992;3:333.

Mellonig JT, Bowers GM, Bailey RC. Clinical evaluation of freeze-dried bone allograft in periodontal osseous defects. J Periodontol 1976;47:125.

Mellonig JT, Seamans BC, Gray JL, Towle HJ. Clinical evaluation of guided tissue regeneration in the treatment of grade II molar furcation invasions. Int J Periodont Rest Dent 1994;14,25.

Minabe M. A critical review of the biologic rationale for guided tissue regeneration. J Periodontol 1991;62:171.

Nabers CL. Long term results of autogenous bone grafts. Int J Periodont Rest Dent 1984;4:50.

Narayanan AS, Bartold PM. Biochemistry of periodontal connective tissues. A current perspective. Connect Tiss Res 1996;34:191

Nyman S, Gottlow J, Karring T, Lindhe J. The regenerative potential of the periodontal ligament. An experimental study in the monkey. J Clin Periodontol 1982a;9:257.

Nyman S, Karring T, Lindhe J, Planten S. Healing following implantation of periodontitis-affected roots into gingival connective tissue. J Periodontol 1980;64:142.

Nyman S, Lindhe J, Karring T, Rylander H. New attachment following surgical treatment of human periodontal disease. J Clin Periodontol 1982b;9:290.

Offenbacher S. Periodontal diseases. Pathogenesis. Ann Periodontol 1996;1:821.

Page RC, Offenbacher S, Schroeder HE, Seymour GJ, Kornman KS. Advances in the pathogenesis of periodontitis: summary of developments, clinical implications and future directions. Periodontol 2000 1997;14:216.

Parashis AO, Mitsis FJ. Clinical evaluation of the effect of tetracycline root preparation on guided tissue regeneration in the treatment of class II furcation defects. J Periodontol 1993;64:133.

Pearson BS, Klebe RJ, Boyan BD, Moskowicz D. Comments on clinical application of fibronectin in dentistry. J Dent Res 1988;67:515.

Pearson GE, Rosen S, Deporter DA. Preliminary observations on the usefulness of a decalcified freeze-dried cancellous bone allograft material in periodontal surgery. J Periodontol 1981;52:55.

Phipps RP, Borrello MA, Blieden TM. Fibroblast heterogeneity in the periodontium and other tissues. J Periodont Res 1997;32:159.

Pitaru S, McCulloch CAG, Narayanan AS. Cellular origins and differentiation control mechanisms during periodontal development and wound healing. J Periodont Res 1994; 29:81.

Polson AM, Frederick GT, Ladenheim S, Hanes PJ. The production of root surface smear layer by instrumentation and its removal by citric acid. J Periodontol 1984;55:443.

Polson AM, Proye MP. Fibrin linkage: a precursor for new attachment. J Periodontol 1983;53:141.

Porvaznick M, Cohen ME, Bockowski W, Mueller EJ, Wirthlin MR. Enhancement of cell attachment to a substrate coated with oral bacterial endotoxin by plasma fibronectin. J Periodont Res 1982;17:154.

Proestakis G, Bratthall S, Söderholm G, et al. Guided tissue regeneration in the treatment of infrabony defects on maxillary premolars. A pilot study. J Clin Periodontol 1992;19:766.

Quintero G, Mellonig JT, Gambill VM, Pelleu GB Jr. A six-month clinical evaluation of decalcified freeze-dried bone allografts in periodontal osseous defects. J Periodontol 1982;53:726.

Register AA. Bone and cementum induction by dentin demineralized in situ. J Periodontol 1973;44:49.

Ripamonti U, Heliotis M, van den Heever B, Reddi AH. Bone morphogenetic proteins induce periodontal regeneration in the baboon *(Papio ursinus)*. J Periodont Res 1994;29:439.

Rummelhart JM, Mellonig JT, Gray JL, Towle HJ. Comparison of freeze-dried bone allograft and demineralized freeze-dried bone allograft in human periodontal defects. J Periodontol 1989;60:655.

Rutherford RB, Niekrash CE, Kennedy JE, Charette MF. Platelet-derived and insulin-like growth factors stimulate regeneration of periodontal attachment in monkeys. J Periodont Res 1992;27:285.

Rutherford RB, Ryan ME, Kennedy JE, Tucker MM, Charette MF. Platelet-derived growth factor and dexamethasone combined with a collagen matrix induced regeneration of the periodontium in monkeys. J Clin Periodontol 1993;12:537.

Sanders JJ, Sepe WW, Bowers GM, et al. Clinical evaluation of freeze-dried bone allografts in periodontal osseous defects. Part III. Composite freeze-dried bone allografts with and without autogenous bone grafts. J Periodontol 1983;54:1.

Scantlebury TV. 1982-1992: A decade of technical development for guided tissue regeneration. J Periodontol 1993; 64:1129.

Schallhorn RG, McClain PK. Combined osseous composite grafting, root conditioning, and guided tissue regeneration. Int J Periodont Rest Dent 1988;8:9.

Schonfeld SE, Slavkin HC. Demonstration of enamel matrix proteins on root-analogue surfaces of rabbit permanent incisor teeth. Calcif Tissue Res 1977;24:223.

Schroeder HE. Biological problems of regenerative cementogenesis: Synthesis and attachment of collagenous matrices on growing and established root surfaces. Int Rev Cytol 1992;142:1.

Selvig KA, Kersten BG, Chamberlain ADH, Wikesjö UME, Nilveus RE. Regenerative surgery of intrabony periodontal defects using ePTFE barrier membranes: scanning electron microscopic evaluation of retrieved membranes versus clinical healing. J Periodontol 1992;63:974.

Sepe WW, Bowers GM, Lawrence JJ, Friedlander GE, Koch R. Clinical evaluation of freeze dried bone allografts in periodontal osseous defects—Part II. J Periodontol 1978;49:9.

Shetty V, Han TJ. Alloplastic materials in reconstructive periodontal surgery. Dent Clin North Am 1991;35:521.

Sigurdsson TJ, Lee MB, Kubota K, Turek TJ, Wozney JM, Wikesjö UME. Periodontal repair in dogs: Recombinant human bone morphogenetic protein-2 significantly enhances periodontal regeneration. J Periodontol 1995; 66:131.

Sigurdsson TJ, Tatakis DN, Lee MB, Wikesjö UME. Periodontal regenerative potential of space-providing expanded polytetrafluorethylene membranes and recombinant human bone morphogenetic proteins. J Periodontol 1996; 66:511.

Slavkin HC, Bringas P, Bessem C, et al. Hertwig's epithelial root sheath differentiation and initial cementum and bone formation during long-term organ culture of mouse mandibular first molars using serumless, chemically defined medium. J Periodont Res 1989;24:28.

Smith B, Caffesse R, Nasjleti C, Kon S, Castelli W. Effects of citric acid and fibronectin and laminin application in treating periodontitis. J Clin Periodontol 1987;14:396.

Stahl SS, Froum SJ. Human clinical and histologic repair following the use of citric acid in periodontal therapy. J Clin Periodontol 1977;48:261.

Stahl SS, Froum SJ. Histological evaluation of human intraosseous healing responses to the placement of tricalcium phosphate ceramic implants. J Periodontol 1986;57:211.

Stahl SS, Slavkin HC, Yamada L, Levine S. Speculations about gingival repair. J Periodontol 1972;43:395.

Tagge DL, O'Leary TJ, El-Kafrawy AH. The clinical and histological response of periodontal pockets to root planing and oral hygiene. J Periodontol 1975;46:527.

Ten Cate AR. Formation of supporting bone in association with periodontal ligament organization in the mouse. Arch Oral Biol 1975;20:137.

Ten Cate AR. The role of epithelium in the development, structure and function of the tissues of tooth support. Oral Diseases 1996;2:55.

Ten Cate AR. The development of the periodontium—a largely ectomesenchymally derived unit. Periodontol 2000 1997;13:9.

Terranova VP. Biologically active factors in the treatment of periodontal disease. Curr Opin Periodontol 1993; 129–135.

Terranova VP, Franzetti L, Hic S, et al. A biochemical approach to periodontal regeneration. Tetracycline treatment of dentine promotes fibroblast adhesion and growth. J Periodont Res 1986;21:330.

Terranova VP, Martin GR. Molecular factors determining gingival tissue interaction with tooth structure. J Periodont Res 1982;17:530.

Tonetti MS, Pini-Prato G, Cortellini P. Periodontal regeneration of human intrabony defects. IV. Determinants of healing response. J Periodontol 1993;64:934.

Torfason T, Kiger R, Selvig K, Egelberg J. Clinical improvement of gingival conditions following ultrasonic versus hand instrumentation of periodontal pockets. J Clin Periodontol 1979;6:165.

Urist MR. Bone formation by autoinduction. Science 1965;150:893.

Urist MR. Bone histogenesis and morphogenesis in implants of demineralized enamel and dentin. J Oral Surg 1971;29:88.

Urist MR, Iwata H. Preservation and biodegradation of the morphogenetic property of bone matrix. J Theor Biol 1973;38:155.

Urist MR, Strates B. Bone formation in implants of partially or wholly demineralized bone matrix. Clin Orthop 1970;71:271.

Weiss RE, Reddi AH. Synthesis and localization of fibronectin during collagenous matrix-mesenchymal cell interaction and differentiation of cartilage and bone *in vivo*. Proc Natl Acad Sci USA 1980;77:2074.

Wikesjö UME, Baker PJ, Christersson L, et al. A biochemical approach to periodontal regeneration: tetracycline treatment conditions dentine surfaces. J Periodont Res 1986;21:322.

Wikesjö UME, Nilveus RE, Selvig KA. Significance of early healing events of periodontal repair. A review. J Periodontol 1992;63:158.

Wirthlin MR, Hancock EB. Regeneration and repair after biological treatment of root surfaces in monkeys. II. Proximal surfaces of posterior teeth. J Periodontol 1982;53:302.

Xiao Y, Parry DA, Li H, Arnold R, Jackson WJ, Bartold PM. Expression of extracellular macromolecules around demineralized freeze dried bone allografts. J Periodontol 1996;67:1233.

Yamaoka SB, Mellonig JT, Meffert RM, Arnold RM, Nummikoski PV, Mealey BL. Clinical evaluation of demineralized unicortical-ilium-strips for guided tissue regeneration. J Periodontol 1996;67:803.

Yeomans JD, Urist MR. Bone induction by decalcified dentine implanted into oral, osseous and muscle tissue. Arch Oral Biol 1967;12:999.

Yukna RA. A clinical and histologic study of healing following the excisional new attachment procedure in monkeys. J Periodontol 1976;47:701.

Zaner DJ, Yukna RA, Malinin TI. Human freeze-dried dura mater allograft as a periodontal biologic bandage. J Periodontol 1989;60:617.

Index